THE QUAD LIFE

Unexpected Times Abound, Reliance on God a Must

JOEL VANDER MOLEN

The Quad Life
Unexpected Times Abound, Reliance on God a Must
Joel Vander Molen

To contact the author: joel@joelvm.com, trainmanj.blogspot.com

Published by
Mary Ethel Eckard

Mary Ethel

Frisco, Texas
Printed in the United States of America

Library of Congress Control Number: 2023912187
ISBN (Paperback): 979-8-9880326-5-6
ISBN (Hardcover): 979-8-9880326-7-0
ISBN (E-Book): 979-8-9880326-6-3

DEDICATION

This book is dedicated to my parents, caregivers, and extended family.
I can never repay all their work and encouragement given to me
throughout my life to continue moving forward.
Most of all, I'm thankful to God for His many blessings
and all He has allowed me to do.

CONTENTS

FOREWORD

"Does he speak?"

The question was well intentioned and came from the dearest older lady, but it certainly provoked an odd look from me. Not so much from Joel. Sitting there in his chair, arms strapped down and trach tube coming out of his throat, it wasn't the first time someone had asked a question like this right in front of him, nor would it be the last. Being his ever-gracious self with a witty and self-deprecating sense of humor, he simply replied "Yeah, it's getting me to stop that's the problem!"

I honestly don't recall when I met him. I was a few weeks into seventh grade and had just moved from sunny California to a small town in Iowa where we were promised snow. As the pastor's kid, I met so many people those first few weeks that he just blended in with the rest. Still, seeing him again at school (and better yet, with his kind greeting to the new kid a year younger than he) it was certainly enough to jog the memory to realize there was some connection there, however brief, compared to the sea of new faces.

Things just went from there. We had similar interests and he introduced me to a few new ones including train watching which, to me, was just a great excuse to hang out with friends (sometimes even overnight) with the added brief thrill of a train occasionally blowing past. I don't remember which of us introduced the other to StarCraft but, being cross-platform, it quickly became our game – he with his PC, and me with my trusty Mac. I dare not think about how many hours our respective phone lines were tied up with the screeching of dialup modems as we slaughtered onslaughts of invading Zerg and, occasionally, each other. I'm told that may even have contributed to the installation of a second dedicated phone line in Joel's house.

He was the friend that any kid would want through those junior high and high school years. We split 40-piece chicken nugget meals from McDonald's, took apart computers (to the horror of his mother), and shared the agony of high school crushes (speaking in code of course so the "parental units" wouldn't overhear.)

But Joel dealt with much more than just the usual teenage angst of trying years. Being a quadriplegic confined to a chair or bed was hard enough. Seeing the burden that represented on those he loved weighed even heavier. There were constant worries about the future – most went much further back than when I met him. Worries about sores that wouldn't heal, breathing tubes that would slip off, lifts that would break down, and most perennial of all, funding for all his care.

It never occurred to me at the time to think him inspirational or brave. He was just Joel, living the life, day by day, that his Creator had laid out for him. Looking back, I don't ever recall him even hinting at any sort of resentment over his injury. No blaming God for a life different from his classmates. If there was ever resentment, it was always accompanied by almost a smug pride and directed not at the Lord, but at those who, in the immediate hours, months, and even years after the accident, had dared to suggest it would have been "better" if he had slipped away that cold morning on the side of the road because the life ahead was too hard and would be too short to justify the pain. Smug indeed, he certainly proved them wrong!

Among the milestones he was never supposed to reach was moving away to college. He relished the chance he had to strike out on his own, even if it ended up being for a short time and dove into college life. I struck out on my own path as well a year later, albeit a few states away. We certainly stayed in touch, but paths started going different ways. Still, with correspondence and even contact with nearly all other friends from high school fading away, Joel remained the constant, though at times, infrequent, friend. The rare trips back to Iowa always included visits to his place and trading stories of adventures and setbacks.

After college, I joined my soon-to-be bride in Wisconsin and, finding myself with much more free time and many fewer friends around than I had in college, was happy to rekindle the friendship via the webcam and microphone (though the camera proved boring and bandwidth intensive before long and hours-long open mics became the norm.) Again, we caught up, again we battled the Zerg, again we talked computers. When the time came to start nailing down wedding plans, my choice for a best man was obvious – who else could it be after I was told in no uncertain terms that there would be NO eighty-year-old groomsmen. Still, I knew it would be challenging bordering on impossible with the wedding being in Canada, but I had to ask, if only so he knew he was the first choice. He was understandably grateful (though I don't know how he'd be surprised) but he, being ever sensibly minded, admitted it likely wasn't feasible. My surprise was his parents who, in a commitment of untold proportions, declared that they would get Joel to that wedding. I am forever grateful to them.

The experience of having my best man with me for those few days in Canada was one of the highlights of my life and a tale told better from his perspective. The skidding down a muddy hill for the bachelor party, the photos in somehow immaculate wheels only a few hours later, the uncertain ramp up the front stairs of the chapel and the careful signing of the marriage certificate with pen in his mouth and his speech at the reception – all things I'll never forget.

But life went on. My wife's career later took us to Maryland and then to Minnesota while picking up a couple kids along the way. The visits were less frequent but still as special – even more so as I started to bring my boys with me. We're both somehow in our forties and while it's been more than a few years since we battled the Zerg, once the boys and those ever faithful parental units are in bed, we're back to sitting up in his room, talking until all hours of the night and sometimes early morning, just as if we were still back in high school.

It's only in retrospect that the impact of Joel's life thus far really hits home with me. Outwardly, no one has better reason for despair with the trials of life. But there's never despair, always hope. Not hope for something so pedestrian as to walk again but a sure hope, a trust and faith in the knowledge that he is not his own but belongs not only with his soul but yes, even in his body, to his faithful Savior. He knows people watch him, some out of curiosity, some out of fascination, some out of pity. To all of them, he shows nothing more than what he is—a child of God living each day for God's glory.

Joel is my oldest friend. I count myself lucky (well, blessed) on account of that. I love hearing stories people tell of themselves. Who can have a better story than him? I was so pleased a few years back to hear that he was starting to record those stories. Reading it over, it's clear to me that however long and close a friendship may be, hearing someone tell their own story will always reveal more. I've certainly had that experience reading these pages ahead and trust that others will end up joining me in the only appropriate refrain…

Thanks be to God.

Thomas Zeilstra
Rochester, MN
May 2023

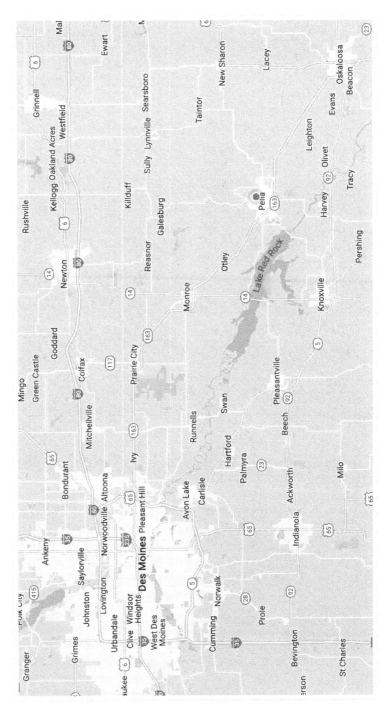

Google Map of Pella and surrounding areas

1

IN THE BEGINNING

In the opening chapters of Genesis, God tells how He created the universe by speaking it into existence. On day six, He created our first parents, Adam and Eve, from the dust of the ground. Starting from these first verses, God's plan for mankind is shown from beginning to end.

This book is my story, and how I have lived through the path God has given me. Starting from the beginning, I can look back and see God's guiding hand through it all.

My parents learned the basics of life from being raised on the farm in central Iowa. My mom, Julie, lived near the town of Sully with her two brothers and two sisters. Her oldest sister was born just before her dad went to serve in the Korean War. After his safe return, the Labermen family resumed life in his wife's childhood home.

Growing up in a family with five kids, everyone had their responsibilities around the house. Julie spent the summer months harvesting and canning vegetables from the garden with her siblings. It was not a fun task, but peeling potatoes for supper was something that helped feed the family.

Learning how to serve God was done both through church and Sully Christian Grade School. To cover tuition, Julie's family raised dogs and sold puppies. It was a unique way to make an income, and it provided for their needs and taught them how to work with what was given. On Saturday nights, if everyone knew their Catechism lesson for Sunday school, they would get a treat of a Tootsie Roll Pop.

At the same time, my dad, Lowell, lived on farms near small Iowa towns with his two brothers and sister. As a five-year-old, he ventured off and played by the coal mines around the town of Tracy. When a farm became available close to the city of Pella, the Vander Molen family moved to better land.

When the school day was complete at Pella Christian, it was time to do chores on the farm. Milking cows meant balancing on two pieces of wood while holding a bucket and watching for it not to be kicked over. Pigs also needed attention with fresh hay for bedding, especially in winter, and the barn needed to be cleaned out. After school was out for the summer, life didn't relax. Fertile Iowa soil provides work all year. Some jobs for Lowell included helping neighbors and relatives with baling hay, detasseling corn, or walking beans to pull weeds.

Growing up on the farm wasn't always work. If the bus was on time after school, Lowell could watch the television before his dad came home. Summer months allowed for handmade boat races on the nearby creek and fishing in the neighbor's pond. The loft of the barn was also fun with trying to swing on the rafters from the front to the back.

As the farm kids grew, grade school lessons moved on to high school with both teenagers attending Pella Christian High. With Julie a year ahead of Lowell, the two met at school and started dating. They had both grown up on the farm, but neither wanted to continue farming in their adult life. This was one of several items that grew their relationship. Most importantly, they both loved God and knew to look to His word for everything.

Julie graduated from high school in 1974 and started work at General Telephone in Grinnell. She was responsible for billing customers and verifying information on a computer with punch cards. That same year, Lowell started a school-to-work program at the Town Crier, a commercial printing company in Pella. Lowell completed school a year after Julie. He thought about attending college after graduation, but the Town Crier was persuasive, and he decided to stay with them, at least for a while.

After an epic road trip out west, Lowell got engaged to Julie in October at the Strawtown restaurant in Pella. His parents said he had to wait until he was 19 to get married. Six months after getting engaged, and five days after his birthday, Lowell and Julie were married. Expressing their love, the two exchanged vows before God, family, and friends. They would be together for better or for worse, sickness or health, for richer or poorer, until death would them part. Even though they were young, Lowell and Julie understood it was a lifetime commitment to each other, whatever would come. The newlyweds spent their honeymoon at Pike's Peak and Estes Park in Colorado. Julie had never seen mountains before, but Lowell loved the high hills. They found a new hotel that had just opened with rooms at $17.00 per night.

The young married couple left their parents' homes and moved into a small apartment near Central College in Pella. Lowell didn't think he could ever get used to "city" milk after growing up with it coming directly from the source. A year later, they purchased a house near the Pella hospital. The split foyer ranch was just barely in the couple's budget, but it was a good house. Lowell's parents helped inspect the purchase and gave their approval. The residence had space for three bedrooms upstairs and an open basement. Going from the garage into the basement was the only level entrance. Entering by the front-door meant going either up or down a flight of steps.

The drive to General Telephone ended for Julie when she started working at Pella National Bank. Through work, Lowell and Julie made friends they enjoyed spending time with. During her free time, Julie also had fun watching her nephews.

Four years passed and God had not allowed the young couple to start a family. After much prayer, they looked to medical assistance to find possible answers. Options were available, but any medical procedure carries risk, and one of the stated possibilities was death if complications arose.

Lowell said that Julie's life and health were worth more than any number of children and decided against medical solutions. Without a family, Julie considered going to college, but plans changed.

On Thanksgiving Day, Julie missed the usual celebrations as she went into labor, nearly two weeks earlier than expected. After spending all night in the hospital, Lowell was annoyed that he was missing football games on television. I arrived the day after Thanksgiving, on November 27, 1981. Lowell and Julie combined their names to come up with mine, Joel Vander Molen. They had waited five years for this day, and it finally came.

I was baptized at just a few months of age into the Christian Reformed Church denomination, where my parents were raised. My dad had become a railroad enthusiast through a friend at work, Richard, and made sure to start me off on the right track. One of my first toys was a train engine that went back and forth on the rail of my crib.

Both sides of my family were direct descendants from the Netherlands and fit well into the community. Every spring, Pella holds a three-day celebration called Tulip Time to celebrate the town's Dutch heritage. In 1982, I was decked out in a miniature Dutch costume and strolled through the streets of town with the other new babies that year.

My first birthday came quickly and was celebrated with my family. Dad's older brother and his wife had their fourth child, Russell, a week earlier and went to the hospital to bring him home after my birthday party.

Life wasn't always tulips and Dutch treats though, as I was often dealing with ear problems. When I reached 13 months, I had surgery to place tubes in my ears to help decrease pressure. On the way home from the hospital, my car seat sat between my parents. I reached out my hand and rubbed the arm of Mom's coat and my eyes grew big. There was a sound I hadn't heard before and I now had more things to explore.

Time continued to march on, and I was soon an active toddler around the house. Running around and playing was much more fun than taking a nap or trying to use that thing called the potty.

I loved to play with the other kids in daycare, but I especially liked it when my cousin Russell came to visit. Dad made a shelving system in the toy closet that I called my "neat." It was good for putting toys right where I could reach them, and Russell and I could also put ourselves in it and play.

Two of our neighbors had girls close to my age, Tera and Kera. During the warm months, the three of us would ride our tricycles around and around on my back deck. My trike squeaked whenever it moved. With the deck next to the kitchen, Mom could work on meals or dishes as long as she heard squeaking wheels. When the noise stopped, she knew to come investigate. I also liked to play outside in my large plastic sandbox. Inside the house, I had large tractors and wagons to use so I could farm just like my grandparents and uncles.

Dad's parents purchased a small grain elevator in town called Pella Feed Service. Along with my grandparents, both of Dad's brothers and sister worked at the grain mill. It was my favorite place to visit and see all the trucks and tractors bringing grain to sell. The train tracks also went right next to, and through, the elevator and I could see the cars parked nearby.

As a toddler, Mom enjoyed reading to me, and I sat on her lap through many books. I was very inquisitive and asked questions with every one of my books. However, it was always the same inquiries, every time with every book. I was also enrolled in swim classes at Pella's indoor pool. The lessons were fun kicking my feet in the water. However, I did not want to jump off the diving board. The instructor and Dad coaxed me, but I did not want to go. Finally, with the instructor's direction, Dad dropped me off the board into the water. The lesson didn't work, but it did leave a lasting impression.

The Trip that Changed Everything

After that summer, November 27, 1984, was my third birthday. As winter continued, I had fun helping Dad shovel snow on the driveway.

On Sunday, February 17, 1985, we had lunch at Mom's parent's house. Grandpa had a little red toy pickup that my cousins and I always wanted to play with, but he didn't let us. However, on this day, he let me carefully use it.

The forecast for the upcoming Wednesday looked to be good. Mom and her younger sister thought we would take a trip to Des Moines for shopping. I was growing out of clothes and the sisters enjoyed spending time together. It would just be the two of them, along with me.

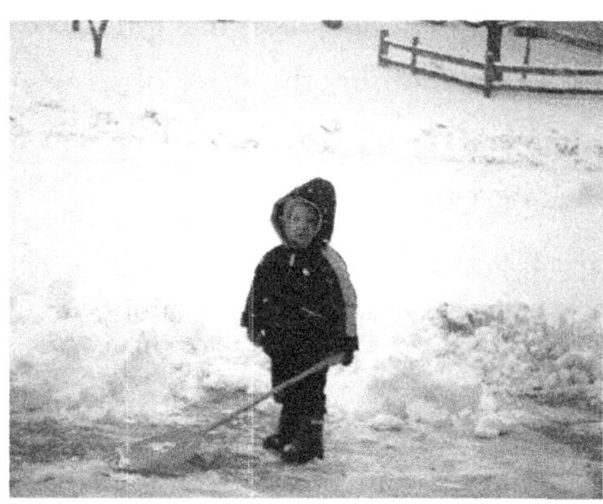

Wednesday came and, after daycare that morning, Mom wanted me to take a nap so I would be ready to ride in the car. I wasn't having anything to do with it though; running around and playing with my toys was much more fun. Dad wasn't planning to go, but decided at the last minute to tag along, so Mom delayed the excursion a couple of hours until he got off work. Around 5:00, my parents, aunt, and I got into Dad's 1976 blue Ford Elite with its long hood. I sat in my car seat in the back with my seatbelt on to help keep me contained, but nobody else bothered with the restraint.

Mom finally got her wish of me taking a rest when I fell asleep en route. As I slept in the car, my family continued driving to "the big city" of Des Moines. The weather forecast for a nice day wasn't completely accurate and it started to rain along the way. The two-lane highway 163 was wet, but not turning into ice. Dad continued to drive on to our destination but slowed down to better handle driving conditions. We were close to Prairie City, over halfway to Des Moines, and all was well. In just a few more miles, the road would change to four lanes and provide more open space if needed.

Not long after passing the town, an oncoming semi came toward us in the opposite lane. As the large vehicle passed by, the wind gusts it created pulled on our car and brought us into the opposite lane. Dad attempted to steer us back to the proper place but didn't make it. There was no time to react before another oncoming truck hit us. Upon impact, the front of the car was crushed, and all the occupants were thrown forward. Dad was thrown into the windshield and knocked unconscious by the jolt. Mom was pinned in her seat by the front dash with her ankles broken as well as much of her lower body and ribs. My aunt was stuck in the back seat, but received no lasting injuries, and the truck driver was not injured. The two most serious problems were Mom and me.

The lap belt caught me and dug into my abdomen, cutting my colon. My upper body was jerked forward, snapping my head, and injuring my spinal cord between the 2nd and 3rd vertebrae in my neck. I was instantly unable to breathe or control any part of my body below my neck.

Mom saw Dad motionless with glass protruding from his forehead and thought he was dead. While in great pain herself, she didn't hear me crying or making any noise from the back. Nobody knows how long I was without air, but God was watching over me. Gordon, another resident of Pella and volunteer fire fighter, was taking the same route to Des Moines and came upon the scene. He worked to assess the scene and determine who needed help. He saw that I was not breathing, but he couldn't work on me where I was positioned in the car. The two-door vehicle had limited access to the rear seats and didn't provide room to help me. Gordon very carefully got me out of my seat, laid my body on the cement, and started to perform CPR.

The lap belt caught me and dug into my abdomen, cutting my colon. My upper body was jerked forward snapping my head and injuring my spinal cord between the 2nd and 3rd vertebrae in my neck.

Despite not knowing what was wrong, Gordon continued to breathe for me while lying on the cold, wet pavement. A nurse came a short while later and provided blankets for both of us and helped monitor my heart rate. When paramedics arrived, they started to prepare everyone for transport. When they were finally able to get to me, Gordon had been providing my air for over 30 minutes.

We were all taken to Iowa Methodist Medical Center in downtown Des Moines. It was a hospital with modern facilities but not a major center for spinal cord injuries. I woke up shortly after arriving at the hospital.

Someone told me we had been in a car accident, but I did not know what was going on around me. Surgery was done to repair the cut in my colon and a tube was put down my throat so I could breathe. A few days later, I was given a tracheostomy tube (or trach) to use with a ventilator. To prevent further injury to my neck, a metal halo was screwed into my head so I couldn't move. The halo was soon removed, though, as it wouldn't provide further help.

Lowell had bruises and cuts on his forehead from the windshield. After a short stay in the hospital, he was released with no permanent injuries. Mom had the first of many surgeries to repair her broken bones with pins, screws, and metal brackets. She lay in bed in traction while I was in the Pediatric Intensive Care Unit (PICU).

My parents were told about my injuries, with the explanation that only time would tell what would happen with my nerve damage. The spinal cord wasn't broken, but it was bruised, and changes could develop. However, decisions needed to be made on what to do for some of my treatment.

Since I was only recently toilet trained, I could continue to use diapers. If I had been fully trained, then alternatives would need to be used such as cathing routines and medicine for bladder control. A routine started with cathing once a day to make sure everything was draining, and digital stimulation was added to help get rid of stool.

For breathing, a recent invention called a phrenic nerve stimulator was available. It gave an electric shock to the nerve and caused the diaphragm to move and make me breathe. However, it was believed that long-term use would cause permanent damage to the phrenic nerve. If a cure became available for spinal cord injuries, it would still be possible that I would not be able to breathe independently due to nerve damage. To avoid further problems, Mom and Dad decided to have me continue to use a ventilator. Options were either an LP-9 or PLV portable vent. The PLV-100 by Respironics was the quieter of the two and what they chose.

The type of trach I was given didn't allow air to pass over my vocal cords or allow me to swallow. A device called a g-tube was put in my lower chest to put food directly into my stomach. I couldn't feel anyone touch me, but I could feel the formula as it went into my stomach. It was cold and did not feel good.

I wanted to talk to anyone that came into my room but couldn't speak because of the trach. Instead, I ground my teeth back and forth with every syllable that went through my head. Every day, Mom would be transported on her bed, on a long, painful, journey through the hospital, to see me. My mouth ground out, "I love you," and I tried to talk with her, but I didn't know why she couldn't understand me. The words in my head came out perfectly through my teeth, but they just did not understand me.

One of my regular respiratory therapists came to check on my vent and took time to help me play. They found a toy that was right for me- foam trains. First, they came in a small package and looked like medicine pills. When they were put in water, they turned into different foam shapes. I watched with excitement as each pill magically turned into a train engine, car, or caboose. After they were all made, she put the train together on the table in front of me, but she put the red caboose in the middle. I kept grinding my teeth trying to tell her the caboose went at the end. Moving my head from side to side, trying to point directions, didn't help. Finally, to my relief, after much frustration, she realized the error and corrected it.

Dad was back working at the Town Crier but came to Des Moines as soon as he was done for the day. Both sets of grandparents were also regular visitors for Mom and me. Our pastor also came to visit us every week. As the weeks passed, it was apparent my condition was not going to change, and my spinal cord injury was permanent. The doctor said, "With the way medical technology is progressing, he'll likely be walking by the time he's ten." My arms and legs started moving a few days after the accident, much to the excitement of my parents. However, it was something called a muscle spasm where my muscles get stiff and move on their own. They can even be a reaction to being touched, but it's not under my control.

My doctors also wanted to try to give me a different kind of trach that would allow air to pass over my vocal cords. My parents were told that I could possibly be taught to speak some words by late grade school. The new trach was put in and a few days later, April 7, 1985, Easter Sunday, I said my first words with the vent. "I'm hungry." Speech therapy visited later that week, but I chatted with them enough that they didn't think they needed to return.

Though I couldn't move, I was still an inquisitive boy. My favorite books were put where I could see the pictures, and a cassette tape of Mom reading it was played as the pages were turned. Just as before the accident, I asked the same questions I always had, and the audio version of Mom answered every one of them. I was happy she talked back to me from the machine, but she sometimes didn't answer quite right.

I could also feel above my neck. Anything that touched my face felt good. When the nurses turned me to my side, I loved when my ear got curled against the pillow. It was something out of the ordinary, but they kept straightening it. My favorite blanket also had to be over my head or right beside me at night. The thin fabric and the silky-smooth border around it felt great to rub on my lips and cheek.

Sitting in my hospital room, my main entertainment was cartoons from the television hanging from the ceiling. I loved watching Scooby Doo, the Smurfs, Sesame Street, and a few others. One of them was the Duane and Floppy show. Floppy was a dog in a box that talked to his friend Duane. One day, those people came out of the TV and to my room.

It was arranged that Duane would come to see me along with his puppet, Floppy. When I saw them, I was terrified. Duane came into my room with that box in his hand. I knew if I looked at the box, that thing would come out and get me. Duane moved around the room to try to get me to look at him, but I knew I had to look away or it would pop out. I moved my head as fast as I could and hoped he would leave. They eventually left and I was safe again with everything back as it should be. Mom wasn't happy at the way I responded to Duane, but I was glad the thing didn't get me.

More Family Tragedy

Summer came to Iowa as Mom and I continued our recovery at the hospital. The PICU where I was had recently been added to the hospital and wasn't very busy. Some days, the nurses would close the unit and take me for a walk outside, pushing me in a wheelchair. Where a street had been, a new building was being constructed next to the hospital. I loved seeing the equipment and watching everything go up. Mom had a manual wheelchair donated by Easter Seals to use in the hospital, and later at home. When Dad came, he took Mom and me around the hospital in our chairs. I got to be in front while he pushed me and pulled Mom. Other times, I would sit beside Rose, the secretary in the PICU. We talked away as she did paperwork.

Throughout the hospital, there were fish tanks in different waiting areas. I liked making regular visits to the aquariums to see the different fish and watch them swim. One tank had large Oscar fish that were fun to make faces at. They were at the same level as my eyes, and I looked forward to visiting them.

In the parking lot, the helicopter was always ready near the emergency department. Each time it left, I could see it take off outside my window. I couldn't read yet, but figured out it was called Life Flight. I got to know the pilot, and he would tip the helicopter to wave at me through the window before leaving.

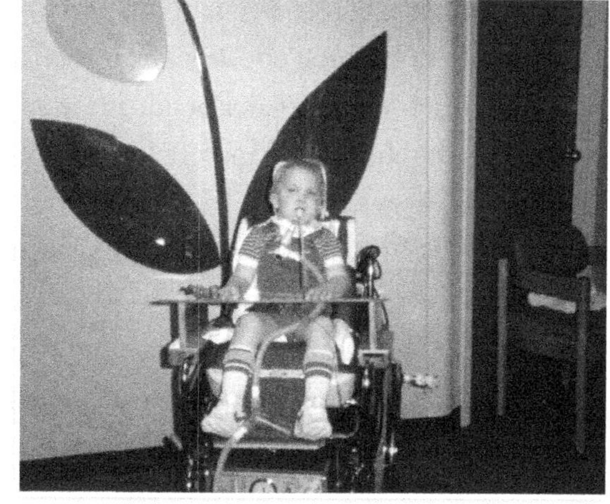

Even with the new trach that allowed me to swallow, I had no interest in eating. When my dad and grandparents came to visit, I would sometimes get in my wheelchair and venture to a waiting area down the hall. We had a great game of crunch contests. Everyone would put a Cheeto in their mouth and see who could make the most noise biting it. I chomped as hard as I could but didn't always win. It sometimes took multiple tries before I got it just right. I was always full from the other stuff I got, but crunch contests were fun.

There were not many rehabilitation options at that time, but I learned how to use a mouth stick to play games and put pegs in holes. Tic-tac-toe was a fun game. I had to pick up wooden pieces with my stick and put them where I wanted. If I was careful, I could beat the person helping me.

Mom had to learn how to walk and stand again. When we were both at therapy, I would help her along by saying, "Shake a yeg, Mommy!" My parents continued to learn how to keep me healthy and take care of me, clearing out my lungs with a suction machine, running the vent and its circuits. In order to keep my feet in good condition, they were told I needed specific high-top shoes to support them so they would not turn sideways.

While Mom and I adjusted to our new life, our families continued to support us as we looked forward to going home. My younger cousin, Russell, went with his parents to our favorite place, Pella Feed Service. While there, an accident occurred that resulted in his death. Dad was a pallbearer at Russell's funeral while Mom and I were in the hospital.

Finally Returning Home

After months of learning our new life, it was time for me to leave the hospital. Looking at the ventilator beside me in my hospital room, I watched as a green light blinked on and off and thought it was pretty. I asked if I could take it home with me. The nurse said she was glad I liked it and it would get to come with me. That news made me even more excited to go home again.

In 1985, it was unheard of for a child with my care needs to return home. My primary physician, Dr. Kelly, thought I should go to a care facility near Des Moines for children with severe disabilities. However, my parents knew God had different plans for me and insisted that I would go home with them. Dr. Kelly objected and warned them that if anything happened to me, they would be held responsible. He also said I couldn't go to regular school and be in the public as I would always be sick. After much debate and hard discussions, my parents got their wish.

Before returning home from the hospital, Dad had an assignment from Mom. All the toys I used to play with, my tricycle, sandbox, and others, needed to be out of sight so as not to remind her of them. When I was told I would be going home, I asked every day, "is this the day?" I told Mom I couldn't wait to play with my big tractors. I didn't understand why she cried when I said that.

Dad purchased a 1981 Ford club wagon van in northwest Iowa. A Crow River wheelchair lift was put in the side to get me up and in the vehicle. He had made a model train layout in the basement but dismantled it so the space could be used for medical supplies. Getting funding for nurses and equipment at home was usually a big hurdle. Thankfully, the Town Crier's insurance policy was the best Iowa Methodist had seen and 24/7 nursing was arranged for me at home.

On September 10, almost seven months after the accident, I finally left the hospital, and we went home as a family. I cried nearly the entire 40-mile trip back to Pella because I didn't want to leave all my friends at the hospital and miss watching the helicopter.

When the van turned onto our street, yellow ribbons were tied around the trees. Dad carried me upstairs to my bedroom and quickly connected me to the waiting vent. Seeing I had my own TV on the ceiling helped me feel better. The trip we had left on so many months earlier was finally over, and everyone was home.

Now we could resume the task of continuing in the life we had been given.

2

TRAIN A CHILD

Proverbs 22:6 says, "Train up a child in the way he should go, and when he is old he will not depart from it."

As a newly injured quadriplegic, lessons and routines that are learned in the first few months and years have an impact on independence. These life skills can become integral to life years in the future.

When Thanksgiving came in 1985, my family was getting used to the new routine of life. Mom continued to get rehab and still had a challenge walking and getting around. Since she couldn't always be available if one of my vent tubes popped off, I had a nurse every hour of every day. As we celebrated the holiday at my mom's parents' house, we had many reasons to give thanks. It had been a hard year, but Mom and I were home from the hospital and doing well. A nurse came with us to my grandparents' house to help with anything I needed, but she didn't believe in celebrating holidays, so she sat in a nearby room. It would take time to get used to having people around who had different backgrounds than my family.

Along with giving thanks, I also had a fourth birthday to celebrate. Learning to open presents with my mouth stick wasn't something I had practiced, but I soon figured it out. But to have room for my stick, my mouth needed to be bigger. I went to the hospital in Des Moines with Mom to rehab. A device was put in my mouth that pushed against my cheeks to stretch them out. It hurt badly and I wanted them to stop, but it went in and stretched again and again. Thankfully the procedure was only needed once. I had a big enough mouth already.

Another thing we adjusted was the way we used our split foyer ranch house. We had one restroom upstairs that was shared by the bedrooms. The other restroom was downstairs and became the designated area for sterilizing my vent tubes, trachs, and other equipment. One morning, my nurse was downstairs cleaning supplies while my parents slept. The tube of my vent popped off and the alarm started to sound 15 seconds later. I lay in bed struggling without air for what seemed like forever, but the nurse finally heard the alarm and came upstairs. This was different from the hospital when I had more people and monitors around.

That year, I started attending preschool a few days per week. A school bus from the public-school system came and picked up my nurse and me and took us to school. It was fun getting on the wheelchair lift and going high up in the air.

Insurance, Caregivers, and Night Shifts

Bills for my nursing and medical supplies continued to come. My insurance had a lifetime maximum of $1 million. If I reached it before I turned 18, they would no longer cover any of my expenses and I would have to use state funding. That meant I would have to live in a facility to get the care I needed. With Mom's experience in bookwork, she monitored billing closely. After about a year at home, she noticed the nursing agency was billing for more hours than the nurses came. After presenting this information to the insurance provider, the agency was dropped, and we were allowed to hire our own caregivers, but nights were still staffed through another agency. If a nurse couldn't come, their supervisor had to cover the shift. This meant finding and training our own caregivers for days.

One evening, women learning to help take care of me surrounded my bed. Dad showed them all of my cares and how to do everything he had learned. Two of them were Patty, who would help during the day, and Leah, who would cover three evenings a week. A volunteer relative would cover one night a week.

That was my last stay overnight for observation.

Every other week, I spent an overnight at Pella hospital to help cover hours and monitor my health. I did not like it at all, not knowing the nurses and not having someone where I could see them. Richard's wife, Dad's train friend from work, was a nurse and worked at the hospital. I liked it when she was there, but not when I was with anyone else.

One morning, my parents picked me up from my regular hospital stay. My hand and foot splints were on, but not correctly. My foot braces had small cups that were meant to go under my heels. Instead of being on my feet, they were on my elbows, causing dark red marks. That was my last stay overnight for observation.

Since we lived an hour from Des Moines, Mom was able to get insurance to purchase two ventilators. One was beside my bed and the other on my chair. If something happened to one, I could go to the other. One evening, I had a drink of milk, and the cup was put on top of my bed vent. Not long after, the bed vent was bumped and the milk poured down the front of the machine. The PLV-100 had a solid front with no openings, except for a small grate for the alarm. The milk went in the hole and stopped the vent from working and started to alarm. Because I was the only home patient at that time, an RT was able to come quickly to deliver another machine.

Starting Kindergarten

In 1987, I followed in my parents' path and started kindergarten at Pella Christian Grade School. I had a power wheelchair that I could control with my mouth. My chin wasn't big enough for the rubber chin control, so I just stuck it in my mouth and moved it the direction I needed to go. At recess, I could drive around the cement pad at school and often ended up having a trail of kids behind me playing "Follow the Leader." In class, I used a large drafting table for my desk that I drove under and sometimes listened to the teacher.

Dad made a wooden board that sat upright in front of me, and my nurse could clip papers on it for me to reach. With a marker in my mouth, I learned how to write the alphabet along with the rest of my classmates.

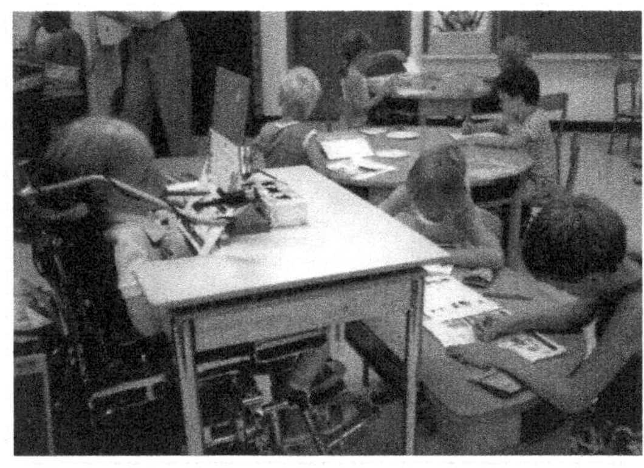

Twice every Sunday, Mom, Dad, and I attended church. The 1930's-built structure had a long flight of stairs leading up to the sanctuary and no other access. A chair lift had been installed at some point, but there was nothing I could use. To get into the church, Dad pulled me backwards, in my manual chair, up the steps while keeping me level. Once in church, I had a designated parking spot at the end of the very last bench.

The sanctuary floor was on a gradual downhill slope to the front for easier viewing. This meant my wheelchair was tilted slightly forward. Although I was doing well at increasing my neck muscles, I had little strength to hold my head back and, if it fell forward, I couldn't move it back again without help. As the hour long service went on, Dad frequently had to put my head back up to my chair's headrest.

As a kindergartner, I had yet to master the nuances of reading songs from a book. I didn't have a table and mouth stick to play with my toys, so all I could do was sit and watch, wait for the sermon, and then Dad would give a piece of candy to the three of us. If I sucked slowly, without biting, I could almost make the Life Saver last the entire sermon.

One evening service, Dad gave me my entertainment piece. I gladly took it in my mouth and secured it between my tongue and the roof of my mouth. As I started the slow battle of dissolving sugar, I lost my grip and the full-size piece of candy slipped into my throat and got stuck. Without making noise and getting in trouble, I tried to tell Dad what happened. My parents conferred with each other before my chair was quietly bounced down the steps. I was soon in the ER at Pella hospital being examined by a doctor. After a conversation I didn't understand, it was decided nothing would be done. The trach had stopped the candy from going too far and the vent was giving me air without problem. The next day in school, it still felt like I had the treat in my throat, but it eventually went away.

During Tulip Time, boys in kindergarten get to ride the wooden shoemaker float. When my turn came, it was a hot afternoon, and I was dressed in my black Dutch costume. Dad carried me onto the float and propped me up so I could sit. The vent was plugged into a car battery and sat beside me, along with one of my nurses in her Dutch costume.

My parents were told that I was unable to sweat and regulate my body temperature, and this day was showing the results. Before the float left, Dad got a wet washcloth and put it under my cap. This helped, but on the parade route I continued to get hotter and overheated. The sun felt like a hot iron blazing on my face that I couldn't escape. The other boys on the float waved at everyone as we slowly toured the parade route. I hardly noticed anyone; all I could think about was the heat and not feeling well. Dad managed to get through throngs of people to refresh my cold washcloth, but it didn't help much.

When the float finally reached the end of the parade, it was near my great-grandmother's house. My parents got me to the small home and removed my clothes to cool me with washcloths and fans. After a long time in the air conditioning, everything returned to normal. This was my first experience with overheating and autonomic dysreflexia, but not the last.

Our house had a level entrance from the garage into the basement, but there were stairs to get everywhere else. Therefore, my power chair had to stay in the basement and I was either carried upstairs to my room or Dad would bounce me up the steps in my manual chair. To help me navigate better in the house and eliminate having to bounce me up all those stairs, my parents found a small porch lift from a family in Sully. The woman who used it had died and her husband no longer needed it. Dad also put a sidewalk beside our house and installed the lift so I could get up on the back deck. From there, I could go into the kitchen and be on the main floor. My bedroom and the hallway were too small for my chair, so I still had to be carried to my room, but it was a shorter trip without having to navigate stairs.

Moving Up in Grades

The summer between kindergarten and first grade was a time of experimenting. Without control of my arms, I couldn't raise my hand in school. Therefore, the Area Education Agency (AEA) tried to find a solution. After testing various flashlights and gadgets, I decided on a small battery-powered light that would sit on my desk with a large switch on my headrest. It was a custom-molded plastic cup that fit around the headrest to keep it within reach. When school started, I was ready to raise my hand. If I got bored, it was also fun to play with, but the teacher tended to notice a blinking light quickly.

One day at school, my class had a substitute teacher helping us work on math skills. She gave every student two dice to flip and told us to add the numbers together. When she came to me, she said she was sorry I couldn't do the activity. "Yes, I can," was my prompt response. My helper, Patty, gave me my stick and I demonstrated how pushing down on the side of the dice made it flip. Patty had to pick it up from the floor, but my dice wasn't the only one there.

Most boys in my class were interested in sports. I couldn't participate in any and had no interest. Some of the kids made fun of me, but they didn't talk to me much. Therefore, most of my friends at school were girls; most of whom sat in front of me.

One day, I quietly sat listening to the teacher, Mrs. Henderson. In order for me to get in my desk, I sat in the back of the row. That meant I had four desks lined up in front of my large drafting table. While the teacher continued, I sat with my chin control away from my face. Patty often helped correct papers and sat beside me working on them. Suddenly, my chair took off forward at top speed. My chest hit my table, pushing it forward toward my unsuspecting neighbors. My friend Jana, sitting directly in front of me, was pinned under my table while she and her desk became part of the rapidly increasing chain. Hearing desk legs screeching on the floor behind them, the other students ahead bailed out of their desks. My chair continued to plow forward, pushing the entire row until everything hit the front wall. The rest of the class and my teacher looked quite surprised at this interruption and weren't quite sure what happened. Mrs. Henderson was about to reprimand me when she realized my controls weren't in reach and I had not willingly made the spectacle. Fortunately, everyone was okay, and class resumed as normal after the desks and students were back to their proper position.

As the school year continued, I discovered I could raise and lower my shoulders on my own. Doing so also made my arms move and, in my mind, I could control them. The next day in school I couldn't wait to show my classmates. I said, "I can move my arms, watch!" A few kids gathered around as I showed my new trick, but they weren't as impressed as I was.

When Leah came at 4:00, three days a week, she would help me through an exercise routine. She made me lift my head off the pillow ten times in a row, while she did various movements with my arms and legs. After my head lifts, I had to do ten rounds of raising and lowering my shoulders. Finally, she would put me in a standing frame and had me stand for a full hour. I didn't like any of it and just wanted to watch the Discovery channel or Nickelodeon on TV. However, she insisted I needed to do it and didn't let me skip anything.

Every day at school, groups of about six kids would go to the reading corner and work on reading skills with Mrs. Henderson's assistant. As my group was in the corner one day, I could feel my arms get stiff and start to stretch. I didn't want my arms to move, but I couldn't make them stop. Instead of them shaking as usual, my left hand came up and looked like I was raising my hand. I didn't have a question, though, and I hoped nobody would notice. Just as quickly as I thought about it, the teacher saw, and surprisingly said, "Yes Joel?" I quickly shook my head indicating that I did not have a question and I wasn't raising my hand, but I was powerless to put it down.

In the first years of school, my class and I worked on learning the fundamentals of reading, writing, arithmetic, and the Bible. Writing with a small marker in my mouth worked perfectly well, but reading was more difficult. When my ventilator gave me a breath, I could speak for a few seconds while air was coming in. After it stopped, the air exhaled through my vent circuits, and I had to wait to speak until the next breath. I could read the words in my head without a problem but reading out loud and having to stop and start every few seconds made it sound like I wasn't comprehending well.

In second grade, my respiratory therapist had me try something called a speaking valve. It made it so that my air didn't go out through the tubes, and I had to exhale through my nose when I wanted. With the first try, I did not like it at all. It felt like my lungs had too much air and I didn't know what it felt like to breathe out. I quickly said no and just wanted to stay with what I knew. But through the next few weeks, I had a hard time keeping up with reading in school and I told Mom I would try again.

After much encouragement, I gave it more of a try and soon loved it. Now I could speak without a pause. If I wanted, I could talk on and on without having to stop. I learned how much air to exhale and still have enough when the next breath came from the vent. It was great for reading, singing in school and church, but not necessarily for my parents and nurses, as I never had to stop talking.

Five years had passed since our accident, and I was still using the g-tube to eat. Every night, my caregiver would connect the tube to the ceiling above my bed and pour in formula. At our family meals, Mom would always fix me a plate of food with her and Dad, but I only ate a few bites. She wanted me to eat more, but I protested that my stomach was smaller than theirs and I just couldn't eat much.

At school, sitting with everybody eating around me, I would take a few bites, but wasn't hungry. Mom tried to tell my doctor to stop the formula for a few days and see if I would eat, but he wouldn't agree. He said it was my only way of rebelling against the life I now had.

One night, my feeding tube was secured above me with my liquid diet going in. I had a muscle spasm and my arms started to flail around as they often did. This time my left arm flew up to the feeding tube while wearing my hand brace. The force pulled it out of my chest, leaving a hole where it had been. The next morning, Mom and the nurse took me to the hospital to see what to do. My doctor said to try leaving it out for a few days and see what happened. Without a stomach full of formula, I started eating regular food. The hole eventually closed on its own, leaving a crater just below my ribs. Mom got her wish that I only ate by mouth. Next the challenge was finding food I liked, which was another large battle.

Just as some experiences from childhood can stay with someone into adult years, so can time with friends. School is often where these relationships start and can continue to grow.

3

PHONE A FRIEND

The book of Proverbs talks about the value of a good friend, as well as warnings about bad ones. Throughout scripture, friends helped each other, and Jesus was called a friend to sinners.

When I came home from the hospital, my parents acquired an Apple IIe computer for me to use to draw with a sip-and-puff system. It didn't work well, so it was sold to a college student. Through the late 1980s, home computers weren't very common. If I wasn't in my wheelchair, which was frequent, I often watched television in bed.

It was common for my cousins to be around the house. Mom enjoyed watching her nieces and nephews and I liked playing with other kids. Mom's older sister had three boys. They were all older than me, but not by much. The two younger boys and I liked playing with Construx building systems. We had their commercials memorized and could recite it in unison.

Every month, Mom's family had lunch at her parent's house. We usually got together in the basement, which required Dad to bounce me down the steps in my manual chair. After we finished eating, three or four of the kids my age would play together. Board games were common, but so was our own form of baseball. Someone would throw a ping-pong ball toward me, and I would bat it with my stick. However, I could only hit it behind me, and the ball pitcher would frequently run out of balls. Once they mastered walking, we trained our younger cousins how to collect the balls that I hit.

When Christmas came, I always asked Grandma Labermen if I could play Santa. When she said yes, one of my cousins would put the present on my lap, then push me over to the correct recipient.

Meeting Kyle

In grade school, I did well in my subjects and got to do extracurricular study time. I had already seen on the Discovery channel a lot of what we covered for science. It was still fun to get out of regular class and impress my classmates with what I learned.

At school, I had a few female friends whom I spent time with and I also knew some boys in my class through church. We would sit together in Sunday school every week and talk to each other, but we didn't do much together socially.

Dad's coworker, Wes, attended our church and lived a few houses from us. His son, Kyle, was a year ahead of me in school, but Wes said to give him a call any time to come and play. One day, I called to see if Kyle could come over. He didn't want to at first, but his parents made him. We started to play with my toys, and it wasn't long before he and I were best friends.

Dad's carpentry skills came in very handy to help me play. I had several small Ertl toy trucks and tractors, but I couldn't reach very far with my stick. For Christmas, Dad put a large round piece of wood on a Lazy Susan turntable. He painted roads and farm fields on the wood and made a replica of the buildings from Pella Feed Service. The board was easy to turn with my stick and my farm equipment could make it around as often as I wanted. I had a hard time keeping my head up, so for me not to hit my chin on the board, a rubber pad was put all around the edge.

It served a dual purpose of protecting my chin and containing my grain spills. Popcorn worked well as corn and split peas for soybeans. Kyle and I often had popcorn in more places than my trucks and wagons, but it rarely went on the floor.

If Kyle and I weren't farming, I could also be found working with Legos. Most people would think hands are required to play with these little plastic bricks, but that was not the case. Through practice, I figured out how to slide bricks up walls and what angle they needed to be. The stick then made a very handy hammer to get pieces pounded in place.

Small cars, planes, and trains called Micro Machines were just the right size and a lot of fun. I could push them around roads in plastic cities easily. A little bit of handy tack on the tip of my stick was just enough to pick up an airplane and make it buzz through my imagined sky. Unfortunately, not everything was stick friendly for play. Mom would go to Toys "R" Us before my birthday and Christmas trying to find board games and things I could do. Some trips got to be too much, resulting in tears of frustration.

Dad made some of my mouth sticks. He used an arrow shaft for the body and a wedge pencil eraser for the tip. For my mouth, he formed a chunk of plastic that was made in the proper shape and inserted the arrow shaft. He could also purchase sticks, but only if we were a medical facility. Since Mom hired our own nurses, our house qualified as a facility, but it saved funds to make them on our own.

I had sticks with a suction cup on the end of a hollow rod that I called a suction stick. I could place the cup on a block, apply a little suction with my mouth, and pick it up. Another version had a pincher on the end. I pushed a button with my tongue, and it slid the end of the stick forward and when I let go a rubber band pulled it back, and I could grab whatever I wanted. The sticks were different lengths, depending on what I was doing. I ended up with a variety of options, but they didn't fit in my school bag. I never knew which one I would need and took several with me. Dad found a plastic tube from work, cut it in half, put a cap on the bottom, and mounted it on my backrest. It was a great location to store sticks, but other kids kept asking why I had arrows with me.

Continuing to write and play with different instruments in my mouth allowed me to stay active with my friends and continue to learn. The only problem came when I started losing teeth. What my mouth and head knew to do for movement had to be adapted every time a new gap came, and I waited for the new tooth to come in its place.

In 1989, the Nintendo Entertainment System was released, along with a hands-free controller. For Christmas, I got my very own, along with Super Mario Brothers. The controller lay on my chest with the vent circuit off to one side. I controlled the arrows with a stick that I moved with my chin and activated the buttons by sipping or blowing into a straw. I could get most of the actions, except those that required extra hard pressure. It was sometimes all I could do to blow enough, but it usually worked. The ceiling-mounted television was perfect to see and play on my own or with Kyle.

Meeting Another Boy

As second grade continued, my parents heard about a boy in northwest Iowa who had been in a bicycle accident and received a spinal cord injury like mine. That summer, my parents and I made the five-hour drive to Sioux Center to meet with his family. His dad was a pastor in the Christian Reformed Church, and his mom stayed home to help with the family. This was the first time I had met another kid who used a vent and wheelchair.

> *It was fun exploring and being with another boy just like me.*

Aaron was a year younger than me and had a younger brother. Our visit started at the home of one of his nurses with some of her kids. Aaron stayed at her house for part of the day before going home to his parents. We buzzed around on the driveway in our power wheelchairs, having short races to an agreed-upon finish line. As we drove around, I noticed the driveway had a great view of the train tracks a few blocks away. The husband of the nurse was a professor at the local school,

Dordt College, and he took us on a tour to see large old tree trunks. It was fun exploring and being with another boy just like me.

On our way back from the college, we got near to the house where Aaron was staying. A large curb was between the street and sidewalk that led up to the home and didn't allow easy wheelchair access. Aaron drove along the edge of the street to the nearest driveway so he could get to the sidewalk and back track to where I was. Not to be outdone, I got a hand from Dad, and he popped the front wheels of my chair over the impending curb. With my chair's large wheels, I drove forward a few inches and expertly powered up the obstacle with my rear tires. Aaron concluded his detour just as I took the shortcut to the same location.

I liked that Aaron and his friends watched the same things on TV as me, and that he also had a hospital bed like mine. Later in the day, after both of us quadriplegics had a break, we met Aaron's parents at his house. He also had a Nintendo controller and was using it to land a plane on an aircraft carrier, just like I did. Aaron's brother helped direct the flight as Aaron couldn't see the screen from his wheelchair. It was fun to know I wasn't the only boy with major medical needs, but we didn't live close enough to get to see each other.

At home, Mom needed help with the large amount of medical paperwork and running the house. Karen started in this role about the time I was five. She and her family had a small camper and were members of a campground near Pella. Karen thought it would be fun for me to come with her and camp overnight.

At the campsite, the adults slept in the camper and the kids in a tent. I wanted to sleep in the tent, but Karen insisted it would be best for me to stay in the camper with her and her husband. That night, with everyone in bed, one of my vent's tubes disconnected. As the machine wailed, Karen looked for the problem while giving me air with the ambu bag. After a few minutes, she found the loose connection and put everything back together. Her plan to have me sleep in the camper proved to be good.

The freedom and fun of summer soon ended, and I went back to school. Most of Pella Christian Grade School was wheelchair accessible, but not all. One small section of the basement had stairs with no indoor wheelchair access. Three classes were in the basement, one second grade and both third grades. Since I couldn't get to the classroom, my third-grade teacher traded spaces with the upstairs second grade for one year. It meant I stayed in the same room for two years, but the school made it so I could attend class.

At the end of October, school held a Reformation Celebration evening where all the students participated in songs and other activities. With my speaking valve, I could easily sing with my classmates.

Halloween was also near, and my friends always got to dress up and pilfer candy from relatives and strangers alike. For Halloween, my dad put together wood, cardboard, and paint to make my manual wheelchair into a costume. Over the years, I went as a train engine, a racecar, and a tractor. My parents would get me in and out of the van, costume and all, and go trick-or-treating to my grandparents' house, teachers, and many others. Somehow, not all the hardly earned candy got back to me.

When he wasn't making costumes, Dad quickly became familiar with working on my wheelchair. My chin control had small micro switches that read what direction I moved the stick. If I went up, the chair moved forward, down was backwards, and left and right went the proper direction. Unfortunately, the switches wore down quickly and he often had to open my control stick, adjust plastic parts, and keep it working. Reverse wasn't used as often as forward, and swapping the components could make them last longer.

Mom continued hiring my daytime and evening caregivers. She assembled a book detailing everything I did, how to do all my cares, and how to clean my equipment. A short list of household rules was also included with items such as no smoking, appropriate attire, and putting my toys away when I was finished playing. It came in handy as night nurses didn't always stay with me very long. Hawkeye Health had to find replacements when one left, but they didn't have too hard a time covering my shifts. I cried whenever a nurse quit, wondering if I had done something bad that made them want to leave.

One of the new nurses always seemed to be mad about something. Dad told me that if she ever yelled at me about my stretching or muscle spasms to let him or Mom know. I said, "If she yells again, I will let you know." I didn't understand why I never saw her again.

Being careful with insurance funds, Mom found that the state would pay attendants that helped children at school. Since I went to private school, the administrators didn't think it applied to me and weren't interested in looking into the program. After a few years of persuasion, Pella Christian started to utilize state funding and covered my assistants while in school. It was a great relief as it helped decrease the cost for insurance and extend my lifetime cap.

Train Watching

Outside of school, Dad and I continued to enjoy trains. On warm weekends, he and I would spend a few hours sitting beside the tracks watching them pass. Just an hour's drive to the southeast of Pella, we could watch Burlington Northern (BN) trains go through Ottumwa and the surrounding area. Going north, the Chicago & Northwestern (C&NW) railway in Marshalltown had much more traffic than the BN, but with a longer drive. On rare occasions, we would take a two-hour jaunt to Ft. Madison in southeast Iowa. There we could watch a very busy Santa Fe mainline cross the Mississippi River and barges navigate the water. Kyle would come with us sometimes and Mom would come along just to spend time with her guys.

When someone loses one of their senses, such as hearing, another one often becomes more acute. Since I basically lost my sense of touch, my hearing was more fine-tuned. I could hear a train horn far in the distance, making my excitement level build as it came closer.

The summer before third grade, we took an overnight rail camping trip along the BN near Albia, Iowa. Dad's friend, Richard, came, along with his two sons. The back seat of the van could lie down and made for a perfect bed for Dad and me. Driving down a class B minimum maintenance road, we found a clearing of grass surrounded by trees, a secondary entrance to a farm field, and most importantly, bordered by rails. As camp was packed up Saturday morning, we watched Amtrak's California Zephyr speed past our location. It was an unusual consist with a private car on the end. Everyone waved to the people on the car's rear balcony as it quickly passed us. About an hour later, a BN vehicle came down the road to our location. The person we saw on the train was the president of the railroad and we needed to move as we were on railroad property. We were in that process already, but it was a fun overnight that I haven't forgotten.

Several months later, on a nice spring morning, Dad, two of my cousins, and I went on a train watching trip near Chillicothe, Iowa. It was a tiny town of no more than a few blocks in size, but the Burlington Northern tracks went through the hamlet. A few miles outside of Chillicothe was the large Iowa Southern Utilities electric plant and a two-lane bridge going over the tracks. Parking on the side of the road near the bridge offered good views of the rails, but not great.

Underneath the overpass, two large embankments held back the earth supporting the structure. They were concrete with about a three-foot flat section on the top. After surveying the land, Dad determined he could get me to the area under the bridge. Carefully parking on the side of the paved road, he got me out on the lift in my manual wheelchair. Tilting my chair back, he then guided me down a drainage path from the road under the bridge and parked me on the level cement. With my brakes on, the four of us heard the occasional car drive over our heads and had a bird's eye view directly down to the tracks. Amtrak even tooted a greeting to us as it flew past our location. After a few hours of watching trains, Dad cautiously pulled me back up the hill and into the van for our trip back home.

Three Weeks in Florida

Mom heard about a camp in Florida called VACC Camp. It was the Ventilation Assisted Children's Center Camp and was held in Miami every spring. Mom spoke with my school, and I did class work ahead of time for the days I would miss. In April 1991, we took three weeks out of third grade to travel to Florida and go to camp.

To prepare, Dad took the wheels off a Radio Flyer wagon and made a shelving system on it that held my bed vent and tubes with my supplies. My parents also purchased a camcorder to make video tapes to watch later. With everything packed, Mom, Dad, and I headed south. Along the way, we went through multiple states, picking up a bumper sticker in each one for my trunk. On Easter Sunday, we drove through the Smoky Mountains with a cassette tape playing piano gospel music in the van. Mom held the camera as Dad drove the curvy roads with music in the background.

Arriving in Florida, we stopped for a few days around Orlando to see some of the attractions. At the hotel, small lizards greeted us at the door to our room. I thought they were fun, but Mom had us try a different location with less wildlife. Everywhere we stayed, Dad would sleep in the same bed with me. If I needed something, I could wake him up and he could turn me every few hours.

My first request was to stop at Gatorland. I had only seen alligators on TV and thought they were neat. The trainer held a chicken in the air and a gator would jump out of the water and snap it out of his hand. April in Florida felt very warm to us with temperatures in the 70's and above. However, this was apparently cold for the reptiles and caused them to be sluggish.

As evening approached, we stopped in a small store that had shirts and other items. We didn't buy anything, but I noticed some weird looking gates on the door when we left. I started driving through, but as soon as my vent got to them, the door started beeping. I didn't know what was going on so I stopped. Someone behind me asked Dad if he had anything in his pockets. He responded no and the voice asked, "Is he wearing anything?" I guessed he meant me, but Dad again answered no. We were allowed to leave, but my vent had set off the security alarm.

While in Orlando, Dad found a train museum. The old rail equipment looked neat sitting under large open-side shelters. Several had stairs to the inside of the passenger cars, but none had any ramps. It was still fun seeing trains far from home.

Kyle and I watched shows from Nickelodeon on TV, so my parents and I visited Nickelodeon Studios, Disney World, Sea World, and Cypress Gardens. My parents didn't fully trust my driving skills in crowds of people, so Dad pushed me in my manual all around the theme parks while Mom tried to keep up with us. After seeing alligators, we spent a day at Disney World. Unfortunately, few of the rides were wheelchair accessible, so we got in at half-price. I loved the elevated train ride into the park and could have stayed on it. The only ride I was able to go on was "It's a Small World." However, at every place, I was moved to the front of the line at shows. The next day at Sea World, Mom pushed me so she could stay with us and take pictures.

Sitting high up at the water displays, I was safe from getting splashed and having a wet vent. The warm Florida sun felt good on my face as we explored the grounds. Unfortunately, my bright red cheeks that night at the hotel told a different tale.

Finally, at Cypress Gardens, all the blooming flowers and trees were beautiful to see, especially coming from chilly Iowa. After our time as tourists in Orlando, we finished the drive to Miami.

Every night at bedtime, I had to have my blanket over my head to sleep. It was the same one I had used for as long as I could remember, and it felt soft on my face. Mom said that it wouldn't look cool for me to sleep with an old blanket at camp. Therefore, as we left the hotel, I had my last night with my regular comfort. I graduated to a pillow and sometimes bed sheet over my head at night.

When we got to VACC Camp, all the grounds were level and fully wheelchair accessible. We went into a tall, white building, and checked in with the staff. Almost immediately, I met another boy, Greg, who was also a quadriplegic on a vent. His younger brother stood on the back of Greg's chair just behind the vent and they drove all over. We were instant friends and could chase each other around. About 10 minutes after arriving, he wanted to show me the grounds. With Greg's brother on the back of his chair, we took off, leaving my parents behind. I thought briefly I should have an adult come in case a tube popped off, but figured Greg's brother could handle it. It was fun driving down the paths through the trees as fast as our chairs would go. We found a small pond that looked like it had neon fish in it, just like my aquarium at home. There was also a ramp system that went all through the trees.

A few minutes after I left, my parents realized I wasn't there. Dad started looking for me in a large area that I could fully access and go anywhere. My group of three escapees started our way back to the main building when Dad found us by the fishpond. For some reason, he wasn't as excited to hear everything I had explored in my 15-minute excursion. I was at least allowed to stay in my power chair for the week.

VACC Camp had about twenty kids that year, all using vents or similar devices. Families also participated but stayed in nearby apartments overnight. The campers bunked in two large buildings with several small beds separated by short dividing walls. My parents flew Leah down to help at night when they weren't around. She had the bunk next to mine and slept during the day after everyone left.

While the kids were busy with an activity, the parents had an opportunity to introduce themselves and get to know everyone's story. My parents started off the introductions. With Lowell being his sarcastic self, he said he was my dad and, pointing to Julie, said she was some woman he picked up on the way down. None of the other parents batted an eye at this revelation, although Mom wasn't amused. Later, another parent asked Dad if my birth mother was okay with him picking up women. Dad kind of had an odd look on his face, thinking everyone understood his sarcasm. The concerned parent was then corrected on Mom's identity. Dad and Mom soon realized that of all the families, they and one other couple who had adopted their child, were the only two parent homes. Due to the increased medical challenges of my fellow campers, divorce was the normal result with usually a mother left to care for the child alone.

For most of the week's activities, everyone was loaded onto school buses and driven to our destination. We went to a parrot garden and watched birds do different tricks as well as some dog and monkey acts. Our group visited another aquarium with whales and dolphins, but with almost everyone using a ventilator, no splashing was allowed.

Greg and I continued to be friends during the week. If I was up in my chair before him in the morning, I would go over to his bed and bump it to wake him up. However, he never seemed to respond to my prompts as I expected him to. I slowly befriended another boy as well. José had very similar abilities to me but was unable to talk. I'd ask him yes or no questions and sometimes guessed correctly at what he wanted to do. Most of the time, we just ended up chasing each other around on the sidewalks, with parents watching.

One of the week's events was swimming. I had been told to avoid water so it wouldn't get in my vent or breathed in my lungs, so this sounded fun. Not all the kids used a vent all day like me. For those with just a trach, they could go out in the pool being held by adults. I was directed to park my chair close to the water's edge so I could stay tethered to my vent. Then I sat on the edge of the pool with Dad holding me up and with my legs in the water. Sitting there watching the other kids wasn't as much fun as being in my chair, but this was the first time I had been in a pool since getting hurt.

On the way back from getting my feet wet, a playground was pointed out that included a wheelchair swing. It took careful driving to get on it, but once loaded I could be pushed and let gravity take me up and down. I tried moving my head back and forth to go higher, but it didn't work well.

The last activity at camp was a boat ride through Biscayne Bay. On the way, our bus driver got lost and we joined the rest of the group over 30 minutes late. It severely decreased our time out, but I loved feeling the boat move my chair with the waves and seeing the bay. I noticed a police boat stayed nearby our entire trip, but we never got pulled over. Instead, it was directing us and was nearby if anyone needed help.

All too soon, we were saying our goodbyes to everyone. I told the counselors it was a fun week and I hoped I could return. They assured me I could, but my parents weren't as positive.

Leah flew back to Iowa while my parents and I started the return trip north. This time, we took a more direct route without many tourist stops. When I got back to school, I gladly showed off my tan to my classmates and had a lot of stories to tell.

The entire trip, my parents only had night help with me for one week. The excursion went well and let me meet more kids like me, but future trips wouldn't go as smoothly.

4

GETTING AIR

Genesis 2:7 says, "And the LORD God formed man of the dust of the ground and breathed into his nostrils the breath of life; and man became a living being."

As Adam and Eve's descendants, we require air to breathe and stay alive. For most people, this comes quite easily from the time we're born. That isn't the case with high-level spinal cord injuries. The vent worked well for many years, but changes came as I continued to grow.

Starting in fourth grade, I was becoming more aware of the world around me and the body I was living in. My class learned a new word, decade, early in the year. During the school year, most of us would be turning double digits in age, or one decade old.

> *Starting in fourth grade, I was becoming more aware of the world around me and the body I was living in.*

Twice every night, I had a chest percussion treatment. A vibrating wand was rubbed back and forth over my chest to help loosen any congestion in my lungs. After each treatment, as per the doctor's orders, my nurse would suction to see if anything came up. I learned to tell when I needed my lungs cleared and only wanted to suction when needed. Externally, I could feel my face, neck, and about the top inch of my chest. Internally, I had full feeling of my throat, lungs, and stomach. I also had some sensation of my major muscles in my arms and legs and could tell when they got stiff. Depending on what exact tiny nerve fibers are damaged, and how extensively, every person with a spinal cord injury has slight differences in feeling and function. Learning to use my senses, I talked to Mom, and then my pulmonologist at my next appointment. I told her, "I don't want to be suctioned after every treatment anymore but only when I need it." If done correctly, putting the tube down into my lungs didn't hurt, but it still wasn't fun. The doctor thought a little, and agreed to my request, which helped me sleep through the nightly treatment and only suction when needed.

One day at school, the marker I was using to write with started running low on ink. Patty noticed that the cap from a small marker fit perfectly over the end of a pencil. To keep the pencil from falling out, she put a little handy tack on the eraser. I could have a smooth surface in my mouth from the marker cap but use a pencil. With this invention, I could write just like the other kids and not have my work look different.

To help me write papers, AEA (Area Education Agency) got a Toshiba laptop that I could use to compose documents for school. I had to use the Caps Lock button to get capital letters, but it allowed me to type with my mouth stick. I hadn't used a computer since about the time I came home from the hospital, but it looked like something useful, and I could also play games on it.

Along with new tools, I learned how to better manage my breathing. I did not need to be suctioned frequently, but there were times I needed to leave class to clear my lungs. With the speaking valve, I could have the vent give me a couple of breaths before exhaling, and it would force any mucus in my lungs deeper down. If I then quickly exhaled this large breath, the junk would move up and make it easier to breath. The air manipulation resembled coughing but allowed me to delay suctioning for a while. However, I had to be careful and not hold in too much air. If the vent had too much resistance when it gave me a breath, it would give a high-pressure alarm and make everyone look at me. I had to learn just the right time to exhale so that I didn't make the vent beep and clear my breathing. It was great when it worked, but it was quickly noticed when I missed my timing. Eventually though, I had to roll out of class for a few minutes to get suctioned.

As the year continued, I started getting headaches frequently and I was taken to my general doctor to try to find a reason. Mom wondered if I was getting enough air and if that could be the issue. The doctor said the area my headaches were in didn't concern him, but to monitor it. Unfortunately, they continued to come and did not stop. Finally seeking another opinion, the second doctor said my head pain could be from not having enough oxygen. My pulmonologist was contacted to see if my vent settings could be adjusted to give a larger breath. However, the size of my current trach was not big enough to handle more air. I had surgery a short time later to enlarge the opening for my tracheostomy and go from a size four to six. I went home after the procedure and expected to feel much better, but instead felt worse.

After one day at home, I was feeling miserable, and my lung hurt. We went back to Des Moines to see what the problem was, and testing showed I had a collapsed lung. The new trach was not only bigger in diameter, but also longer than my old one. The added length made it so the device went into one lung and completely blocked the other. The next few days were spent in the pediatric ICU in Des Moines. My new trach sets had to be cut to the length of my previous size for both lungs to get air. Even with the adjustment, it took a while for my lung to inflate again and my breathing to return to normal.

This was my first stay in the hospital since the accident. Even after a few years away, the PICU was still familiar. The nurse's station was right outside my room, but Mom or one of my grandparents were almost always with me. When I was on the vent, it didn't feel like I could get enough air in my lungs. If it was taken off and someone used my ambu bag, the manual version of the vent, I felt like I was getting more air and felt better. The doctor said not to bag me, as the vent would help more. However, as soon as he left the room, Grandma Vander Molen put her back to the door and would bag me until her hand grew tired.

Now that I could breathe again, the rest of the school year went well, at least for breathing. As the end of the school day came near, I couldn't wait for the final bell to ring. I would race through the halls to get to the 5th grade classroom door and try to find Kyle when he departed the room.

Unfortunately, enthusiasm with a heavy wheelchair doesn't always work well together. My teacher, Mr. Klyn, stood by the exit as students made a dash for freedom. As I went through the door, I noticed a bump, but didn't think much of it. After I found Kyle and talked with him, I returned to my classroom. The bump I felt was Mr. Klyn's foot under my wheels. Karen made sure to remind me to be careful with my driving and to apologize for my actions. I felt bad for running him over and for getting the reprimand and I had tears flowing. When the bus came to take us home, I was certain I would get in trouble again after a report of my school day was given. However, Karen felt I had already learned my lesson, and nothing further was needed. I had several moms around me, and I couldn't get away with much.

Wednesday Night Cadets

In church, there was a group called Cadets that every boy from fourth through eighth grade attended. It met Wednesday nights during the school year, and we worked on Bible study, as well as badges for making models, camping, Scripture memorization, and much more. Cadets met in an old house next to our church, but it had steps to every door. Before my turn to join came, a long ramp was built to one door so I could just roll up and in. The boys in my group and I had fun with our counselor, Daryl, and learning all kinds of different projects.

Dad would drop me off at church, along with Leah, for the 90-minute meeting. She would either stay in the same room with me or sit near the door in an adjacent area. I liked spending more time with other boys from church, but I also got bored quickly. At the end of the year, we raced customized pine wood derby cars. Of course, I had mine made to look like a train. After racing was complete, each boy received points for attendance during the year, badges completed, and racing. Every year, I used my points to purchase fishing supplies that I always hoped to use.

Summer Adventures

Patty's husband, Erwin, grew up on a farm which his parents still owned. He also had a collection of Ertl farm toys, like my Grandpa Vander Molen. He made a ramp so I could get into their house. It didn't happen often, but I liked going to Patty's house and playing with their toys and her kids. They were a few years younger than me, but that was okay.

A couple of times, in summer and early fall, Patty took me to Erwin's parents' house to see their farm. They needed to move a wagon out to the field for a combine to fill. With Erwin driving, the two carried me into the tractor and sat me on Patty's lap. She used the ambu bag to give me air for the entire trip out to the field and back so I could ride in a John Deere tractor.

Since the trip to VACC Camp went well, my parents decided on another adventure for the summer between fourth and fifth grade. This time, we would drive out west to see Yellowstone National Park and trains along the way. No nurses would join us this time though; it was just the three of us.

In preparation, Mom and Dad packed my supplies and I got new trach sets as well. They were all customized to my size requirements and should work well. My Shiley trach had two parts, an outside trach and an inside tube called an inner canula. The inner section locked into the outer trach to make an airtight seal for my vent. The inner canula was changed at least daily and the entire trach was changed every other week. My newest set was put in just before we left so it would not need to be changed while we were away.

The trip started with a familiar drive toward Des Moines, but then continued to new areas. Going west, following train tracks, we went through an area called the badlands. Dad stopped at a place where we could all get out of the van and look over the area. The name seemed correct. I saw a lot of hills of rock with nothing growing on them. Later that day, we stopped at Mt. Rushmore. Mom had hoped to arrive earlier, but it was early evening when we got to it. Trees had returned, but a big rock stuck up in the middle of them with four president's faces carved into it. I had heard a little about the place, but it was cool to see it as the sun started to set. I noticed a big pile of rocks under the faces that Mom said came from the carving. I wondered why they hadn't cleaned them up, but I didn't ask.

Just like our Florida trip, Dad laid beside me in bed at night in the hotels. If I needed help, I could just say something or try to bump him with my head or make my body stretch. Dad regularly woke up and turned me, but I kept having trouble sleeping.

We made sure to stop and ride a tourist train in the area before continuing west. Then, the three of us made our way to Cody, Wyoming and looked forward to entering Yellowstone. The next day found a different plan. It was mid-June, but the gate we were near was closed due to snow. The Buffalo Bill Museum in town was open, though, and made for a distraction and helped to fill the day. Mom hoped we could get in the park the next morning, but the gate still didn't open. Therefore, my parents decided to try for another entrance, and we drove around the park to try to get in through a gate in Montana.

As we drove through the desolate areas of northwest Wyoming and southeast Montana, I kept falling asleep. Somewhere between sleep and being awake, I dreamt I was at home playing Nintendo with Kyle. Mom and Dad could hear me saying, "jump Kyle, jump," as the two of us played in my head. However, my parents wondered what was going on with me. Dad managed to drive around the expansive national park and make it to the northern entrance a few hours before it closed.

Even in June, Yellowstone was not as warm as I would have preferred. Even with jeans and a jacket on, I did not want to get out of the van. All I could feel was cold air on my face and I didn't feel well. At some locations, I won the argument and Dad got out to see a waterfall or something without me or Mom.

We stopped at an accessible boardwalk that went along some different things in the ground. There were small bright blue ponds with yellow edges that I thought looked good for people to swim. Other areas had red, yellow, and other colors of water that had steam coming off them. At one point, we came to an area on the walk that had a cloud of steam going over our path. I knew my vent couldn't get wet, but I couldn't go back and didn't have anywhere else I could go. I wasn't sure what to do, so I put my chair in the fastest gear I could and sped through the mist. When I got to the other side, everything was still working correctly, and I made it unharmed. Dad just kept filming with his video camera while I wondered if I would keep breathing.

Next, we went to see what Mom said were paint pots, which had another path I could drive on with no steam hazards. The ground looked like mud after a rain, but areas kept bubbling up. It sounded like when I blew in a straw with milk, but I didn't see anyone blowing.

Our destination was to see Old Faithful. Driving through the park, we could see some geysers in different locations beside the road. Dad pointed out there were a lot of dead trees from a fire a few years earlier. I didn't know what fire he was referring to but did think there were a lot of them.

After driving and more sleeping, we came to a big building that had some stuff in it. I saw on one wall a paper clock that said the next eruption would be at a certain time. A few minutes before the expected eruption, the three of us went back out to the clear, but cold, outdoors to watch the event. It went off later than the wall clock said, but it went higher than the other geysers we had seen. As water spouted in the sky, I watched small streams come from it and trickle under the viewing area we were on.

As we left Yellowstone, Mom and Dad were wondering if they should take me to Salt Lake City or some major hospital to see what was happening with me. They were growing more concerned about me falling asleep during the day and not always making sense when I talked.

That night in the hotel, Dad checked my vent tubes, connections, and my trach. He noticed air was leaking between the crack of the trach and inner cannula. When I was awake, I breathed in larger breaths to talk, but more air leaked out when I slept. He took a Band-Aid from his bag and wrapped it around the gap between the two parts. The simple solution stopped the leak, and I slept well. With the problem fixed, we started driving toward home. We followed the train tracks in Wyoming and could see an Amtrak train on a cliff in the distance. Our route coincided with it, and we got to the station in Green River shortly before the train. Dad unhooked my chair from the van's seatbelts, and I drove out onto the lift just as the train was arriving at the depot. I stopped my chair on the platform and Dad started lowering me to the ground, however, the wheelchair didn't follow my command. Once again it took off at top speed without me in control and only inches to the edge of the lift. Dad quickly noticed what was happening and fought to keep my chair from popping over the safety ramps and to the ground. Resembling a bucking bronco, he held back all 400 pounds of the chair with one hand and operated the lift's controls with the other. Once I was safely out of the air, Dad hit the off switch to stop any movement. We missed seeing the train up close, but everyone was safe.

A day later, we arrived in Omaha and went for lunch at a fast-food taco place. I sat a few feet away from the order counter and looked over the menu. The manager came from behind the counter and, simultaneously, my chair took off straight for him. Dad was standing just behind me and took one large step and managed to hit my chair's off switch, making it come to a screeching halt. With very large eyes, the manager looked at Dad and said, "What would have happened if you didn't do that?" With half a grin, Dad replied, "He would have run you right over." With a pale look on his face, the taco manager gave a quiet response and went on his way.

The remainder of the trip home went without problems, but my parents were glad to be back in Iowa where they had help to take care of me. It was the last time just the three of us took an extended trip.

Dad worked on everything he could and shipped out various components for testing, but my power wheelchair continued having problems. Finally, just after starting fifth grade, my entire chair was sent to Buffalo, New York to be serviced. That meant I had to use my manual wheelchair and get pushed everywhere. It was annoying that I couldn't move on my own, but I hoped it wouldn't last long.

Back to School

Along with different wheels, my class could start taking band. My classmates tried different instruments to see what they liked best. I was offered items from the percussion section and things that used sticks. School required students to have taken piano lessons to join percussion, but this was waived for me. The bells, or xylophone, worked best and I soon had my very own set to play. With the mallet in my mouth, I could give a quick hit of the note to make it sound. I learned to read music along with my classmates and enjoyed playing with everyone; but practicing at home wasn't fun.

For the first time, I was no longer in extracurricular classes. My grades had been dropping and I was having more trouble studying. As the school year continued, some lessons started to become more difficult. I studied for several nights for an upcoming science test, but my final mark was below passing. After receiving the grade at the end of the day, it was hard to keep the tears from flowing. Mom assured me I had done my best, as she had seen me study, but it still didn't feel good. I could look at the material, but I could not remember or always understand it.

Very few children with my physical challenges ever went to regular school. The AEA followed me to see what I might need help with, and how class went. One morning before school, Mom told me someone was going to be in class to see how I interacted with other kids. They would be told she was a student teacher, but it wasn't true. Throughout the day, I wasn't sure if I was doing what I should be for her. In warm months when I had my regular chair, I could go outside during recess. I sometimes played Red Rover, dodge ball, or duck-duck-goose with the other kids. I could tap someone's back with my footrest to pick them as goose or drive out of the way of balls. However, it was cold and snowy outside, so I didn't go out on the playground. A few boys from church who were in my class stayed back and we played with some toy skateboards we were given in Sunday school. We did it regularly, but I hoped it was what the observer wanted to see.

Along with academic problems, it was getting harder to take care of me in our house. Every day, I had to use the lift outside to get in and out through the back door and then park my chair in the kitchen. To get into bed, Dad or my nurses had to carry me down the hall to my room. I wasn't very big, but I was growing and something needed to change before I got heavier. My parents looked at the possibility of adding on to our current residence and remodeling, but limitations made this option impractical. Therefore, they decided building a completely new house that I could easily get around in would be best.

As winter 1992 turned into 1993, several different plans were evaluated and a building contractor from church was hired for the project. An empty corner lot was available several blocks north from our current address. It wasn't on a dead end, or just down from Kyle, but would meet our needs. It had enough slope to allow for a walk-out basement and was in the budget.

My parents spent many nights working through plans, deciding how to lay out rooms, and affordability. I lay in bed in my room somewhat listening to them and waiting for what seemed liked forever to get a response to requests for help. Sitting with an increasingly annoying itch on my face or the wrong channel on TV, I kept telling myself, "This too shall pass."

Finally, over halfway through the school year, my power wheelchair returned. Before shipping it east, Dad said the problem was in the main control box. Fortress insisted that was not possible and therefore needed the full chair. The conclusion was that the main control box was indeed causing the issue.

In class one day, Mr. Kimble, my fifth-grade teacher, came to me as the students worked on an assignment. He wanted me to push down on his hand with my stick as hard as I could. I wasn't sure why but obliged to his request and then he promptly left the room. We were studying U.S. government, the House and Senate, and discussing our class laws. As I continued helping with our project, I saw him get a long dusty board and set it up under his desk with some other scrap wood. A short time later, Mr. Kimble redirected us to the next lesson of the day, fulcrums. He told us that if a lever is used with a fulcrum in the middle, a downward force can be used to move heavy objects. Then he called me to the front of the room and told me to bring my stick with me. I parked beside the dirty board which I noticed was a height I could reach. Mr. Kimble had me push down on the wood and, with just my stick, his desk slightly tilted up! I was impressed that I could move a big desk on my own.

My Time of Fame

Just before the arrival of spring, a local television meteorologist contacted Mom about doing a story on Kyle and me. Pam Daale was a paraplegic and had seen me a few years earlier when visiting school. The station was doing a segment on friends of people with special circumstances and wanted to use us as part of it.

The camera crew came to school and recorded me getting on the bus to go home and Kyle riding along. With me in bed, the crew interviewed Kyle in my tiny room. The bright camera lights were really warm, and I liked how my room glowed. Kyle told the reporter he hadn't really wanted to come at first, but his mom made him. After a few visits, he started seeing me as just another kid and liked coming over. Now, we were best friends and did everything together, at least when our parents allowed.

A few weeks later, we were on ABC 5 News as part of a segment on Pam's heroes. Nobody else in my school had been on the news and it was great to talk about it. One of my writing assignments later that year used my time of fame as the subject.

For Tulip Time in May, all students in Pella, from kindergarten to fifth grade, marched in the afternoon parades. Every class would march together, holding hands, with everyone dressed in Dutch costumes, or something resembling one. My power chair didn't go the same speed as the parade, nor was it always trustworthy, so I had to be pushed in my manual. Sometimes my classmates would help me, but usually my nurse pushed me around the parade route with the other students. Fifth grade marked the end of the tradition for me and on to more grand participation.

More Summer Excitement

The school year eventually came to an end with another summer of fun ahead. After looking at city codes, budgets, and what we needed for a house, final blueprints were made, and house construction began in early summer of 1993. Leah and I could walk over to watch progress in the evening and Patty would drive me over in the van to see construction equipment working. Along with construction, I had other activities to look forward to.

Before I went to VACC Camp in Florida, Mom heard about another camp in the Midwest, but it was only for kids that lived in a certain hospital in Indianapolis. Now, CHAMP Camp, standing for Children Have A lot of Motivation and Potential, was open to all kids with vents.

Unlike Florida, parents did not stay with the kids, but Patty was going along to help me during the day. As we made the twelve-hour drive to Columbus, OH, the basement was dug for our new house. After a long drive, we dropped Patty off at the camp's grounds near Ashley, Ohio for training. My parents and I stayed in Columbus overnight so they could drop me off the next day. Everyone had an allotted arrival time on Monday, and we waited at the hotel until time to leave. An hour later, we were back to Recreation Unlimited for an arrival in a steady downpour.

We came to a circular drive on the main gate and were greeted by a mob of adults screaming, "Joel!" The three of us looked at each other wondering what I was getting into and nearly kept driving around the circle to make a quick retreat. Dad stopped the van and got me out to the waiting crowd. More people started unloading the back of the van with all my supplies as Dad made sure his and Mom's suitcases weren't also taken.

Mom and I were ushered into a small room for getting checked in and we were introduced to Dr. Chuck. He responded that he wasn't a real doctor and just played one on TV. He wore a t-shirt that was printed to look like a physician's lab coat and shorts. No matter who he was, he and a nurse took my blood pressure, medical information, checked to make sure I didn't take any medications, and then went to the bunk cabin. Mom kept waiting to meet the actual doctor at the camp, but was surprised Chuck was it. After a short time, my parents left, but stayed in a hotel about 15 minutes away, just in case.

The grounds were much more open than in Florida with less trees and paths that went in large circles. The rain provided great puddles on the sidewalk to roll through as we were shown where my stuff had been taken. All the boys were in one cabin and the girls in another. My bunk was between two other campers: one was James, who was also a quadriplegic, and the other George. James and I became friends almost as soon as we met. He sounded like Donald Duck when speaking, but I could usually understand him.

The week started off cloudy, cool, and wet, but activities continued as planned. One of the first activities was an obstacle course through the woods. As my trail group approached, we had to leave the cement path and go through the grass. Another camper was ahead of me, and I hesitated to get off the sidewalk. I knew the grass was wet and my wheels would get dirty. I thought, "Dad won't like me getting my wheels muddy." Then I remembered the cabins had concrete floors and I would not be home for several days, so drove ahead with my group after my short internal debate.

Some of the obstacles had physical challenges and others mental. One had a ramp up to a balance board. To get through, I would have to park my chair just right so the board would stay level. I crept up as slowly as my chair would move and was guided by the counselors. A little too far forward, I would tip ahead, but not far enough didn't work either. After a few minutes of determination, I got it just right and sat perfectly balanced.

Other obstacles required campers to get out of our wheelchairs and have a counselor or two help us across. I was put on someone's back as he carried me through a rope course. Another counselor used my ambu bag during the challenge so I could get air. I wasn't comfortable doing activities that made me get out of my chair, but I went along with the group.

What I liked best was fishing in the small lake. Surrounded by trees, a floating dock went several feet into the water and provided a platform where I could sit and see my bobber. The camp had a fishing pole that strapped to my chair's arm rest. Hooking it to a battery and motor, I could hit a button with my chin to make the line reel in. I couldn't cast or catch anything big, but it was still more than I had done before.

By Wednesday, I determined this would be my only year. The activities and people were okay, but not quite that fun for the long drive. It was also pool day for my group. Unlike at VACC Camp, all the kids got in the water, or away from the edge at least. Patty and another counselor got me out of my chair and laid me on a blow-up floating lounge type mattress. They put towels and other items behind my back to prop me up. Then, one person would bag me while another moved me around like a barge. It was fun to get off the sidelines and out in the water with everyone else. Counselors were eager to be targets for water guns and to control them for anyone. Lounging in my swimsuit, I just couldn't get comfortable on my mattress, despite many attempts to adjust. I didn't stay in the pool very long and was content to sit in my chair poolside with Greg, another camper.

At supper, I heard that our evening group activity would be a dance. My eleven-year-old mind went swirling. I didn't know how to dance; did I have to pick one of the girls to dance with? As my thoughts raced with excitement and apprehension, I also kept feeling cold. With several days of damp weather and little sun, I never felt like I could get warm. I wanted to avoid sitting under a fan in the cafeteria, but there wasn't a choice. All the available tables that I could get to were under the objects circulating air.

As Patty helped feed me supper, we noticed my right arm kept shaking, shivering, and felt cold. We went back to the cabin after eating and took my temperature; it was 93.3°. A little later, I was lying in my bunk with blankets over me and Dr. Chuck came to check me out. He didn't believe the thermometer and took my temperature again. It now read 93.0°.

The medical team decided I would stay back from the dance in my bed with warm towels and wash cloths, as well as turning off the cabin ceiling fans. After the dance apprehension and all the excitement of getting checked out in an unfamiliar area, tears started to come. Patty stayed with me, supplying warm wash cloths, and the uneasiness went away quickly. The warming regime gradually got my temperature back to a better number, so I was ready for the next day.

Thursday was the last full day of camp and included closing ceremonies by Lake Crumb. It had been a good week of fishing, arts and crafts, obstacle courses, swimming, and pranks between cabins. After I received my reward of top fisherman, I was ready to be done with camp. However, upon returning to the cabins, a squirt gun battle ensued between the boys' and girls' cabins. I couldn't operate the gun, but several counselors were willing to squirt anywhere or anyone I wanted. A trio of girls had been behind several of the week's shenanigans, and I made sure they got extra wet. After about 20 minutes of battle, my cabin declared victory and we worked toward going to bed. This final part of camp completely made up my mind that this was a great place, and I couldn't wait to come back next year.

After camp, I spent the rest of summer checking on the progress of the house construction and playing with Kyle. With all the rain, it was difficult to keep the basement and everything dry. As the walls went up, various ramps were made so I could get in and see the different rooms.

Just after her 4:00 shift started, Leah and I went up the street a few houses to see if Kyle was home. It had been a hot day, and I hadn't heard anything from my friend. When we arrived, we went up the driveway and rang the doorbell. Nobody answered the door, so we left to go home.

Most of Kyle's driveway was level, but the end had a steep incline and small bump to the street. I couldn't hold my head up going forward, so I backed down the hill as I had done before. When I got to the bottom, my rear wheels dropped off the bump and I was suddenly looking straight up into the sky. My front wheels kept going up until none of my wheels were on the ground and I was pointed up. With my chair laying on the vent in the back, Leah managed to get my front wheels back on the ground. I learned that cement swells on hot days, making bumps bigger and flipping my chair backwards.

Summer 1993 ended with a record flood in central Iowa, making house construction difficult. After a few short months, sixth grade and the start of junior high were upon me, along with more changes to life.

5

THE PRESSURE MOUNTS

James 1:2 says, "My brethren, count it all joy when you fall into various trials." This passage refers to being tested in our faith as a Christian, but trials come in many forms. Growing up with the added challenges of quadriplegia had times in life that were quite difficult.

Junior high at Pella Christian Grade School went from 6th-8th grade. Just as in lower grades, we stayed with our same classmates all day. However, we now had set periods and needed to change rooms for each subject and use lockers for our books.

After fifth grade, Mr. Kimble suggested I get a smaller table so my classmates could get closer to me. With using more classrooms, my parents purchased a few overbed tables. They were on wheels and could easily be moved when I wasn't in a room, but I could roll my wheelchair under them and have enough space for anything I needed.

New classroom arrangements became familiar easily. I learned to navigate the halls around other students and locker doors without hitting anyone, usually. As teen years approached, my growing body also started to adjust. Sitting in my chair, I wasn't comfortable unless my hips were moved to one side. With this position, I felt stable and could use my mouth stick or pencil easily, but it also made the rest of my body sit at an odd angle and caused my spine to curve.

A few months after school started, the new house was nearing completion. Unlike the current house, every doorway was level, without stairs, and I no longer needed a lift. My room and neighboring laundry room had sliding pocket doors so the hall would be free of obstacles. Finally, on November 20, 1993, one week before my twelfth birthday, it was moving day.

As Dad, his brothers, and much of our family picked up furniture and boxes, I tried to stay out of the way as much as possible. I sat in a corner near where the dining room table had been and felt the sun on my face through the window. I enjoyed the warmth and a sense of calm compared to everything going on around me.

After a few loads, it was time to use the lift to exit the split-foyer house for the last time. The porch-lift I used for so many years had a built-in hole in the new house so I could use it to get downstairs. I could also go around on the sidewalk outside and use the walk-in doors during the summer.

The commute to the new house went quickly and I drove from the garage right onto the main floor. Navigating around boxes, I parked beside one of the large windows by the fireplace. The sun came through the glass and perfectly warmed my face. It felt like a warm departure and greeting saying everything would be okay.

The first night in our new home, I laid in bed looking around at my new view. Lying flat in bed frequently, I knew my old bedroom ceiling well. I now had new bumps to get familiar with while my cares were being done. Just as before, there was a chair directly beside my bed for the nurse to use, and my TV was on the ceiling for easy viewing.

I thought about the old house and how it was the last house I was able to walk in. I thought about the orange kitchen carpet that had come loose from my spinning in circles. Mom came to check on me and asked how my day went. A tear escaped from my eye when everything hit me, all at once. She brushed it away just before the night nurse came, trying to find all my supplies for her shift.

Shortly after moving, Mom's job at Pella National Bank was eliminated, so she started working at Pella Feed Service with Dad's brothers, sister, and parents. The accounting work was different from the bank, but it allowed more flexibility to be at home and work on insurance claims and paperwork.

A few months later, Dad and Richard planned to go on a train trip to Glacier National Park and do some hiking. Before he left, Mom made sure he installed a new lift system so she and the nurses could get me in and out of bed more easily.

I thought the Barrier Free lift was neat, as it had a steel beam on the ceiling with a small crane that picked me up with a sling. After adding extra cross-bracing in the attic, Dad drilled holes in my ceiling with large bolts coming through them. As I laid in bed, he, along with Kyle, positioned the long 20' track above me, which was nearly the entire length of my room. Dad and Kyle got it in place, bolted it to the ceiling, and put the lift on the track. When the battery was charged, Kyle took the inaugural test flight through my bedroom. The sling came between his upper legs and pulled tight. He advised caution when placing it and pulling me up so that nothing sensitive got crushed.

Along with new housing, our church also had an update. To get into the sanctuary for worship, everyone had to first ascend a long flight of stairs. Every week, for morning and evening service, Dad pulled me in my manual wheelchair up every step. After church, it would be a careful descent to the front entrance. After several years of this practice, an elevator was installed in the southeast corner of the building. It was a tight squeeze, but I could stay in my power chair and easily go from the outside to the sanctuary, and to the basement for Sunday school. I was initially the primary person to use the lift, but some of the elderly members also utilized it.

Sixth Grade

At the start of every school year, my nurse and I would show my teachers how to use the ambu bag. If my vent quit working and my assistant was gone for some reason, my parents wanted to have a backup. It was a very unlikely sequence of events, but we went through the procedure, just in case.

Sixth grade continued with reading assignments such as *To Kill a Mockingbird* and with science experiments, including incubating chicken eggs. As I sat in class, Karen stepped out through the back door to use the restroom. Shortly after she left, I heard the vent tube behind me pop off and I no longer received air. With my speaking valve in place by my trach, I had learned how to move my neck and throat to breathe on my own. Conditions had to be perfect, but I could go on my own for a short time in an emergency. Karen also taught me that if something happened, I needed to stay calm and not panic as it only raised my heart rate and made the situation worse.

As soon as I heard the tube come off, I started my breathing routine, but I knew the alarm would start to sound after 15 seconds of no air. Growing up with mainly the same classmates, I knew a few I could use to try to help if needed. Just as the alarm started, I gulped in a larger breath and called for one of the boys, Levi, a few desks ahead of me. He had been in school with me since kindergarten and was also with me in Cadets and Sunday school. I thought he may be able to figure out how to reconnect the tube.

Levi headed to where I directed him, as Mrs. Jungling began to look panicked as she realized what was happening. Unfortunately, the tube came apart at one of the trickier places to get reconnected. Even though I couldn't see it, I knew my vent circuits well and what he was seeing. Levi couldn't reattach the tube, so he sat down while my vent continued to scream. Just as our teacher got to the front door to get help, Karen appeared. With her eyes the size of dinner plates, Mrs. Jungling said, "Joel needs you!" Karen looked over to see me grinning from ear to ear, but then heard the vent's alarm as she got closer. She quickly slipped the rubber connector back in its place and I felt a welcome breath of air fill my lungs again. The entire scenario only took a minute or two, but I did as I had been taught and was thankful everything went well.

Another day, as I sat in my manual chair just before lunch, Karen wanted us to leave early to get our trays before the crowd came. I told her to go ahead, I would be okay. She gave me a strange look but went to get lunch. When the bell rang, my classmates filed out in front of me as I sat unable to move. When almost everyone was gone, I got the attention of the girl I had been waiting for and said, "Will you push me?" She complied by putting her books on my lap and shuttled me the short distance to our homeroom where we would be eating lunch. Karen returned shortly to find me with a large grin plastered on my face and wondered what had happened during her brief absence. Just because my body didn't react to my thoughts or commands, did not mean typical teenage hormones had stopped.

Junior high was also the first year my class joined the marching band. Kyle had been in band for a year already and I was glad to join him, but I could not drive my chair and play the bells at the same time. This meant on days when we practiced marching, I had to use my manual chair.

When Tulip Time came, I was ready to play with the band as we marched around the streets of Pella in our wooden shoes and band uniforms. Our band played in three of the six parades over the three-day period. On sunny days, the light reflected off my metal bells and nearly blinded me. I was happy to see turns coming so the light came from different angles and did not reflect into my face. Patty pushed me along the parade route as I gladly played with the rest of the band.

Summer Break and CHAMP Camp

A few weeks after school let out, it was time for my second year at CHAMP Camp. Unlike my first experience, this year at camp was typical late June weather, sunny and warm.

The activities had changed a little from the previous year and included horseback riding. The saddle was modified to include a holster for the respirator and a battery to power it. Getting up on the large animal was a team effort, but one that had been practiced several times.

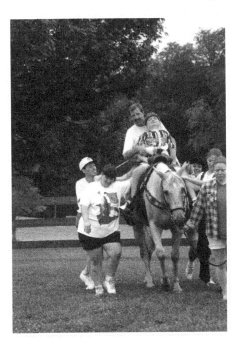

I sat straight up in the customized saddle with my head strapped to keep from falling over. Switching from my vent to the one mounted on the horse was done quickly so as not to cause alarms and frighten the animal. I didn't like the way the camp's vent gave me air, but since it wasn't going to be long ride, I didn't have Dave, the camp founder and RT, mess with it very much.

With final adjustments, I was soon off on my first horse ride. One person led the horse around a circle while two other counselors walked beside me. In case the animal got spooked, a quick release switch was at hand to get me off the bucking bronco. Unable to move, I swayed from side to side, forward and backward, with every step the horse took. They were small movements, but I thought it was a bumpy ride and the horse could use shocks. After two times around the paddock, I was ready to dismount and hang up my non-existing spurs.

Along with fishing, I now loved getting in the pool and floating around on the air mattress and getting sun. One counselor used an ambu bag to give me air and the other acted as a tugboat and moved me around the water.

All too quickly, the week was over and it was time to head home. I loved being with the other kids and enjoyed most of the activities. It was the only time I wasn't an outsider just watching kids play. My parents had a fun vacation as well, but I only heard a few of their stories as Patty and I slept most of the way home.

As the months progressed, I kept having trouble sitting upright and leaned heavily on my left elbow. After time, the pressure resulted in a sore and open area on my arm. This was something my parents and I had not dealt with before and I was recommended to a plastic surgeon, Dr. Rouce, in downtown Des Moines.

We tried different adjustments to my arm rest, but nothing seemed to help. As I began seventh grade a series of surgeries on my arm also started to close the hole and try to prevent more serious problems.

Seventh Grade

School required more work with writing papers and larger assignments. Typing with my mouth stick worked fine, but the AEA thought I needed an alternate method of writing as they thought my mouth would get tired. Before school, they evaluated me on a computer that was set up to use Morse code. It had two keys, marked with a dot and a dash, and a code for every character on the keyboard. With my stick, I could quickly go between the two keys and code each letter. During testing, I started remembering what code produced certain letters.

The new year also meant having new teachers. Mr. Kimble moved up from fifth grade and was now the 7th and 8th grade math teacher. For English and literature, my instructor would be Mr. Muether. My reputation as a rail enthusiast preceded me and, in the first day of class, Mr. Muether said he would be testing my knowledge, as he also liked trains.

The Morse code system I tried was installed on my Toshiba laptop, but instead of hitting two keys, I had to use a straw to sip or puff for a dot or dash. Doing a spelling test in Mr. Muether's class, he let everyone know what the beeping was all about. Also, if anyone knew Morse code, as he did, they weren't allowed to cheat from my answers.

After two weeks of huffing and puffing to blow the schoolwork down, I gave up on the system and continued to type with my stick. A series of eight dots and dashes would give me a period, two spaces, and capitalize the next letter. Four keystrokes produced the same result faster with less effort. It would have been easier with just hitting keys, but it took too much time and effort to use sip and puff.

As English class continued, we had a few weeks of keyboarding with proper finger placement and technique. Since stick placement wasn't in the course, I was allowed to copy articles from *Trains* magazine to improve my typing. Looking back and forth from the magazine to my keyboard helped my typing speed, but not as much as my classmates.

A few months after school started, we were given the main large assignment for the year. Each student had to research someone and write a biography about them. I finally settled on Charles Lindbergh, as he had a lot written about him already. It was interesting learning about the early pioneer of flight, and I received an A+ on the small book. Despite the warning from the AEA, I had no trouble with using only my mouth stick.

Awake for Surgery

School activities helped distract me, but I continued having elbow trouble. I needed to have another surgery, but Dr. Rouce said I did not have to be completely sedated. Since I couldn't feel my arm anyway, the anesthesiologist just gave me enough medication to prevent muscle spasms while staying awake. A new child-life specialist talked to me before the procedure and wanted to see what surgery was like. She came to the operating room and held up a *Trains* magazine for me to read while my arm received work.

A cloth drape was between my head and arm so I couldn't see what was happening. I could feel my arm jerk every now and then as the doctor and nurses talked about car payments and upcoming weekend plans. After surgery was finished, I didn't have to stay in recovery as long as usual and was soon on the way home. Not long after getting back to Pella, I was out again to another doctor, the dentist. I told Mom I wasn't excited about two major appointments in the same day, but she said I missed less school this way.

My last baby tooth was finally gone, and I would now be starting with braces. However, when I ground my teeth together to communicate shortly after my injury, it fused two of my adult teeth together. One of them had to be removed before the straightening process could begin. With arm surgery and tooth extraction, I was glad when the day was over, and I could stay in my bed for the night.

I tried HAM radio club with Mr. Muether, but I didn't pass the licensing tests, so he started a model train club. It met on Friday after school for about half an hour. The small group consisted of me, a few boys from my class, and anyone else who wanted to come. We usually worked on model train cars, engines, buildings, or talked trains. I liked spending time with other boys centered around a subject I loved.

Seventh grade continued with the three-headed monster of diagraming sentences and the junior high school play. The musical *Oliver* was put on with Mr. Muether as director and Mr. Kouy in charge of music. I didn't care to memorize lines, but a part was made just for me as one of the lost boys, Hot Wheels. I only had one line and otherwise had to sit and get pushed around a circle. Play practice got to be a familiar routine as everyone learned all the lines and where to stand or sit. Both directors were strict and wanted everyone involved to do their best.

During the show, Kyle stayed with me backstage while my parents stayed in the audience. If I needed suctioning or major help, he would get them. Otherwise, the two of us were okay on our own. From our roost, we could see the actions on stage as we quietly chatted about Kyle's props of a shot glass and large wooden cane. Our discussions distracted us and, soon enough, the cane dropped to the wood floor with a loud crack. The back-stage director quickly found us and gave directions on being quiet. It was a fun experience, but not one I cared to repeat.

The Wednesday Night Cadet Cadre

Cadets continued at church most Wednesday evenings during the school year. I didn't like going out on cold winter nights and tried various excuses to skip going, but Mom usually made me, and Dad would drop Leah and me off at church.

There were three other boys in my cadre who I saw at church every week and at school daily. I hung out with them some at train club, but not as often as with the girls. Daryl was our Cadet leader and worked at Vermeer Manufacturing in town. The company built baling equipment, tree chippers, and other related devices that were sold worldwide. One of our badges was designing and building model rockets. Daryl took us to his office at Vermeer and let our group design our craft with the computers. He made a special pointer with a rubber tip so I could plot out the design with his direction. It was neat to make the blueprint on the computer and then see it printed out on large sheets of paper.

A few months later, he was able to get Vermeer's pilot to take our cadre on a plane ride around Pella. Dad and Daryl got me positioned in a rear facing seat, propped up with pillows, and my vent on the floor. With Dad beside me, the other boys and I got to see the area around home from the single engine prop. Corn silos that looked so tall from the ground hardly seemed noticeable. The vent didn't have any trouble with the higher altitude, but we were soon back in the hanger at Pella Municipal Airport. It was the only time I had ever been in an airplane, and I thought it was fun.

At school, in Mr. Muether's English class, we worked on writing letters and how to properly layout address information, dates, and everything to communicate effectively. With his help, I wrote to several companies that had train related products. A few were train model brands and one made scanners that could monitor railroad frequencies. I told my story about being a quadriplegic from a young age and enjoying trains.

My classmate's goals were to get a reply from a letter sent to a corporation. While they got letters, it wasn't long until I started getting packages at school. A box full of a dozen model railroad kits from Accurail was one of the first deliveries. Another delivery came from Bearcat with a ten-channel programmable scanner I could put in the van. With every package, Mr. Muether would ask me to meet him during recess or after school while waiting for the bus and he would show me the delivery. I was thankful for his help and the extra attention he gave me. A hobby shop in Ottumwa also offered to design and assist in building a model train layout in my basement, but Dad declined and opted to build one on our own, eventually.

The year quickly came to an end, but not before more surgeries on my elbow. Just before summer started, I visited Dr. Rouce to see the results from the latest procedure. As he unwrapped the bandages on my arm, both the doctor and nurse got a look on their face that was somewhere between surprise and horror. I looked from my side of the arm and could see yellowish goo on the wrapping as it was removed. The surgery site in my arm had become infected, going to the bone, and required heavy antibiotics for several weeks. I received a new device called a PICC line that had a tube going directly into an artery. The line was connected to a small pump that had a container with antibiotics. I had to be on the pump all day, every day, and the canister of liquid changed daily so it wouldn't run dry. It was a very involved process that would go on for half the summer, including during camp.

This would now be my third year of traveling to Ohio for a week of fun, but I had more complications than usual. The time ahead looked uncertain, but God had His plans for everything to work.

6

TO THE TOP

There are many times in life when you get to the top of the ladder and quickly go back down again. Going into eighth grade, I was at the top of the grade school and junior high pile. Jesus said in Matthew 19:30, "But many *who are* first will be last, and the last first." The puffed head of being in this position would only last a year, one that would go quickly.

With my added hardware, I took more people with me to camp. Patty came as a general counselor to help with the other campers and Leah would be my primary assistant. The antibiotic needed to be in a cool environment for storage and changing canisters. Every day during our break before supper, Leah and I would go to the only air-conditioned place at Recreation Unlimited. Another counselor would often join us, but we got the task completed easily.

New at camp this year was the tree climb. Way back in the woods, a pulley system and sling had been set up to hoist campers 25 feet up in a tree. A ventilator with a 50-foot-long tube sat on the ground to provide air for those of us on a vent 24/7.

After bouncing through a dirt path, my group got back to the tree. My friend, James, and I waited our turn as some of the other campers went first. There was little breeze sitting in the middle of trees. Eventually, the two of us started to get too hot while we waited. Since neither of us quads could sweat, a counselor carefully poured a cup of cold water over James' head. The tactic helped him and I couldn't wait for my turn. Leah was concerned that the water would cause problems for the PICC line dressing, but the other counselors, mainly medical professionals, assured her it would be fine. The ice-cold liquid was a shock to my scalp, but it felt good running down my face and helped cool me off.

Eventually, my turn came, and I got strapped into the system and set up with the vent in the woods. As I went up, one of the counselors climbed the tree beside me with my ambu bag in case something went wrong. When I reached the top, I looked around to see the tops of everyone's head far below me and a bunch of leaves. I didn't know what to expect, but it was the first tree climbing experience I could remember. With my third year at camp, I was getting familiar with the regular activities. I looked forward to fishing and the pool, but always tried to get out of arts and crafts. I also enjoyed seeing my friends again, both other campers and counselors. One of the girls, Holly, who had been at camp my first year, had passed away. She had the same injury level as me and I was sad to hear she died.

Summer continued after camp with the train club meeting in my basement. The unfinished walls didn't matter, all we needed was a table and chairs and we had a great time. Patty and Mr. Muether took me to watch trains in Marshalltown a few times as well, but it was great being with other kids.

Our group picked a Friday evening to camp overnight by the tracks near Albia, Iowa. It was the same place I had camped with Dad before, down a dirt road to a former field entrance. Dad came along with Mr. Muether and the four boys in the club. As one of the boys attempted to pound stakes in the ground for a tent, he quickly realized the rubber mallet he brought was not the best tool for the job.

Dad and I would sleep in the van while the others used the tent. I had an extra car battery for my vent to run all night and I could stay with the group. All too soon, the summer of camping was over, and school began again.

Another School Year

With the new school year and six surgeries later, my elbow was no longer having issues. I now sported an elbow pad on each arm and had less range of motion in my left arm. However, my back continued to twist, and doctors wanted to do surgery to put rods in my spine to straighten it. The procedure would require me to be flat for several weeks afterward and my parents were told it would increase my chance of getting pneumonia. Therefore, they chose to delay the procedure as long as possible.

By October 1995, the school year was going well, and I was free of major problems. At church, our pastor went on to another congregation in northwest Iowa and a replacement had been found from California. Pastor Zeilstra came with his wife and three kids to Pella. His oldest and only boy, Tom, was one year behind me in school. As I went from math to English between periods, I noticed the new pastor and Tom standing in the doorway to Bible class. I only saw their backs, but I knew I would see them more in church.

The door into junior high was directly beside my home room, but it had a large bump to get over. The school bus dropped me off directly in front of it and if I hit it at the right angle, I could pop my wheels over the hump and go in. My chair made for a good place to put my backpack and everything else, so Patty didn't have to carry anything. With my book bag, computer, and bells on the back of my chair, along with the vent, portable suction, and ambu bag, I expertly popped my wheels up into the door. This time, though, they didn't go back down. I was now looking straight up at the overhang of the building with my chair laying on the vent. After getting righted again, we decided I shouldn't carry everything on the back until I was inside.

Every class has its unique qualities. My class had the gift of gab and regularly got in trouble for talking too much. It wasn't uncommon for us to stay in during noon recess and read as a punishment. It was the only recess we had and was an effective deterrent to talking. I usually was excused, though, as noon recess was the time I had to tend to personal needs. Since I was only recently toilet trained when I was injured, my parents decided to just continue with doing padded briefs. Once a day, a tube would be inserted into my bladder to make sure everything was coming out. The process was called cathing and the system worked for my needs.

After lunch, my classmates would go out for recess while my caregiver and I went to the small nurse's room. It was basically a large closet with a bed in it so a student could lay down for a while if not feeling well. I would park my chair beside the bed and get picked up by hand where I would lay on the bed, have my pants changed, do some stretching exercises, and get back into my chair. The process usually took most of recess, and I missed out on social time.

In junior high, I was growing, and it was getting harder to pick me up from my chair. The track system in my bedroom worked well at home, but something had to change at school. A new night nurse, Rhoda, started helping while I was in seventh grade. Her daughter had spina-bifida and some similar needs to mine. Rhoda suggested looking at a different cathing schedule so I would no longer need briefs.

One of my regular doctor's visits was to a urologist. In early grade school, I heard Mom explain my routine to him and said I was incontinent. I didn't know what it meant, but thought it was fun to use a big word. As I got older, I understood better and started taking over the conversations from Mom. We discussed different cathing options and the doctor had me start a medication called Oxybutynin. It would relax my bladder muscle to make it bigger and not squeeze. I would also increase cathing to three times a day. I had taken medications before for bladder infections or other problems, but those were only temporary. This was the first time I started taking anything multiple times a day with no end in sight.

The new routine started partway through eighth grade and, checking my pants at noon, I found them to be dry. After a couple weeks of success, the day came that I went to school with just regular clothing. I didn't get much out of class that day as I kept glancing at my crotch to make sure I didn't spring a leak. Everything went as expected and the cathing routine became normal. I was drained just before school at 8:00, when I got home around 4:00 in the afternoon, and again at midnight. It made the school day easier, and I preferred not using briefs.

Soon after arriving home from the hospital in 1985, I started using a standing frame. I would be laid on a flat table with straps put over my chest and knees before the entire table was tilted up by a crank and put me in a standing position. There was a small tray in front of me so I could play with a few things, but not much. All I could do was stand in one place and not go anywhere.

When Kyle was over, we would make up some form of entertainment while I stood around, but it quickly got boring. Now that he was a high school student with a busier schedule, he wasn't around my house as much, which made the standing time even less fun.

By eighth grade, I was tired of it and wanted to stop doing things I didn't think were important. I had a different rehab doctor and I tried to do my own talking when visiting with him. He said standing for one hour three times a week wasn't enough to do any good. I didn't need to hear anymore and gladly stopped the routine for other activities.

Pre-Winter Activities

Before winter set in, the train club took a Friday evening excursion to Des Moines. With Tom and a few of my female friends along for the trip, we took two vehicles to the city for supper, a visit to Hobby Haven, and a brief stop to watch planes at the Des Moines airport. Over an hour away from home, my vent started alarming, indicating it had a low battery. Patty started the van, got the vent's plugin for the vehicle's cigarette lighter, and everything was good.

The drive back to Pella went well and I enjoyed showing Tom the sights of the big city. Near Pella, the vehicles separated while dropping off kids at their homes. We dropped off Tom, but turned off the van as he crawled around my wheelchair to get out past the chair lift. My vent loudly alarmed of low battery when the engine turned off, but we expected it with the van not running. When the passenger left, the van was turned on, and my vent completely died and stopped giving me air. We were about five minutes from my house, but I was having trouble breathing on my own. Patty quickly drove us home down empty streets in the late evening light. As we reached highway speeds on residential streets a few blocks from home, I considered our remaining passengers.

Honking the horn as we pulled into the garage did not alert my parents for help as they weren't home. With little air, I explained to one frightened boy behind me how to operate the ambu bag and remove my vent tube from my trach. He managed to give me a few breaths while Patty got the van's lift unfolded, and my chair unstrapped so I could get out. The short trip from the garage to my room was a blur, but I was glad to get hooked up to my bed vent and get air again.

When the new house was built, one of the requirements was to have a level driveway. Unfortunately, the basement wasn't dug deep enough, and the result ended with a large slope on the driveway. Dad always worked hard to keep it clear of snow and ice, but small areas would sometimes stick.

My power chair continued to have problems, and I still had to sometimes use my manual to go to school. In very early spring, the school bus came to pick me up. Karen started pushing me down the driveway, and I heard her yell something. The next thing I remember was waking up in bed with Mom and Dad beside me, and Karen quietly crying. The left side of my head was sore, but I wasn't sure why. Dad looked at me for a few seconds, then asked, "What's your favorite railroad?" I answered Conrail, and then Mom talked with Karen telling her I was okay.

I was told that as Karen pushed me down the driveway, she slipped on a piece of ice and fell. She yelled to the bus driver to catch me as I rolled down the hill, but she couldn't reach me fast enough. My chair hit the curb at the edge of the street and flipped me over on my left side with my head barely missing the bumper of the bus and hitting the pavement. While Dad came home from work and Karen got me in bed, Mom called the hospital to see what she should do. After regaining consciousness, Dad's question was to assess my alertness and see how I was thinking. My parents didn't take me to the hospital as I seemed okay, and I returned to school later in the day. Sitting in class, my head was sore, and I had trouble concentrating, but I assumed it would pass.

Tulip Time and Eighth Grade Graduation

Tulip Time came along with playing in the marching band. I wanted to drop band for eighth grade, but Mom convinced me to stay in for my last year of junior high.

For the first day of the celebration, the band wasn't playing in the afternoon parade, and I thought it would be a good time to show the new kid, Tom, around the sites. He seemed nice in Sunday school, and we talked a little at school. Karen and I met him near church, then showed him all the floats and food booths around town. We sat and watched the afternoon parade until the tulip vendor came. The vendor sells tulips to anyone, but only for a kiss. My perplexed friend made little fuss as Karen pulled Tom to the street to purchase a flower for his sisters.

Partway through the parade, dark clouds started coming as we left our viewing position and went a few blocks to the Town Crier. Heavy rain started a short time later canceling the rest of the parade. Tom wasn't expected home yet, so he got in the van with us and came to my house. I showed Tom my room and we talked for a while before my impromptu house guest figured he should call his parents. Partway through the conversation, he turned to me and asked, "Where am I?" Not long after, the pastor arrived to retrieve his wandering son.

This would be my last year marching with the band in school at Tulip Time. Patty or my parents usually pushed me through the parade route, but I liked having other kids help me. One of my night nurses had two boys, of six total, that were close to my age. On some Friday nights she would bring one and we would have a game night until the early hours of the morning.

I asked if her oldest son, Jesse, would be able to push me in the parade. He went to public school, but she agreed it was fine and my band teacher got an extra uniform for him. I liked not always having an adult help me, even though they were only a few feet away. The band marched Friday afternoon and Jesse pushed me along the route just as we had practiced. With only a few blocks to go, an ambulance came up behind the band and needed to get through the street. Jesse wasn't sure what to do, so we went to the right side of the road while the band went left.

With my bells on my tray in front of me and mallet in my mouth, we were now parked alone directly next to a bunch of tourists. Patty had been watching Jesse and me, but she also got separated and went the opposite direction from us. I played what I could hear the rest of the band playing and gave the guests their own mini concert. When the road cleared, we rejoined everyone else. Thankfully, my vent's tubes all stayed connected and we didn't add to the entertainment.

The next few weeks went quickly toward the end of the school year. Our eighth-grade class trip was to Adventureland near Des Moines. My classmates took the school bus while Patty and I followed behind in my van. This was a popular, and only, amusement park in the area, but I had never gone. After everyone got through the ticket line, the rest of my class ran off to various roller coasters, the silly silo, and more. Patty and I roamed around the grounds and saw some of my classmates on different rides, but I couldn't do any of them.

A small train went around the park that looked like fun, but it didn't have a place for my wheelchair. Toward the end of the day, Patty talked with a couple of my teachers and figured how to get me on the train. The school principal, a teacher, and Patty worked together to carry me to a seat and get me sitting upright. I was bagged with the ambu bag while the train made its lap around the park. After a day of watching everyone else have fun, I was happy to finally get on a ride and get a different view.

Just a few days later, it was time for graduation. I was in the same black gown as the other boys in my class and waited for my name to be called. Graduation was at a church, and everyone was supposed to go on stage, get their diploma, and go back down. A ramp was set up so that I could get up to the stage and all my classmates had to take the same path as me to receive their diploma. After a long wait, I heard "Joel Vander Molen" and rolled up the ramp toward the principal. With a pat of my hand and a diploma on my lap, I was now an official graduate from grade school. I was the first student with a wheelchair to graduate from Pella Christian and I was thankful for the accommodations the school made to help me.

May 31, 1996 was the end of what I knew for school, and now I was on to the big world of high school. Through God's care with my parents and many caregivers, I defied what doctors had said eleven years earlier. I did not have major trouble with illness from the other kids and was able to stay with my class.

As summer started, I continued to watch trains with Mr. Muether, Patty, and some of the boys from train club. Mergers were changing the rail industry and it would be an interesting summer in many areas. I also was heading to another week of CHAMP Camp and new adventures.

However, other changes were coming for my transportation along with new challenges my family didn't expect.

7

ALL IS NEW

"All scripture *is* given by inspiration of God, and *is* profitable for doctrine, for reproof, for correction, for instruction in righteousness, that the man of God may be complete, thoroughly equipped for every good work." 2 Timothy 3:16-17

God has given us His word so we can be thoroughly equipped in every way to serve Him. In my life, that includes nurses, ventilators, wheelchairs, and education.

My power wheelchair continued to have problems and parts were getting hard to find, so my parents worked toward finding a new chair that would meet my needs. The only option available that filled my requirements was an Action Arrow. It had large rear wheels that were driven by a belt system. I had seen other kids at camp use chairs like it, but they were starting to get phased out. One challenge was that the church elevator was small, and I could only fit if I wore certain shoes. Therefore, I could not have anything longer than my current Fortress model.

After the new chair was purchased, it was sent to Colorado to be completely rebuilt so it could be the length I needed. A few months before I started high school in 1996, my new wheels were also ready.

I had a lot of things to learn about how to drive again. With my first wheelchair, I selected one of three gears, and it moved at a set speed. The new chair could go faster or slower just by moving my control stick further up or down. Different modes were set to certain maximum speeds and torque, but I could adjust what I wanted without stopping.

Another change was that the seat could tilt and recline. My controls had different modes and I could choose between driving or seat functions, all with my chin. I never had the option to move my seat before and had to remember to change my position throughout the day. There was also an on/off switch and gear selector that I could control myself.

When the therapist dropped off my new wheelchair at the house, he showed me all the functions, but I couldn't reach the on/off button. He searched through his van and found a green shaft from something, drilled a hole in it, and stuck it on the toggle switch. I now had a green stick to change gears and turn the chair on or off and a white one to drive with.

Dad and I talked about the problems my first chair had with taking off on its own without me controlling it. The therapist had heard about that happening with other chairs. It had been found that radio signals and some types of phones interfered with the electronics and made the chair take off. I was assured that it would not happen again and was shown where a rubber damper had been put in place just for that purpose.

Summer Camp 1996

CHAMP Camp 1996 was a great way to learn how to drive my new set of wheels. James, and a few other friends, said my brand-new wheelchair looked like older models they had already used and replaced. I didn't care as it worked well for me and was an upgrade from what I had.

It was now my fourth year at camp, and I knew the week's routine well. Patty and her husband came as counselors, but not just to help me. They worked with younger kids, and I received care from the other counselors.

Most of them worked in some field of healthcare, but not everyone. I knew my medical routine and could usually explain my needs.

Being around adults all the time at home, I tended to befriend counselors more quickly than other campers. Melanie was an energetic lady who got along well with everyone. I could explain to her how I suctioned, cathed, got positioned in my chair, and my morning and evening routines. Early in the week, I needed to have my daily cleaning done around my trach. It was then I learned Melanie was a speech therapist and was comfortable with most cares but opted to have a respiratory therapist work with my trach. I assumed she was a nurse and was surprised with this news, but I still liked her help.

Brenda, one of the girls, had started coming to camp the previous year. She could walk on her own for short distances and only used breathing support at night. Not long into the week, she asked me to the dance and started writing letters to me during the year. Now, with a new chair, she liked how I could control it better and sit more easily. On talent night, Brenda shared a poem she wrote about me and how I drove around in my Action Arrow. At the end of the week, I was more familiar with the new controls. Brenda made sure to give me a peck on the cheek before departing for another year. I assured her we could write letters through the mail, and I would plan to see her again. I was ready to get home and become an official high school student.

Entering High School

Most high school freshmen are excited to earn their driving permit and drive their parents' car. I got to start with new wheels and to get familiar with new school routines. I was able to choose a few of the classes I wanted to take, instead of having everything already selected for me. I decided not to take band or choir, but I did sign up for Spanish and art classes. I also was not required to take physical education since I couldn't participate anyway.

My locker was at the very end of the freshman hallway. This way, I could get to it and not have to squeeze beside neighbors. Along with my classmates from Pella Christian Grade School, students from four other Christian schools joined my class. A lot of faces were familiar, but several were new.

During lunch break, I sat near my locker talking with my new neighbor, David. He was previously home-schooled and was starting regular classes for high school. As we talked, a group of seniors came around the far corner and loudly announced, "More freshmen." They slowly sauntered by everyone looking at the new class and we stayed by our lockers trying not to be singled out.

Just as in grade school, my main group of friends consisted of all girls.

Just as in grade school, my main group of friends consisted of all girls. Our group quickly grew to six: Jenny, Jenny, Jana, Jenae, Valerie, and Kelli. Kyle was already a high school veteran, a sophomore with a busy schedule. Even though it wasn't cool to be seen with a freshman, we still spent some free time together.

The bedside tables from grade school came along with me to the new building, as well as a few additions. I no longer had the large drafting table and only used the small mobile desks. My new teachers quickly adopted them for use during lectures but let me use them when I was in the room.

I was used to study hall from junior high, but then it was just my classmates. In high school, it was one large room where everybody in school came. With homework, it was easier and faster to tell my caregivers what to write for answers. However, that didn't work well in a room full of people. I talked with the school guidance counselor and made it so that my assistant and I would go to an empty classroom instead. Frequently, I was assigned the home economics room, but it changed every semester. Patty, Karen, and I got to know the teachers well by having just us in the room. Unlike grade school, there wasn't a place to get me out of my chair during lunch break, so I had free time to socialize. Often, whoever was with me during the day would stay in a certain nearby classroom and I could be alone with my friends.

Every October, teachers at Christian schools around Pella had a few days training time in northwest Iowa. Students didn't care about the reason, we just liked getting out of school. Some families would take advantage of the four-day weekend and go on short trips. The break occurred every year since I started school, but my family never did anything special. This year, however, my parents decided we would take an overnight train-watching trip to Wisconsin.

Mom asked the nursing agency not to schedule anyone on Friday night of the fall break. We looked forward to getting away with just the three of us after a few years off. When Friday finally came, it was a rainy day with a forecast of light rain and cool temperatures for two days. Dad wanted to stay home and skip the trip completely, but since I wouldn't have a night nurse anyway, Mom convinced him to go.

Before leaving Pella, Dad stopped at Zylstra welding with my chair's headrest. One of the connection points from the chair's frame to the head support had broken and needed to be fixed. Dad went in and left Mom and me in the van to wait. While he was gone, I had no choice other than to hold my head up. I didn't think it would be a problem until several minutes had passed. My neck started to get sore, and I realized I utilized the support more than I thought. After about ten minutes, the part had been welded together, replaced on my chair, and we were off.

After driving much of the day and watching trains, we stopped at a Cabela's store in Prairie du Chien, Wisconsin. I had heard about them before but was impressed with the multitude of stuffed animals and sporting displays. Roaming around inside was a nice change from being in the van for multiple hours through gray skies and wet roads.

The busy Burlington Northern Santa Fe railroad followed the Mississippi River through several small towns in western Wisconsin. As the sun set, Dad found a parking lot in Prairie du Chien that was adjacent to the tracks and the Mississippi River just beyond them. He parked the van beside some semi-trailers and set up the back seat that would be our bed for the night. Mom was concerned about not having bathroom access, but we settled in, with one parent laying on each side of me. It was close accommodations, but we were rail camping as a family.

I enjoyed the trains that interrupted my sleep during the night. As the sun started to rise Saturday morning, we packed up and headed for home while following the tracks. Mom wasn't sure about our trip, but it was a good interruption to my start of high school.

Freshman year continued into the winter, and I mainly hung out with my group of girls between classes. Kyle and I got together some, but he was busy with sports after school most days and didn't always want to be seen with a freshman.

As my body adjusted to teenage hormones, my muscle spasms and stiffness continued to increase. Any touch on my skin or hitting a bump would make my back and neck tighten so that all I could do was move my eyes. In Spanish class, I sat in the back corner of the room, and I had to move out of my spot before the next class came in. Just as I started to move, I would stiffen up and get stuck and have to try to navigate out while a new class tried to enter.

After talking with my doctor, I started on a medication called Baclofen to try to reduce the spasticity. The pharmacist told me to decide how much to start with and I was quickly up to taking a pill four times a day before noticing any difference. He was surprised that I needed so much, but at least it helped enough to get me clear of the classroom.

Willy the Wheelchair Technician

I loved that my new chair's headrest had buttons that allowed me to move my control stick. Pushing the right side moved the controls away from me and the left brought it back. With my back continuing to curve, I couldn't always move my head to reach both buttons. Sitting straight continued to get harder, so my parents and I took several trips to Ft. Dodge in northwest Iowa to see Willy the wheelchair technician.

As we traveled north on one visit in late fall the roads became questionable, with high winds and snow flurries. Just as the van went over a bridge, we crossed the county line, and the road suddenly went from dry to damp. A gust of wind started pushing us toward the median of the four-lane road as Dad wrestled with the steering wheel. The first attempt didn't work, but as we neared the gravel between the road and median, the wheels stuck, and we were once again pointed in the right direction. With visions of our accident in her head, Mom questioned if continuing chair work was worth the drive, but we pressed on.

Arriving in Fort Dodge, Willy put me in a device where the backrest had small beads in an air-tight sack. As I sat, he would push beads to give support in different places to allow me to sit straight. One adjustment would help one area but make something worse elsewhere. It took multiple attempts to remove air to lock the beads in place and try to get me upright. Mom watched my mouth to see if I was straight or not. If I was trying to sit correctly, my head would move and often my mouth would look crooked. Even if I felt straight, my body showed otherwise.

After multiple attempts and frustration, Willy was considering switching careers to working in fast food. However, a solution was made so that I could use my chair as intended and sit correctly.

The Second Semester of Freshman Year

I soon celebrated my 15th birthday and enjoyed gifts and cards. Mom's older brother and his wife had a delivery I couldn't forget. A new baby! Levi decided to share my birthday as well, and I looked forward to watching him grow.

As freshman year continued, I started to develop another pressure sore, but this time it was on my butt. I tilted during breaks and study hall as much as possible, but it still continued to grow.

Just as in junior high, I went back to Dr. Rouce to see what could be done. The solution was to have muscle taken from my leg and put it in the hole to fill it up. My orthopedic doctor also said that my back's curve could be contributing to the sores. My parents decided I should have surgery to fix the sore, while trying to get me to camp in June, and then put rods in my back to straighten the scoliosis.

Surgery for the sore would happen in spring, but I couldn't be in my chair for several weeks afterward. Then I would start a very slow process of increasing my time in the chair again. For the last few months of school, I would have to do my work at home and have a tutor to keep up with my classmates.

For the second semester of freshman year, I took an art class that included designing and building a house. My design was approved in class, but I had surgery before finishing. After one week in the hospital, I returned home to a new air mattress on my bed that allowed me to sit some, but lay flat most of the time.

In the evening, Leah and I worked on building the house by shaping walls out of thin white foam. Windows were cut out and then they were attached to the base using straightened out paper clips and glue. The project was completed on time and taken to school to be turned in. However, since I didn't physically build the model myself, Mr. F (as the class called him) never gave me a grade for it. Leah took it to use in her Sunday school class of preschoolers where it didn't survive long.

Another class I took was word processing. We were to use software called Microsoft Word and edit text. I did what I could on my Toshiba laptop but had several sections I had to write "unable to do." With technology changing, my parents decided to get a new desktop computer, which came from Gateway in a large cow print box. It included a new operating system called Windows 95 that was completely different from my laptop. In addition, we got more new technology, dial-up internet. I could send email, do my homework assignments, and play a flight simulator game. It was originally set up in the front room of our house for anyone to use. Tom came over and I showed him how I flew planes, and he seemed to like computers.

After surgery, I wasn't allowed to get up in my chair and had to stay in bed for six weeks. Dad reinforced one of the bedside tables so that the computer's monitor could be on the top and the tower on the bottom.

Another table held the keyboard and mouse so I could then do schoolwork and play games lying flat in bed. Unfortunately, I was unable to reach all the keys and couldn't fly planes. I needed just a little more reach to get the top row of keys. I asked Patty to tape another mouth stick on top of my regular one so that it stuck out further. She didn't think it would work and wasn't worth trying, but I convinced her anyway. Now, to reach the other keys, I flipped the stick over in my mouth and used the extension. For everything else, the regular setup worked well, and the combination served its purpose.

Lying in bed, I could only watch out my window as spring bloomed, so Dad laid the rear seat flat in the van and positioned me to see out the window. The world went by sideways, but it was a different view. The three of us went to Marshalltown and parked so I could see the rails from my flat vantage point. I followed the doctor's orders but got out of the house.

My month of being down was finally over and it was time to start sitting. I could do 30 minutes at a time one to two times a day for a week, then increase by another half-hour each week.

The process was started in enough time to get to camp in late June and be able to experience summer again.

8

STRAIGHTEN UP

Luke 13:10-17 gives an account of a woman who was bent over and unable to straighten up on her own. Jesus freed her from this infirmity by simply laying His hands on her. While we don't often experience miraculous healings like this today, God has given us medicine and tools to help with modern infirmities. Technology was not as advanced in 1997 as today, but it was still able to help.

Rod surgery for my spine was scheduled to take place shortly after CHAMP Camp. When it was complete, my 89° curve would be decreased, and I wouldn't fit in my current backrest. We returned to Willy to get molded for another back support, but this time he had to guess what I would need.

We made our annual trip to Ohio for another week of fun. The time at camp was when I could be a regular teenager and not be the only one on a vent and using a wheelchair.

It was fun seeing James and my other friends again. The tree climb had now been replaced with a 50-foot tower that included a vent with a 100-foot tube on it. I was the only camper that used a PLV-100 for a ventilator, and I thought the LP-10 sounded noisy. Getting on one for the tower climb felt odd as it gave air differently, but it did the job.

Ascending the tower was done just like the tree climb from previous years, but higher off the ground. When reaching the top, the question always asked was, "How do you like the view?" Suspended in a sling 50 feet in the air, I felt more breeze than on the ground. Looking around, I could see a lot more trees and further off in the distance. It was fun getting above everything and out of my wheelchair, but I didn't stay in the air very long. Other campers wanted to climb the tower or get hoisted up like me. I was also ready to get connected to my regular ventilator again and breathe normally.

Every day at home, I started my routine by washing my hair and having a bed bath during the night. Part of camp is getting to skip baths and be a regular kid. Swimming in the pool counted as one wash and all the campers got run through the shower the day before returning home. I had used my parents' whirlpool a few times, but it was hard to do without having a lift. When my turn came for the shower, it was a three-counselor team to help me. Getting my shirt off in the chair was easy, but shorts took one counselor holding my shoulders up as I tilted back and another to slide them off. As I sat naked in my chair, the counselors debated the best way to put me in the shower and get me cleaned.

Two people picked me up to lay me on a bench in the shower, and a third used the ambu bag to give me air. It was a different experience using a shower, and a lot more work. We thought it would be easiest to get me dressed laying on the shower bench, but in the process my damp posterior rubbed on the wet bench. After getting clean, I hoped to join the other boys with a poker game. It was the last night of camp, and the teenagers were allowed to stay up late for poker and possibly pizza. Unfortunately, by the time I got back, the impromptu party was disbanding, and night routines had already started.

It was hard to leave my friends the next day, but it was time to return to Iowa and another surgery.

By this time, surgery was a familiar process, but rod placement was much more extensive than anything I had previously done. Several weeks before, I made a few visits to the Iowa blood bank for them to take blood that would be used during the procedure. To give blood for myself, I had to answer a series of questions about many details of my life, some rather surprising. Since Mom was with me when I was questioned, I had to answer them all a second time without her listening. None of my responses changed, but it was still policy.

As the surgery began, my body relaxed completely with the help of the anesthetic. While knocked out, I didn't breathe as I normally did and let too much air escape through my mouth. To stop the leak, the anesthesiologist put in a cuffed trach to seal off my throat and keep oxygen in. Seven hours after the procedure began, rod placement was complete. In that time, I grew six inches taller, but the surgeons were only able to get down to a 30° curve instead of completely straight.

> *When the pulmonologist left, Dad looked at the nurse and said, "That wasn't done right, was it?"*

I was taken to the Pediatric Intensive Care Unit for recovery and for the anesthetic to get out of my system. Dad stayed in my room for a while as I drifted between sleep and semi-awake. A pulmonologist and nurse came to take out the cuffed trach and replace it with my own. The doctor tugged on the device in my throat to pull it out, but it wouldn't come. She continued to pull harder, eventually bringing my top half off the bed. Finally, the trach yanked out with the balloon cuff, designed to be deflated for removal, fully inflated. It was all Dad could do to not punch the doctor as she kept yanking on my throat to remove the tube. With a bleeding trach stoma, my regular trach was inserted so I could get connected to the ventilator again. When the pulmonologist left, Dad looked at the nurse and said, "That wasn't done right, was it?" She answered with a quick "no" and promptly left the room.

Over the next week, I stayed in the PICU and started being awake more as I recovered from the procedure. A few teachers from school visited as well Pastor Zeilstra and Tom. Mom and I watched Independence Day fireworks through my hospital window before finally being able to return home.

Getting up for the first time with a straighter back felt good, and it was a relief that Willy had guessed well with the new back support. When I got to the van, though, I had a new problem. With my increased height, I could no longer sit upright without hitting my head on the door. As Dad put the van's lift platform up, I tilted my chair back so I could fit. Once inside, I had to stay tilted so I didn't hit the ceiling. In this tilted position, the view out the front window wasn't very good, but I could still see a short distance down the road.

Summer continued and I did not develop pneumonia after surgery as the doctor feared. However, another pressure sore developed where my skin had rubbed in the shower at camp. By August, I once again needed another flap surgery to close the area, making three surgeries in less than a year.

Every month, Mom ordered supplies that I needed for my daily care. I needed gloves, bladder catheters, suction catheters, cleaning supplies, trach ties, and much more. With being home in bed so much, it was a great time for me to start taking more responsibility and keep track of everything on my own. Mom showed me the forms she had for the nurses to make a supply inventory. She could then keep count of how much of each item was on hand. Most supplies had a regular amount used every 30 days. Cathing was three times a day, every day, so I used 90 tubes a month. Along with that there were also sterile swabs, betadine, and gloves. A few extras were also needed in case something was dropped or I was having AD and needed to use more.

In addition to ordering supplies, I also needed to check that everything was received and billed to insurance correctly. One instance mom found was a box of 100 swabs that was supposed to be $6.00 but was charged for $600.00. In those times, it also required calling insurance to get the charges corrected. It took a few months to learn, but it soon became part of my routine to do after school or during breaks. A few things came close to running out, but they usually arrived quickly after ordering.

The Beginning of Sophomore Year

When school started for my sophomore year, I was still on bedrest and not able to get up long enough to go to class. I decided what courses I wanted to take, and a tutor needed to come help me. Mr. Muether wanted the job, but the grade school principal's wife became my at-home instructor. She was able to help with geometry and my other subjects, but not Spanish. I tried going through the book on my own but dropped the subject a few weeks after it started.

Finally, by October, I was able to be up long enough so I could return to school. Sitting in class instead of having a tutor was great, but it was odd starting classes well after everyone else. In order to get home earlier, Patty and Karen drove me in the van so I didn't need to wait for the bus and was able get out of my chair more quickly.

Despite tilting during study halls, a pressure sore returned in November, a month after returning to school. Dr. Rouce said not to do surgery, but he put me back on bedrest for another six weeks. That meant Thanksgiving and my birthday would be spent in bed. After several weeks of already being flat, I started getting irritable and depressed.

Unknown to me, Mom organized a birthday letter campaign. I received notes from my nurse's relatives all over the country and letters from most of the student body of Pella Christian High. By my birthday, I had boxes of cards from many more people than I knew. Turning 16 is a milestone for everyone, but it's one I won't forget.

The slow sitting routine started again with 30 minutes in my chair per day for a week and increased 30 minutes every week. I couldn't do much in this time, but it was a great excuse to get to the basement and

Turning 16 is a milestone for everyone, but it's one I won't forget.

work on our model train layout. It didn't get much attention otherwise, but it was fun to do for short periods.

A new night nurse, Mary, had started working with me a few months earlier. She had three boys that were a few years older than me and a younger daughter. Mary knew how to celebrate birthdays and, when I was able to sit a little longer, she organized a limo ride for my 16th birthday. Every Saturday night, it was common for teenagers to drive around the square for hours at a time or "scoop the loop," as it was called. Kyle and a few boys from church joined me as we circled the square in style for an hour.

By Christmas, I could be up for about 90 minutes at a time. It allowed me to briefly attend our family celebrations. It was a short time to eat and open presents, but I could go out again. As Dad loaded me into the van for one party, he commented how most boys my age had their driver's license and car. Mom saw tears come to my eyes as the unwelcome reminder hit me, and she quickly changed the subject.

When January 1998 arrived, I was back in school to finish my sophomore year. I started Spanish again and loved being with my group of girls during breaks. Now that Tom was also in high school, we started to hang out more when we could. My Gateway computer had a problem with its video card and a replacement was sent by mail. Tom and I gladly opened the computer's tower to remove the faulty part and replace it with the new one. Mom came home to see computer parts on my bedroom floor with two happy teenagers looking at them. She decided to look away and soon everything was in working order again and we could continue our technology escapades.

Tom and I often played games with each other online, which meant blocking the phone line to use the internet. It wasn't long before my parents decided to get a second phone line. In response, Tom could come over with his Apple laptop, use the second line for his computer, and we could play through the world wide web while sitting a few feet apart.

As my second year of high school progressed, my parents and I started thinking about what to do after graduation. It was thought that college would be the best step, but we didn't know what would be possible and where I could go. We started working with Vocational Rehabilitation (Voc Rehab), a government branch that helps people with disabilities find work. The counselor I was given helped us to see if college would be beneficial and what would be required for it to be an option. I wanted to be able to live on campus in the dorm, if possible. It would be a lot of work to complete, but it helped that we were starting early.

To start the process, my family would need to see what it would take for me to live on my own. Finding nurses to cover me 24 hours a day would be the first, and largest, barrier. Along with that, I needed to have an accessible dorm that I could easily use along with my medical supplies. Without my parents around, I would also be responsible for taking care of all my needs, including training. I learned some of these skills at camp, but that was also a different situation. To help me prepare and set realistic goals, an occupational therapist from ASK Resources would start working with me. Amy, the therapist, was ready to help, but knew I had to learn a lot to be ready before I could be on my own.

Summer came again, and it would be another busy few months. I did not have any more pressure sores, but I was planning to go to camp and then to Craig Hospital to get help with my wheelchair.

My parents and I had great plans for the summer, but we had learned to expect the unexpected.

9

BURNING ADVICE

James 4:14-15 cautions not to boast about future plans as we do not know what a day will bring. Instead, we should say "If the Lord wills, we shall live and do this or that." In planning for summer 1998, we had certain expectations of what would happen. What occurred was not planned and serves as a reminder to treat each day as a gift.

Living in a small community with a high-level spinal cord injury, my parents, nurses, and I learned how to take care of my needs somewhat independently. However, with the frequent pressure sores I had dealt with since starting high school, Mom and Dad thought it would be good to get my wheelchair evaluated and see if anything could be adjusted.

Craig Hospital, near Denver, CO, was known to be an expert facility for spinal cord injuries. When I was originally injured, some doctors thought about transferring me from Des Moines to Denver. However, since Mom couldn't travel, it was best for me to stay near her. Mom had to work with insurance to approve care outside of Iowa, but it was eventually granted. The hospital said it would be best for me to stay as a patient for a few days so that I could be assessed, and we wouldn't need to bring any of my nurses. Mom reluctantly agreed to this and set a visit date for just after I returned from camp.

We had used the same brown Ford van since I came home from the hospital in 1985. It worked well and had allowed my family to take many trips. However, I could no longer sit fully upright in the van since getting my back straightened. Tilting was better for pressure relief on my skin, but I could hardly see anything out the windows, and it was difficult to reach me from the front if I needed something. Dad found a white Chevrolet van with a high-top. Once inside, I could sit upright instead of having to tilt. We weren't sure it would be a good long-term option, so Dad used boards as a ramp to get me in and out and we only used the vehicle for long trips.

Two days before our scheduled departure for camp, Mom's dad had a heart attack and was flown to Des Moines for emergency surgery. Going to camp usually meant my parents dropped me off and then went on their own vacation. Mom didn't want to leave with grandpa's health uncertain, so I also thought about staying home. However, my cousin Luke was home from college for the summer and volunteered to ride with Dad and me to help as needed.

Driving out to Ohio was very familiar, staying overnight in either Dayton or Delaware, Ohio before going to camp near Ashley. Even though I knew the landmarks along the way, I still enjoyed seeing the scenery. Sitting up straight in the white van was nice, but I could primarily only see the inside of the raised top. Directly in front of me was a television that I didn't care to watch while traveling. My view of the road ahead was only two to three road marks and nothing else. After a full day driving through multiple states, Dad, Luke, and I stayed at a hotel until my scheduled arrival the next morning. It felt strange being in a hotel room with Dad doing my cathing and changing clothes while Luke looked the opposite way.

Arriving at camp, I was excited to show it to Luke. We were greeted with the usual fanfare of my name being shouted and cheers. Since he wasn't using it, we took grandpa's cell phone in case the three of us needed to be reached. Without it, we had no way of communicating back home. Just as I got off the boards, the phone rang. I imagined it was someone calling to say grandpa had died or was in worse shape and all of us needed to return home. However, the call was Mom checking in to see if we arrived okay.

As my supplies were unloaded, I heard several comments that my brother had come with me. Since Luke and I had similar features, it was hard to convince anyone we were only cousins. After I was deposited at Recreation Unlimited, Dad and Luke drove to Columbus airport and rented a vehicle with better gas mileage. They drove the 13 hours back to Iowa to check on grandpa and be with the family.

The camp routine was fun again, but it was starting to feel like a repeat each year. In any case, I enjoyed getting to be a "regular" teenager for a week and training new counselors to the camp way of life. An unusual activity for the year was a type of wheelchair dodgeball.

My trail group consisted of boys from my cabin and some of the older girls. We all played on an open tennis court, avoiding balls, and having fun together. The sun felt great, but the counselors insisted I put on sunscreen. James absolutely did not want any but allowed it on his scalp due to his new buzz cut. I reluctantly got lathered with the stuff and went on enjoying the afternoon.

That night, with my face sandwiched between pillows, it felt like I sat in the sun too long and got a slight sunburn. My cheeks were a little tender against the fabric, but it wasn't anything I hadn't experienced before. By morning, I saw I had a burn everywhere I had exposed skin, including my feet where my sandals didn't cover. This wasn't my first sunburn, but it felt more substantial than previous ones. After all the boys were up for the morning, I saw James had a sunburn as well, but only on the top of his head. As we sat waiting for the horse ride later in the day, James and I sat in the shade of the barn instead of in the warm sun as we usually did. Getting more sun exposure hurt my face, and likely everywhere else. Looking at my right hand near my thumb, I noticed one small spot still hadn't been crisped by the sun's rays.

I loved fishing at camp and using their chin-controlled rod and reel. At the end of the week, each camper could choose what activity they wanted to repeat. Most of my friends went swimming, but I went down to the lake with my tackle box. Unfortunately, even sitting in the shade of a tree, my head was sore when the sun hit me. I reluctantly joined other campers inside at arts and crafts.

Grandpa recovered well and returned home from the hospital while I was away. Both of my parents came to pick me up after the week of camp. Mom was very displeased to see my red skin. Normally, I fell asleep within minutes of leaving the campgrounds, but the van's air conditioning hurt when it hit my face. I let Dad leave it on for a while but couldn't tolerate it for long. It made for an even longer trip home than usual, but I was glad to get back.

A few days later, I visited my primary doctor and was diagnosed with first- and second-degree burns. Inspecting the sunscreen more carefully, Mom noticed it had expired well before the trip. The combination of old product and my fair skin resulted in the burn and was the reason the spot that was missed looked fine.

More Unexpected Events

About a week after returning from Ohio, my parents and I headed to Denver for a few days at Craig Hospital. This was the first time since going to Yellowstone that we travelled multiple days without a nurse. Since I would be a patient, there wouldn't be any nights I needed help. We prayed everything would go well and the visit would be successful.

The 700-mile trip out west went well, following train tracks as much as possible. I was soon getting checked into the hospital for my seating evaluation and anything else the experts could help with. My skin was now starting to recover with damaged portions flaking off in chunks. I explained what happened the last few weeks and about enjoying my time at camp. I easily answered questions about the history of my spinal cord injury and health in general. When the nurse asked about how many times I had pneumonia, my answer was twice.

Nurse, "Two times in the past year? That's pretty good."

Me, "No, two times in my life."

The look on her face was a mix of shock and disbelief. It apparently was rare for quads at my injury level to have few lung problems. Questions continued with how often I have any pain. I answered, "Only when I think." The nurse expressed sympathy, saying that having such a problem must be horrible. I found myself explaining my odd sense of humor to my interviewer and was assured humor fits in well at the facility.

My room resembled a combination hospital room and apartment. As we entered, there was a regular hospital bed with monitors and a suction machine on the wall. It also had a large restroom with a roll-in shower that looked interesting. Further in was a dividing wall to a carpeted area with a pull-out sofa bed, small kitchen, table, and chairs. This was a room someone with a new injury would go to when learning to live on their own. Mom and Dad would sleep on the pull-out bed while hospital staff helped me at night.

Mom and I went through my daily cares with the nurse. Part of my routine was doing passive range of motion (PROM), or stretching exercises, several times a day, and turning every two hours at night. We were told they only did exercises once a week and preferred to use medication to help control spasms. Turning at night also wasn't done by the nurses, but I would be on a mattress that automatically turned me. My parents and I weren't sure how well that would work, but thought we try it for our stay.

My chair evaluation wasn't for a few days, but the hospital had more events planned for me. Working with occupational therapy, I was shown different kinds of mouth stick options, but there was nothing I hadn't seen before. Some of my computer games required discs to be changed in the machine's CD tray, and I wondered if I could do it on my own. The therapists thought a pincher stick might work, but I knew it would pick up the disc in the wrong direction. They continued the presentation by showing options for stick holders. Something would sit on my table, and I could put my stick in it and give my mouth a break but be able to pick it up when I wanted. Some solutions required magnets to be glued to the stick so it could connect to a metal stand. I wondered how heavy the stick was with the attachment and how hard it was to retrieve.

A demonstration model was sitting in front of me with what looked like new stick ends on it. I doubted they had been changed since the previous person tested it, so I didn't want to put it in my mouth. While the therapist talked with my parents, I attempted to grab the stick between my lip and chin to give it a tug. Just as I was about to try my test, Mom returned her attention to me and promptly announced not to pick up the stick as we don't know where it had been. That was already my plan, but I aborted my test.

As the first night came, I laid in bed as my parents and I were told about the turning system. It wouldn't flip me at a 90° angle like I preferred but would slowly move me from side to side. After 30 minutes, I didn't notice any movement in either direction. I had been given a straw call light system to page the nurse and I gave it a puff to voice my concern. She said the bed went very slowly and I may not always notice the change.

The next day, I was scheduled to speak with a psychologist. I didn't really know what to talk with her about, but she asked general questions about how life was going and any concerns I had. As a teenager, she thought it would be good for me to watch a video about how quads can have adult relations. I had already gone through sex education class in junior high and the previous year in high school. I knew the workings of everything but hadn't thought about it as if I was to get married someday.

Mom and Dad reluctantly agreed to let me watch it and, later in the day, I was in an oversize closet watching the video on my own. After a lengthy discussion on logistics to get help if needed, the room's door was left slightly open so I could get assistance. After the video finished, I opened the door and said it was complete. The staff didn't know how I could open a door toward me. I demonstrated how I hooked my shoe and footrest on the door, and then drove backwards and turned to open it. (Until this time, I drove my chair by putting the control stick in my mouth. I didn't have enough chin to drive with when I was little, so I just got used to it. However, I thought I may encounter newly injured quads and should show correct driving skills and switched to using my chin instead. It took effort to remember, but I thought I should be a good example.)

When I wasn't being studied, my parents and I took a few excursions in the area. Since I was a hospital patient, I had to have plastic bracelets on my arm with my identification information. We strategically put them under the Velcro straps on my armrest so I didn't look like I had escaped. One trip was to Caboose Hobbies, a model train store I had heard about for as long as I could remember. It was fun browsing their unique engines and model displays but wasn't quite as big as I expected.

By night three, I still didn't notice the mattress turning me. A technician looked at the bed and noticed it wasn't turned on. He flipped a switch and it started making more noise, but I still couldn't tell that it was turning.

As soon as I was upright, incredible pain shot through my lungs and my vision started to shimmer.

The next morning was the day we had come for, to get my chair tested. Dad did my morning routine and passive range of motion, but my lungs hurt every time he moved my legs and I spasmed. I tried to tell him to stop, but I knew I also needed stretching. When he finished, he did the normal routine of picking me up and putting me in the chair. As soon as I was upright, incredible pain shot through my lungs and my vision started to shimmer. When he connected the vent to my trach, I struggled to croak out one word, "Bed!" Dad was reluctant and suggested waiting a few minutes to see if the feeling would pass. Mom could see my face was pale and I was nearly ready to pass out and agreed with my request to go down again.

The pain slightly subsided when I went flat, and Mom went to find help just outside the door. The responding nurse found my oxygen saturation was low and connected my vent to oxygen. After a doctor's evaluation, I was soon rolled down the hall and across a bridge to another part of the hospital. My bed was parked in a room that had more patients and beds separated by curtains. It was determined I had a collapsed lung and discovered the automatic turn feature on my bed had never been activated.

After multiple nights of not turning and drier air than I was used to, my lungs couldn't handle it.

To help reinflate the lung, I had to have deep suctioning, much more than usual, and drink lots of water. The different suction procedure was uncomfortable, and I wanted it to stop. Mom could see how it made me feel and had to step behind the curtain to not watch. One of the nurses held her hand on my cheek so I could feel her touch and concentrate on feeling something other than my lung. The meeting we had waited for would not happen, at least for now, and my stay was going to be extended.

Shortly after arriving to the new room, I was put on a regular air mattress and would get manually turned every two hours. It was what we had originally requested, but the hospital thought technology was better. Now they agreed that my family's method worked best. I also needed suctioning much more, but Mom and I noticed the nurses didn't use sterile gloves. Mom asked why they didn't and if we could please do so. The nurse said using clean technique was just as good and they didn't have the equipment for sterile suctioning. Now we understood why the nurse at check-in was surprised I was healthier than expected. Seeing how lung care was done, it would lead, from our experience, to frequent infections. In compromise, an enclosed system was added to my trach so that the catheter wouldn't need to be touched. However, it also would not get changed each time I needed my lungs cleared.

As I laid in bed later that day, I took in my new surroundings. Four other patients were in the same room with me, including a teenager who had recently been injured. His bed was directly across from mine with no barrier other than several feet of space. I could easily see his bed and hear most conversations. Just like when I was initially injured, he was unable to speak.

In the general patient room, I was improving quickly with continued suctioning, increased water intake, and regularly getting turned. I was allowed up in my chair again after a day, but I was hesitant at first. The only other thing I could do was lay in bed and quietly watch a television on a flexible ceiling mount. The limited channels weren't very interesting, except one playing the movie *Independence Day* on a continuous loop. Even just going to the hospital cafeteria with my parents was a nice break.

I had been scheduled to be home by July 4, but instead was in the hospital with an unknown discharge date. On the evening of the holiday, several patients were brought to the top of a nearby parking garage where a small band was playing. As the sun light faded into dusk, we could see fireworks all around from different suburbs near Denver. It was the most amazing display I had seen and never knew which way to look. When celebrations were complete, it was time to return to bed.

The next day, I was allowed to return to my original room. As Dad helped transfer the last of my things through the hospital, the family across the room with the teenager stopped him. They had seen me talking and had questions about our experience with spinal cord injury. I had somewhat hoped to get the opportunity to help but was glad to hear he could offer some assistance.

After much delay, the time finally came when I could leave the hospital. My parents called home a few times to let my nurses know what was happening and when I may return. As we packed to leave, we were able to talk briefly with someone about my chair. The technician said there were a few things he could do to adjust my seat and allow better repositioning. If we could leave my wheelchair with him a few days, he could get it fixed. Since we were leaving in a few hours, that wasn't an option. We came all the way to Denver to work on my chair, but it would stay the same as when we came.

When the van was packed, we detoured through Estes Park before heading east. It was fun driving through the mountains and above the tree line, but all three of us were ready for home. Late in the evening, Dad stopped by a railroad track in central Nebraska. He didn't want to get a hotel and move my supplies in and out of the van again. It would also require setting up the boards to ramp me out and in the vehicle. Instead, the three of us would camp by the tracks overnight, laying in the back seat to sleep. The single track in front of us didn't seem to be a major line, but it ended up being very busy, and we got very little rest.

The next morning, we made the final push home and were happy to see Pella again. I had stayed in the van for over 24 hours, and my parents only got out for bathroom breaks.

It had been a busy summer and, in a few weeks, my junior year of high school would begin.

10

LOOKING UP

In Psalm 19, David declares the law of the Lord is perfect, reviving the soul. David knew trial and tribulation very well but relied on God for comfort. The teen years can be a difficult time for most people, but especially those with major disabilities. Fitting in to the social crowd is hard, and I learned to look outside of myself for comfort.

Junior year of high school started after a summer of unexpected events. It was great to be with my group of girls again and begin the school year the same time as my classmates. At the start of the year, it was nice enough to sit outside during lunch break. The young ladies would sit on a bench and, if I parked in just the right spot, my large rear wheel made for a good footrest for one of them.

A few of us had gone to the Iowa State Fair together in August and I enjoyed spending extra time with one of the Jenny's in particular. She had come a few times during my periods of bed rest to help with notes and studying, and my parents quietly left us to ourselves, to a point at least.

Tom and I also spent more time together, especially playing a computer game called Starcraft. Using our dial-up internet, we could play together even if not in the same house. His dad, the pastor, had times he wanted to have peace with no phone calls, so it was a perfect time for us to get together online.

Dad researched lowering the floor and adding a wheelchair lift in the white high-top van. He found that it was possible to do with the Chevrolet, but it wasn't advised. Crash studies showed that Chevy vans with lowered floors crumpled like an accordion during an accident. Therefore, it wasn't worth the cost to put in a lift and floor modifications. The van was sold after using it for two years, primarily for long trips. The search for another vehicle that I could use and fit inside started over.

School was becoming a challenge for me in different subjects. As a junior, I could choose about half the courses I wanted to take, with the remainder being required. One I enjoyed was journalism and writing for the school newspaper, but subjects such as history and algebra didn't go very well. Patty and Karen took notes in class that I would study before tests. However, I could go through them for hours, typing them out on my computer, and still not remember the answers. I could tell the exact location in the notebook where the answer was located, third page, on the right, about halfway down. However, I couldn't remember what the section said in order to answer the question.

To engage more in class, the AEA had me use a small computer that could be used as a word processor. It helped to write everything down, but it took too much attention to write and listen, and I ended up missing more of what the instructor said.

Junior year also meant more meetings with Voc Rehab and looking at education possibilities after high school. I thought I wanted to go into computer programming, but wasn't sure which school would be a good choice. Dordt College was a Christian school in northwestern Iowa that a lot of kids from Pella Christian attended. We started by looking at the campus and seeing what could be done for nursing care if I moved five hours away from home. Central College in Pella was also an option, but I didn't want to stay in town after graduation.

Junior year also meant more meetings with Voc Rehab and looking at education possibilities after high school.

College Prep English started off the year preparing us to take the A.C.T. It was a national test that helped determine college eligibility. We covered common questions, how to study, and what to do if time ran short. After taking sample tests online and studying in school, test day came in October.

In Pella, testing was done at Central College. It would take too much time for me to write the answers myself, so I had to tell my assistant what to mark. This meant I got to be in my own room with a monitor to make sure I didn't cheat. Halfway through the testing, a 15-minute break was given to everyone. I tried to eat a granola bar in my personal room, but my monitor promptly said that food wasn't allowed in test rooms and would not allow my snack. I decided to skip the rest of break and went ahead and finished my exams ahead of everyone else.

Mom was concerned that I hadn't studied enough and had warned that if I had to take it again for a better result, the test expense would be up to me. My results came back with a score in the low 20s and I felt it was acceptable. The results went off to Dordt, Central, and a few other colleges I liked.

Tom and my group of girls were my primary friends all through school. There were a couple of boys from church who were also in my class, but they mainly stayed with their group of guys, and I didn't talk with them much.

At noon every day, there were three bells for lunch. Classes were released to the cafeteria at different times to try and avoid long lines and have seating available. In the cafeteria, there were four long rows of tables with attached seats. Students generally sat within their grade level. Freshmen took one row, sophomores another, and so on. There was some intermingling depending on seat availability, but not much. With the chairs attached to the tables, I could only sit at the end of the rows, but that also blocked the main aisle.

There were two tables separate from the main rows. Seniors generally sat at one of them and the faculty and staff used the other. The teachers only used half of their space, so this became the overflow area for students and it was where I usually parked for lunch. I either joined who was already there or my group came and sat with me.

One day as I drove toward my regular table, a group of boys from my class were already there. I saw one of them every week at church and talked with them some at school. I got excited when seeing them and looked forward to having lunch with the guys. However, as soon as they saw me coming, they quickly got up and sat at a table I couldn't use. I stopped in my tracks a few seconds with disappointment, feeling abandoned, but continued to my corner. I enjoyed having my friends and spending time with them but would have liked to be with the guys as well. I was at the last lunch bell that day, so my friends had already been through the cafeteria and I ended up eating with only Patty.

After I ate the food-like substance for lunch, I was back with the girls again in the hall. Sitting high up in a power wheelchair while the girls sat on the floor didn't always work for conversation. If they were on one side of the hallway, I would sit opposite them so I could see and chat. One day, as everyone sat on the floor beside me, I could hear them and just see the top of their heads, so I repositioned a few feet away to the opposite side of the hall to see them better. Jenny screamed in surprise as I moved, and I stopped as fast as possible. Her fingers had been directly beside my wheels where I couldn't see. I felt horrible that I may have hurt her, but thankfully they were clear of danger.

After lunch was a break period for games or time to relax and then back to class. One bell rang to indicate the end of break and three minutes later, another sounded to start class. If we weren't in our seat by the second bell, we were counted tardy. The first bell sounded, and everyone started to saunter in different directions toward their classrooms. I finished what I was doing while Patty got my books, and I headed toward Algebra class with Mr. Hessing.

One of the senior classmen yelled down the hall, "Thirty seconds!" He frequently did this as a joke well before the time, but as I turned the corner toward the long hall to class, it was nearly empty. My chin reacted by pushing my chair to full speed and I arrived outside the classroom before the bell rang. My wheels squealed on the tile floor as I applied full braking at my destination. To my surprise, the door to the room was closed and I couldn't get in. As I pondered my predicament, the bell chimed to be in class. A few seconds later, the door opened, and I entered the room, along with a few others. I parked under my table and Patty joined me a short time later with my books. Mr. Hessing started reading off people with tardy notices and third on the list; "Joel Vander Molen." I briefly considered protesting that I couldn't get in because the door was closed but thought I would take the blame instead.

Patty didn't say anything, so I responded with, "What I had to." I wasn't lying but didn't give away what I did either.

The next day was detention. After lunch, I had to go to the Spanish room during break instead of being out with everyone else. The room was nearly full, but it was a good time to get some reading finished. When I got home from school, Mom asked her usual questions of how the day went along with, "What did you do during lunch break?" Patty didn't say anything, so I responded with, "What I had to." I wasn't lying but didn't give away what I did either. A few more probing questions led to telling the whole truth, and nothing but the truth. Mom didn't say much, but wanted to be sure it was the last time I received detention.

Forensics and Speech

Just before Christmas break, one of the English teachers approached me about joining the forensics club. It was a group of students that competed in activities such as short skits, poem reciting, speech, and other skills. It sounded interesting, so I decided to audition for speech. I needed to make up my own presentation, on any topic, and fill a certain amount of time, but not exceed my limit. I was allowed to have notes but with limitations on how many. With my guidelines understood, I picked a topic I knew well- trains. My speech topic would be about an organization called Operation Lifesaver that worked to raise awareness about safety around railroad crossings.

The regional competition came in late February. None of my close friends were on the team, but I at least knew everyone that represented my school. Some, like me, were competing as individuals and others were in group events. Whoever did well would go on to state competition a few weeks later. Most of the other club members had done similar competitions before, but this was my first time.

Both of my parents went with me to Grinnell High School where area schools gathered to compete. Once my time slot came, I entered the designated classroom and used a music stand to hold my notes. A judge sat in the center of the desks directly in front of me. Behind him, my parents and a few other observers sat along with most of the other forensic club members from Pella Christian.

I started off just as I had practiced and made sure to look around the room at my audience and not stare at my notes. As I looked toward another team member, she gave a short smile and wave of encouragement. Instantly, memories of my classmate's subtle pranks to our journalism teacher came to mind and a big grin spread across my face as I droned on about death statistics at railroad crossings. My eyes darted from the audience to the back corner of the room as I continued speaking and tried to regain a professional look. I finished the presentation without missing anything, but avoided looking back in my classmate's direction.

After finishing, Dad helped give my notes to the judge who asked me a few questions. The friendly examiner said I did well with looking around, but wondered if I could move my eyebrows. I hadn't heard such a request before, but demonstrated I could. He said I should try varying my tone and attempt moving more to keep interest. I thanked him and cleared the room for the next participant.

For the next two hours, I continued to check where I thought scores were posted. I sat with my parents in the school cafeteria while other people waited, unsure what to do. Finally, a team member told me reports were in, but I didn't do well enough to advance. It was disappointing but expected for my first attempt. I was glad I tried and enjoyed the extracurricular activity.

My Profession of Faith

Also during my junior year, I professed to be a Christian and to follow Jesus as Lord and Savior. As part of the Christian Reformed Church, I was baptized as an infant; but as a teen, Pastor Zeilstra encouraged me to make my profession and take the next step in faith, especially since Tom already had. I did believe as a Christian and my need for repentance, so decided to go ahead. Part of the process was being questioned by the church council. Along with quizzing about my faith, they would ask me about knowledge related to a church doctrine called the Heidelberg Catechism. My class had gone over it in Sunday school, but during the previous year when I had mainly been in bed. The pastor offered to take me through a crash course, but he said it was only offered for me.

Before long, I was in a corner of a room at church surrounded by more than a dozen older men of the congregation, most of whom I had seen weekly all my life. After several inquiries about my understanding of sin, repentance, and church doctrines, the council needed to discuss and vote. The room was tight for me to get in and out of with my wheelchair, so Pastor Zeilstra motioned to skip having me depart. As I stayed in place, everyone voted to affirm my membership without discussion. A few weeks later, I answered more questions in front of the entire church congregation and was thankful to be an official member of the church. I didn't know where God would lead me but trusted in His direction for the life I had been given.

A Three-Day Retreat

As spring started to arrive, so did the Central Iowa Teens Encounter Christ (CITEC) retreat. It was a three-day event held at a church and school in Prairie City. I hadn't heard of it before nor would have considered attending, but Jenny wanted me to go, so I said yes. All the other participants would stay overnight in sleeping bags, but it was arranged that I would go home for nights and return in the morning.

Upon arrival, everyone had their watches confiscated for the event as we would be on God's time. I needed to know when it was time to do my afternoon cathing and remember to tilt, so I got to keep my watch, but it was covered by one of my arm straps so nobody else could see. Along with Jenny, Kyle also attended the retreat, but I didn't know any of the other faces.

The entire group of teens had full group meetings in an old gymnasium. Afterward, we would meet in groups of 5-6 people in a nearby church. Commuting the few blocks in between, I could barely get my chair up to its normal speed and I thought my batteries were getting low. I knew I had a lot of driving ahead, so I tried to reduce any superfluous moves. As I slowly drove along, Patty and I caught Kyle as he was about to pass. He was obliged to help push and increased my speed, but sternly said he would not be pushing me the entire weekend. At our destination, I looked closer at my chair controls as our team leader talked. I noticed I had it in the wrong gear, one with a slow top speed. I quietly flicked the switch with my chin and was thankful the problem was easy to solve.

Friday evening went quickly, and I went home to Pella for the night. Early Saturday morning, Patty came, and we went back to Prairie City for another day. In the large group meetings, we talked about how to serve God better and draw close to Him. Part of the activities included writing a letter to our parents and thanking them for their support. I tried to quietly dictate to Patty as I didn't have my writing board, and everyone else wrote silently around me.

I listened to everything and participated in the small group discussions when I felt I had something to share. It wasn't uncommon to see someone in tears as they realized the weight of sin and God's gift to us. Saturday evening, a surprise dance night wrapped up the day. As I tried not to run over anyone in the noisy gymnasium, my vent suddenly stopped. I knew the battery was low and Patty had already

As I tried not to run over anyone in the noisy gymnasium, my vent suddenly stopped. I knew the battery was low and Patty had already switched from the external power to the vent's internal source.

switched from the external power to the vent's internal source. With all the noise, I didn't hear the warning alarm of low battery.

Looking through the crowd while trying to breathe, I found Kyle nearby and attempted to yell, with little air, that I needed a wall outlet immediately. He and I navigated to the wall by the kitchen where we found Patty, who could help, and a plugin for my vent. With my chair vent plugged into the wall, I sat tethered on the sidelines watching everyone else. Jenny noticed my predicament and came over to talk. She wanted to make sure I was getting everything out of the retreat and learning how to improve being a Christian. I assured her I was participating and learning and was thankful I went.

Sunday wrapped up the weekend retreat with a church service and participants giving short messages to an audience of parents. I was deemed quiet, speaking when needed, and steady in my faith. With the conclusion of CITEC and no major problems, my mind went to the next social event on the school calendar.

Junior/Senior Banquet

Juniors and seniors had what was called the Junior/Senior banquet every April. Everyone got dressed up in gowns and tuxedos for a formal dinner and show. Afterward, there were several hours of games at a local gymnasium. Most high schools called it prom, but Pella Christian used the unique name.

Getting in a tux was a challenge, but Patty and my parents managed to stuff me into the rented clothing. Before the banquet, Jenny reminded me we were just friends, but I wasn't always good at following rules. I got her a corsage for her dress, which she reluctantly received. Sitting at the table with my group of girls and caregiver felt normal. The after-dinner show was put on by my classmates and mainly made fun of the seniors, but it was still entertaining.

Patty and I briefly went home between activities to change clothes, tend to medical needs, and get ready for the rest of the night. Back at Central College's recreation center, a plethora of different games and raffles for prizes had been set up. I loved being able to stay up and participate with everyone and even play a few games.

The festivities finished around 1:00 Saturday morning with a raffle drawing for different prizes. I won a new camera, film not included, from the prize drawing.

The school year ended with looking forward to an extremely busy summer ahead. This would be the last season before graduation and would be a final opportunity for making summer memories.

11

FINAL FREEDOM

Growing up, most kids can't wait to become an adult and have the freedom to do anything they want. This somewhat changes through the mid to late teens in learning adult responsibilities. In 1 Corinthians 13:11, Paul talks about putting childish ways behind and having new desires as adults.

The summer of 1999 was my last few months before entering my senior year of high school and graduating into adult life. My parents made sure we did not waste it before responsibilities changed.

Just as summer started, Mom's oldest sister gave me a call. The local newspaper in Sully, The Diamond Trails News, needed an extra journalist. She had given them some of my articles from the school newspaper and the editor liked what I wrote. I didn't know what the job would require, or how to do an interview, but went ahead and met with the lead editor.

Mr. Davitt took me back to a small office while Karen sat outside the room. He asked what I liked to write, how I came up with articles, and what games I played. I simply answered with what I did in school and home and thought the interview was a simple process. He said I wouldn't need to come in to write, just email my ideas for approval and then email the finished article. Mark told Karen I answered his questions better than college graduates and he looked forward to seeing my work.

Other than writing, I had three vacations in the short summer months. First was my usual week at CHAMP Camp in June. After that was something called the Iowa Youth Leadership Forum, or YLF, and finally a train trip to the west coast.

After two summers of trouble at camp, Mom was adamant that I should not go. She made certain to remind me that I could not get a pressure sore and be able to do everything that was planned. Dad helped convince her it was good for me to attend camp, and we were soon off to Ohio.

Before summer break, Patty told us she would be moving on to different work, and camp would be her last week with me. She and her husband drove separately from my parents and me as they would be leaving before I did.

It was a fun week with all the counselors being extra careful with applying sunscreen on me. There was a new activity in the woods that required campers, with counselors' help, to build a shelter and see if we could get in. Mostly everyone in my cabin used wheelchairs and had little to no arm control, so we sat around with nobody knowing what direction to take.

I remembered I had been selected for YLF later in the summer. It was touted as a camp for high school students with disabilities that showed good leadership. I figured I should demonstrate the skill and started directing how to position sticks and different ropes we had been given. A few other campers added ideas as well and by the end of the activity, we had a complete stick lean-to. Only one of us could fit in at a time, but it did meet the specifications.

One of the other boys I became friends with was Greg. He and I grabbed one of the newer counselors, Dave, to help us with a prank. Dave was a Methodist minister but was getting to know the medical routines well. Our threesome found Patty's car in the parking lot, the only one with Iowa license plates, and applied a generous amount of silly string to the windows.

Swimming, fishing, a tower climb, dance, and the other activities were part of the very familiar camp routine, but I enjoyed spending time with friends. James didn't return, but I still had George, Terry, and more campers and counselors that I got to know well.

Thursday night came quickly with the closing campfire, awards, and final pranks of the week. The younger campers went home on Friday morning, but the teenagers got to stay until Sunday for the adolescent retreat.

Just as I got down in my bunk for the night, I watched as my neighboring campers finished their routine. Patty came over and said she noticed the extra car decorations. I found myself covered in silly string a few seconds later.

Caregivers had quit before and it made me wonder if I did something wrong. This time felt closer as we had gone through so many years together.

As Patty said her goodbyes, tears dripped from my eyes at the thought of no longer having someone I grew up with. Caregivers had quit before and it made me wonder if I did something wrong. This time felt closer as we had gone through so many years together. I officially had one mother, but having grown up around adult women, it felt like I had many more to help guide me in life's challenges. Losing one who had been with me for so many years felt like losing a parent.

The adolescent weekend had few scheduled activities, and we could choose what we wanted to do. After a busy week, some decided to sleep the afternoon away. George was the only boy that wanted to rest, so he was temporarily relocated to the girls' cabin for a few hours. I got in some extra fishing and enjoyed being on my own without my regular caregivers around, before heading back home to Iowa.

Rhoda had started helping at night in junior high. With Patty gone, she switched to working during the day. Rhoda already knew my medical cares but not my day schedule. Summer was usually a calm time to learn the daytime activities, but it was soon time for my second camp.

I learned the Youth Leadership Forum had originated in California, but Iowa was now starting their own chapter. This was the first year for it and I wasn't sure what to expect. The information said I needed to be open and talkative, or else I may not get to stay. The week-long forum was held in Ames, Iowa on the campus of Iowa State University. There weren't many college students during the summer, which allowed forum delegates to be housed in the dorms. Instructional classes then met in a different building on campus.

This was my first time staying on a college campus having just two of my nurses from home with me, one for nighttime and the other for daytime. The sessions included information on how to be independent in college with a disability and practical life applications. Halfway through the week, the group was put on buses for a trip to the state capital in Des Moines.

I was the only delegate that used a vent and very few of the others used wheelchairs full-time. I got to ride in the large Greyhound bus with most of the other teenagers. I wasn't aware that some of the large buses had wheelchair lifts, but I was soon hoisted up about six feet in the air before reversing into my position. A few of the regular coach seats had been moved apart to allow room for me. I was used to CHAMP Camp where the other campers had similar medical needs. With this group, I didn't quite feel like I fit in.

At the capital, legislators talked with us about disability concerns at the state level and how to advocate for our needs. After hearing politicians, we were taken on a tour of the building. Growing up in Iowa, I had seen the golden dome of the capital, but the inside was fun to see. It was interesting to see the expansive library and hear the history of how ornate wooden benches were made for judges.

As the week continued, I made sure I kept talking with the counselors and other delegates, as I thought was required. When a reporter from The Des Moines Register came to write an article about the forum, everyone directed the journalist to me. The delegates thought I would be a great one to be interviewed, since I was deemed the talkative one.

Experiencing campus life was a challenge and a learning experience. The small dorm rooms were a place for a few beds and some small furniture. I had to use communal bathrooms in the men's section with only female caregivers. Mary came to help at night, and she figured out a method to get water for my bath and other night cares. We made it work, but I knew I would need to be selective of my dorm at college, especially the bathrooms.

Similar to CHAMP Camp, YLF concluded the week with a wrap-up of activities and accomplishments. As parents heard stories, one evening event made the top of the list. One of the counselors was playing music in the hallway before an activity. A hearing-impaired delegate turned around and said, in sign language, that she was being too loud. The moral to the story: when someone who is unable to hear says you're noisy, it's time to adjust the volume.

Through all the activities, I thankfully stayed free of skin trouble. In between trips, I made up a list of article ideas for the newspaper and sent them to be approved. A month later, I didn't hear back from the newspaper editor or anyone else. After further persistence, I received a green light to pursue my proposals. Interviewing people for different articles was fun, but more time-consuming than I imagined. I was still able to get material out between excursions but needed to be careful with time management.

From Chicago to Sacramento via Train

August's train trip was quickly approaching. I had always traveled by van and didn't have a big concern about how much I packed. That wasn't the case with the train though, as everything would need to be carried by hand a few times. My parents got everything down to the bare minimum to cover the excursion. My bedside vent used a humidifier to keep me from drying out at night. Instead of bringing a gallon of distilled water for it, bottled water from convenience stores would have to work.

Dad's co-worker and fellow railfan, Richard, his wife Alice, and their youngest son would join us. Dad and Richard had taken Amtrak a few times before on hiking trips and Alice, a nurse, had helped me some nights as well.

In early August, the six of us drove to Chicago's Union Station to start our adventure. We got to the station with little time to spare before boarding. I hadn't seen Union Station before and sat looking at the high decorative ceiling and busy travelers. Dad directed us to a deli in the station for a quick lunch before departing, but none of the sandwiches looked appetizing.

The first leg of our trip was on Amtrak's Empire Builder, from Chicago to Seattle. I had an accessible sleeper room with an upper bunk, two chairs that folded down to a bed, and a small bathroom. There was also enough room to park my chair beside the bed and have my vent plugged into an outlet. My room was the full width of the car with windows on both sides. I couldn't see out very well while sitting in my wheelchair as I was a little too tall and far away, so Dad would take me out of my chair and sit me on one of the regular seats, but on my chair's cushion.

Alice would help take care of me at night and my parents helped during the day. They had a roomette just down the hall in the same car where Alice could rest after her shift.

We left Chicago in early afternoon, and I watched Wisconsin and part of Minnesota roll by my window before it got dark. I liked sleeping on the train, the motion felt like being rocked asleep.

Halfway through the country, the train had an extended stop in Minot, North Dakota for fuel and servicing. It was a long enough break for all of us to get off the train and wander around. Just sitting in my room, I didn't see a need for footwear and stayed barefoot. After Dad replaced my seat cushion and plopped me in my wheelchair, Alice put my shoes on to go explore the station.

An old Great Northern steam engine was on display, and I could imagine the days when it was working through the northern United States. The day of our stop was extremely windy, and the breeze kept blowing my jean shorts wide open making a bit of a peep show. I tried to drive with my back to the wind but was afraid of hitting someone.

When the train's engines were refueled and the passenger cars serviced, the conductor yelled "All aboard!" Passengers headed back to their appropriate car and I navigated back to the sleeper. The accessible car I was in had a folding ramp that I used to get in and out. It was a little steep, and the corners inside were tight, but it worked well enough.

As the train started moving westward, Dad got me repositioned back on the train's seat with my chair cushion. I had Alice take my shoes off and, as my left foot came back into view, I saw a purple big toe that had been curled over. Later on, we also noticed another one had been broken at the same time. I was surprised by the sight and was thankful I had a dislike for footwear. If I had kept the shoes on, I likely would have needed an emergency hospital visit and would have one less toe.

During school, I had started reading one chapter of the Bible every night. I didn't take my table and book board with me to read on the trip, but Alice asked if she could read for me. I was in the early chapters of Genesis and, as I heard about God's creation, I watched it fly by my window through North Dakota and eastern Montana. Oncoming trains were just a blur, but it was an experience I wanted to keep in my memory.

The second morning on the train found us in western Washington. Overnight, some cars had been removed to go to Portland. Now, we were in the Cascade mountains and getting close to the coast. Later in the morning, the train reached its final stop in Seattle. Getting off the Empire Builder, Dad quickly found the accessible minivan they had rented for our time in the area. It took a while to get organized, but eventually, our group started to leave the station with two vehicles.

I had eaten the included breakfast on the train but was feeling lightheaded and had to find lunch quickly. Fast food didn't look any different in Seattle than it did in Iowa, but the traffic on the roads was much more than I had seen before. After lunch, we drove east, back into the mountains, to our hotel in Skykomish, Washington.

Skykomish was a town smaller than Pella and was in a valley between several high hills. Most people wouldn't consider it a vacation destination, but it was close to the longest railroad tunnel in the country, the Cascade Tunnel. Dad and Richard had visited the area a few years earlier and acted as tour guides. Before bedding down for the night, our entourage found a cool curved railroad bridge near town. The Foss River Bridge is one I wanted to see, but the mosquitos seemed to congregate on us as we sat between towering fir trees. We hoped to wait long enough to see a train, but the pests soon drove us away.

It felt good to sleep in a stationary bed again, and the bottled water from the local gas station worked fine in my vent's humidifier. Early morning in the valley was brisk with a mist in the air. Immediately behind our accommodation was the Skykomish River with fog reluctantly leaving the cool water. The hotel didn't have breakfast, but as we left our rooms, our group was met with the lonesome sound of a train horn echoing off the hills. The men of the group quickened our pace to get closer to the rails for a better view.

There were two places to eat in town, a bar and a small restaurant. After watching the train, we took a seat around a couple of tables at the cozy restaurant and started to look over the menu. As usual, Mom sat on one side of me and Dad on the other to help me eat. With the menu laying open in front of me, I read through the breakfast options as our waitress started taking drink orders. She first got the opposite side of the table, then moved on to us. After Mom made her choice, the server pointed her pin toward me and said, "Does he drink water?" By 17, I had become used to stares in public and questions of every sort and had many sarcastic replies, but this was a first.

A little flustered, I quickly replied, "I'll take orange juice, please." I noticed the surprised look on her face that I could speak and respond appropriately. I guessed small town waitresses didn't see teenagers using a wheelchair and a ventilator very often.

After breakfast, we toured the rails of western Washington and found our way to the famous Cascade tunnel, spending time at both portals. We had just gone through the 7.8 mile bore the day before, but it was fun to see trains disappear into the ground. On the east end, a fan system was used to help flush the tunnel of diesel exhaust. It also helped indicate when a train was coming. The former Great Northern route wasn't very busy, but we stayed for several hours to try to see trains in both directions through the landmark.

After touring the rails, our group headed to a hotel in Seattle. Before the day ended, our tour included watching planes land at Seattle/Tacoma International Airport where I had landed many times in my flight simulator at home. I was excited to see my first Boeing 747 land before we took off for the night.

Our final full day in Washington started out with clouds and rain that were typical for the area. I had hoped to see the Boeing manufacturing plant, but none of us knew exactly where it was or how to take tours. Instead, we found the Boeing plane museum. Mom could walk short distances okay, but long excursions would quickly cause great pain in her lower joints. Therefore, she stayed by herself in the van while the guys went on what she hoped would be a quick tour of the museum. Unfortunately, it took a few hours and was larger than what I had expected.

The two families went our separate ways for the remainder of the day. Mom hoped to see the Space Needle and have supper at the spinning restaurant. Dad thought it was too expensive and we got to the tower much later than planned. Watching the sun set over Puget Sound and large ships docked by the shore was a beautiful sight to see as the city lights became bright below us.

I liked most seafood, so Dad took us to a restaurant close to the water that he and Richard visited years earlier. Ordering crab legs for the three of us was a fun experience. The waiter started by covering our table with paper and putting a large bowl in the middle. Several crab legs and cups of butter were dumped on the paper, and I watched as my parents dug out the meat with tiny forks. I looked forward to trying the delicacy, but thought it tasted rubbery. I could at least say I tried them in Seattle directly by the water.

Overnight in the hotel was scary with fire alarms constantly going off. I was stuck on the third floor with no working elevator during the sirens. Mom called the front desk to see what the problem was, or if we could change to a room on the ground floor. Thankfully, everything was resolved without any issues.

Touring the Seattle area was fun, but none of us cared very much for cities. Boarding the train, I again had a handicapped sleeper room. This time we were on Amtrak's Coast Starlight as our excursion continued south to Sacramento. The scenery outside my window changed from thick pine forests to more dry scrub in northern California. After just one night on the train, we were close to our next destination.

My parents chose to stay in the coach section for this short leg of the trip. Looking around, Mom noticed some men with bandages on their arms and wrists, but they had odd lumps in them. She and I had been around enough medical facilities to know bandages shouldn't look like that. Several miles before our station, the train stopped in an uninhabited area for several minutes. The conductor announced that a stalled freight train in front of us was the issue and we would be moving soon.

When we finally reached Sacramento and detrained, Mom saw police officers escorting a man from the train with a large wrap on his arm. However, the lumpy bandage passengers got off while laughing at the detained individual. Mom suspected the lumps were likely not medical related and probably not anything legal.

Our visit to California was only going to be for one day and did not include a vehicle. Our group of six carried the luggage and walked to a hotel close to the tracks. Lugging my bed vent, humidifier, chair charger, vent battery charger, and other medical equipment, besides clothing, was a challenge. However, I transported backpacks and whatever else I could. Mom packed my supplies knowing this part of the itinerary and had planned ahead.

After unloading in our hotel rooms, Dad, Richard, and I went to the Sacramento rail museum while the other half of our group did their own thing. I liked seeing the Southern Pacific cab forward steam engine and other relics. It would have been fun to see one still in operation, along with some of the other engines. However, I wasn't as interested in railroad history as much as Dad and Richard. They enjoyed collecting railroad lanterns and other memorabilia, but I preferred modern equipment.

After the museum, we went through old town Sacramento for a brief tour. Roaming around, it looked like an old western movie with small streets and boardwalks for sidewalks. As I rolled along, I noticed there were several people on corners playing music and getting donations from passersby. I hadn't seen this before, but thought it was interesting. Some had signs saying why funds were needed, but most didn't.

The dads spotted an antique shop and wanted to see if it had any railroad lanterns, but the only entrance to the small shop had a short flight of stairs that prevented me from entering. Dad said they would just quickly run in and would check on me through the window, pointing toward the dirty glass. Before I could say much, they popped inside, and I was left on the boardwalk on my own. From inside, Dad tapped on the glass, and I nodded that I was okay. As the minutes passed, I slowly drove in small circles in front of the window so I could still be seen. I parked by a post supporting an overhang and tilted my chair back to try to look like I had a purpose for sitting outside alone.

As I waited, someone came toward me on the boardwalk, so I moved over toward one side to give them more room to pass. As the woman approached, she slowed her walk and gave me a curious look. Already starting to feel abandoned, I gave my usual smile, nodded, and said hello. The woman then asked, "Where's your cup?" I was used to stares and odd questions, but my mind spun, "What cup is she talking about? Dad, why did you leave me out here?" I then realized she thought I was one of the people on the street looking for money. I thanked her for the offer, but explained I was waiting for someone inside. The potential donor looked perplexed but continued on her way.

After what seemed like an eternity, the guys returned from browsing the antiquated item store and we continued with the day. When I told him of my encounter, Dad laughed and said I should have taken something to help fund the trip. Mom wasn't amused or pleased with me being left alone on the boardwalk.

The final leg of our excursion started the next day by boarding the California Zephyr. The train was a few hours late, so I joined Alice with a quick tour of a nearby mall. I was intrigued to notice it looked like a regular mall in Iowa, but it didn't have doors between the outdoors and inside. It was easy for me to enter without assistance, and I thought it must be nice to not have to worry about cold winters and keeping the facility warm.

Back at the train station, a municipal bus stopped to load and unload passengers. As soon as it was stationary, the large vehicle squatted closer to the ground. I was parked near the end of the bus and the driver wanted to know if I was getting on. Mom, closer to his location, answered that I wasn't. I wondered what it would be like to use municipal transportation in a large city but was ready to get home.

Going up the ramp into my sleeper car was becoming routine and Dad quickly had me back on my perch of the train's seat to watch palm trees give way to mountains. The next morning, our train was stopped in Salt Lake City, Utah. Several announcements stated there had been a derailment in Colorado and we would be taking a detour between Salt Lake City and Denver and miss all station stops in between the two cities. This meant we wouldn't see as much mountain scenery, but we saw a lot more rail traffic than the regular route. Since we didn't make any station stops, I stayed in my makeshift chair until late evening while the desert went by my window. I had planned to get out at Denver's union station, but the Zephyr didn't arrive until midnight. I was already lying in bed for the night and decided to stay put.

Dawn came for the last time on the train with my view outside the window showing familiar corn fields and rolling hills. As our final stop came close, we noted our train watching locations as they quickly entered and exited our view. The train arrived in Ottumwa five hours later than scheduled, but we were thankful to be near home.

While we were gone, Dad's older brother and his wife took the train to Chicago to pick up our van and bring it to Ottumwa for us. When Dad got to the vehicle, he found a shattered windshield and a note from his brother. Just outside of Ottumwa, a rock truck pulled out in front of him and sprayed rocks all over the front of the van. The ailing vehicle got us home but soon went in for repairs.

The once-in-a-lifetime trip was fun and now complete. I concluded that the west coast was different than the Midwest I knew so well.

Thankfully, I managed a busy summer without getting any pressure sores, and I looked toward my final year of high school.

12

SENIORITIS

In 1 Timothy 4:12, Paul writes to Timothy, "Let no one despise your youth, but be an example to the believers in word, in conduct, in love, in spirit, in faith, in purity." By senior year of high school, most teenagers feel like they know everything and are ready to conquer the world. I wasn't much different and didn't always look to the examples God had given me or act as I should.

After graduating from junior high, I finished the Cadets program at church and moved to young adults. This was the Wednesday evening group for all high schoolers with meetings varying between fun nights and Bible study. I didn't go every week but did attend most of the time and had fun hanging out with the other teens from church.

During my first three years, adults from the congregation volunteered to lead us. Some weeks met at church, and other weeks we met at some of the leaders' houses. One leader had a walk-in basement with a level entrance that allowed me to get in. It was rare that I could get into anyone else's house, but it was a nice change of experience.

Entering my final year of young adults, no full-time volunteers were found to lead the program. All the teenagers from church gathered at my house, with a parent coming along to monitor. For our first week, the parent thought it would be best for one of us to be appointed president and lead the meetings. A few names were given, then everyone closed our eyes and voted by raising hands, or, for me, shaking my head. When the votes were in, our chaperone declared I had won the lead role of the group. I had few close friends in young adults and was generally one of the quiet participants, so I was surprised to be voted president, but I was willing to try.

More positions were decided upon with Tom voted as secretary. Since he never went anywhere except church without his Apple laptop, Tom was an easy pick. One look at each other and we knew the two of us had a lot of work ahead.

After several weeks of meeting and me coming up with a Bible study, a permanent volunteer was found to help. Before winter came, I organized a car wash fundraiser for the group. We set up at the local Walmart and spent all day cleaning vehicles for anyone that came. Going between vehicles and organizing teams, I managed to keep my chair dry. Most car owners left happy, except one elderly lady who tested every window seal with a tissue, but after another round of drying, she seemed satisfied.

Preparing for My Future

As my school years progressed, required courses decreased and the number of electives increased. Before the school year began, I had to choose the courses I wanted to take. Mom said she had always done accounting work for her jobs and my paperwork, but never took a class in it. She said I had to take accounting as one of my courses whether I wanted to or not.

Computers always came easily for me, and I wanted to go into computer programming in college. Computer math, an introductory programming course, was an easy choice in my schedule. I also took another year of journalism, Spanish, and a required course on U.S. government along with a few others. Tom was also with me in journalism and computer math, making them much more fun. One of my other classmates decided to take journalism again as well. Since his grade point average (GPA) was higher than mine, that automatically made him the editor, even though I worked for a real newspaper.

Shop class had a course on computer aided drafting that sounded interesting, but it had a prerequisite of other shop classes. I couldn't physically build or work on things like Dad, but I was still interested in it and thought it would be fun. However, I didn't try to see if I could take the class without the previous courses.

With my schedule complete, I was ready for another year of school, after visiting potential college choices.

Seniors were allowed two days off during the year to make college visits. My parents and I managed to visit Dordt College during the summer. We liked the accessibility of the campus, and I looked forward to attending. While at Dordt, the proposed nursing agency also met with us and discussed what I would need. The company warned that they were unsure if they could find enough people to cover me all day every day but were looking for nurses. We also did an official tour of Iowa State University in Ames as Voc Rehab said they work well with students with disabilities. I didn't like the dorm during YLF or going to a school that was more than twice the size of Pella.

My senior year started off well after getting settled into new classes. Rhoda hadn't been with me to school before and came with Karen for one day to train. At lunch, I was on the first bell and got to the table before the girls. Rhoda had met a few of them during the summer but was quickly introduced to everyone.

It was stereotypical that high school seniors always made fun of freshman, but it wasn't very common at Pella Christian. However, Tom's sister was now a new freshman in school. During a break in journalism class, he and I made a sign, "To me, freshman are speed bumps." I displayed it on the back of my chair during lunch and made sure to show Tom's sister. Her nickname became "Speed Bump" and the sign made for good decoration in my locker.

The start of the year also meant a few weeks of warm weather for outdoor games during lunch break. I would watch activities and enjoy the sun before going back inside. The only accessible entrance to the outdoor play area was through the freshman hall. My friends and caregiver usually went in the door closer to my classroom and I drove through the halls to join them a minute or two later.

As I headed in from the bright light to indoors, my eyes adjusted, and I could see people standing around. I expertly navigated through the gaps around groups of students and avoided hitting anyone. About halfway down the hall, I hit a large bump that I figured was likely someone's foot. The jolt jammed my control stick into my lower lip and teeth, shooting pain through my mouth. After nearly six years of braces, I had finally gotten them off and hoped I didn't damage anything. I assumed the bump was my fault, so I said, "Sorry" as I rolled along and continued to class.

A few days later, my mouth finally stopped hurting, and I once again headed back inside through the freshman hall. About 30 feet ahead, I could see a group of boys nearly filling the hall. They were talking quickly to each other and one boy on the edge kept looking over his shoulder and grinning as I approached. I headed toward the narrow gap between the boys and the wall and saw a large white shoe purposefully sticking out in my path. I prepared for the bump and as my rear wheel raised up to go over the shoe, I stopped directly on top.

Dad and I had gone to the Iowa State Fair the previous summer and found a cattle scale I could drive my chair on. The total weight was over 450 pounds. My chair also had a rigid frame and didn't flex with bumps. It made for a rough ride and, when one wheel was up on something, the weight didn't distribute well to the others. Therefore, a large portion of that weight now sat on this freshman's foot.

I sat looking straight ahead, lightly leaning on my controls, and remembering the previous jolt from days earlier. After about 20 seconds, I looked up at the young man whose face was now starting to contort and change colors. I said in a stern voice, "Don't do it again." I drove ahead slowly, and he quickly limped back a few steps, dropped to the floor, and leaned on a locker while looking at his shoe. As I rounded a corner, I could hear his friends ask in a surprised tone what I told him. I was soon out of earshot and was unable to hear further discussion.

Nothing was said to anyone outside of our little meeting that day and I never had any further problems. I regret my decision to act as I did and should have brought it up to a teacher. The guidance counselor, Mr. Van Kooten, had his office a few feet away from where the scene played out. Unfortunately, we can't undo decisions that have been made.

Thankfully, most students behaved well and some were even helpful. Even with medication, my muscle spasms (stretching as I called it) continued to cause problems when driving my chair. My headrest had two buttons, one to move my control stick away and the other to move them back. Driving between classes, my neck became stiff, forced my head back to my headrest, and hit the control's away button. With the stiffness continuing, I couldn't move my head or reach the other button. My nurse was still behind me getting books, so I sat in the middle of a crowded hall, unable to move, like a big bump on a log.

I caught the attention of one student, but they just kept walking. A freshman stopped next, and I explained where to find the hidden button in my headrest. Once he found it, I was able to get the controls and move again. I made sure to thank the student for his help and made it to class. A few days later the same scenario happened with getting stuck. Just after my controls were fully away from me, I felt the same hand behind my head to help solve the problem. I was thankful for encountering helpful students.

Turning 18 and Registering for the Draft

A common part of senior year was getting professional pictures taken. They could then be handed around to classmates to share and put in the yearbook. I wanted to get some photos taken near the train tracks, however, the Iowa Interstate Railroad decided to abandon Pella and started removing the rails that had been in place for a century. By October, only a few sections remained, but I was able to sit by one section of track for pictures.

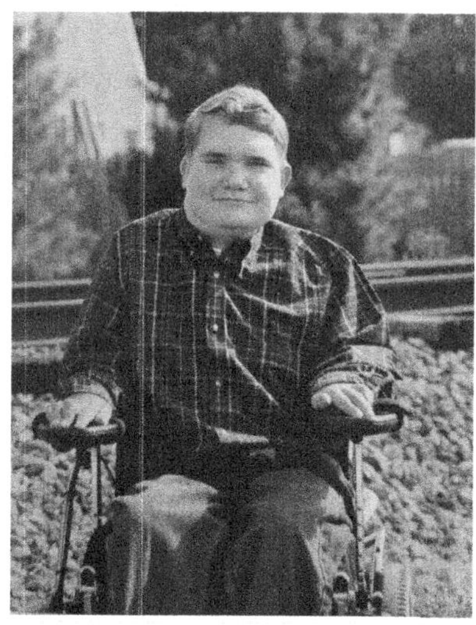

Mom wanted to have a few photos without my vent tubes or trach showing. To accomplish this, I would get positioned where the photographer wanted me and turn my head at just the right angle. Dad would disconnect the tube from my trach, put the shirt over it, then move away for a few quick shots before returning my air. Attempting to smile and look happy while not breathing wasn't fun, but it worked.

Before winter set in, the accounting class took a field trip to Des Moines. We went to a school called AIB College of Business. It was on a main road near the airport I had passed many times but never noticed it.

Our class was put in a small classroom to hear about the school and what majors they offered. Accounting was one, as well as information technology, court reporting, and several more. I noticed the room we were in was in the same building as the dorms. The campus looked nice, except for being built on a hill. Since I was working on arrangements to attend Dordt College, I didn't think I would ever see the campus again.

November came, and with it my 18th birthday. School was off for Thanksgiving on Wednesday with my birthday on Saturday. It had been a few months since Patty left, but she offered to have me stay overnight Friday and Saturday at her house. One of the camp counselors, Big Brian, and his wife came from Indianapolis to help me celebrate. I had never stayed overnight at someone's house before and wasn't sure how it would work. Brian and his wife arrived around 3:00 in the afternoon on Friday.

Then Patty's family, Brian and his wife, and Jenny and I were going to go to Hobby Haven in Des Moines.

My afternoon cathing time was at 4:00. As the hour got closer, I was sure Patty would remember and we'd do my "afternoon stuff" soon. About halfway to Des Moines, I realized we hadn't done my cares or brought anything with us. Patty's husband and Brian went back to Pella in one vehicle while the rest of us went on to the city. Late in the day, Patty and I ended up doing my bathroom routine in a dark parking lot in the van. My first attempt at a fully independent weekend didn't go well.

On Saturday, we went back to my house, and I showed Brian the train layout Dad and I had made. The project slowly progressed during high school, but it now had two tracks going around the room with some sidings and buildings squeezed in. A grain elevator with "Pella Feed Service" on the side was the main focal point. Overnight was at Patty's house again with Mary coming to help me. Sleeping in the home's living room was different, but we managed to get everything done. I rarely heard from anyone at camp during the year and I was thankful Brian's family came.

After turning 18, I knew I had to register for the draft, as any male in the United States must do. I heard there was a new option available for registering on the internet. It felt pointless, but I did my civic duty anyway. The thought of joining the Air Force or other military branch sounded like something I would have been interested in. However, I knew I would never be able to do so with my physical limitations. I could fly planes with my stick on a simulator, but real aircraft would not be as easy. I later found out my registration would be entertaining.

It wasn't a government requirement, but I also signed up for intramurals. During lunch break at school, students could sign-up for intramurals. Depending on the time of year, touch football, basketball or other sports were popular. During the winter, checkers and chess were also options. I played checkers with my cousins and did fairly well. I tried the sport in junior year but lost my first game and didn't realize I could continue playing until losing twice. I decided to give it another try for my last year at school and see how I did.

To play, Karen, Rhoda, or a teacher took one of my bedside tables from the computer lab and set up the checkerboard on it. My opponent had to sit on a high stool to reach it, but it worked. My group of girls usually didn't come to watch me play, but one day they did.

All year, they had been joking about putting my chair in manual mode and pushing me in the girls' bathroom, but they never acted on it. As I concentrated on my checkers opponent's moves, I considered my strategy in clearing the board of his pieces. When I needed to jump a piece, I slid a checker around the opponent's piece. Pushing it off the board, I balanced the defeated checker on my stick and dropped it in the holding container. After several minutes of competition, I rose another notch on the leadership board. As the game was progressing, I noticed my friends around me, but didn't give them much attention.

With the game complete and my table cleared, I hit the button for my controls to come to me and then tried to drive. Pushing my chin control, I heard the motors respond, but my wheels didn't move. Jenny and the girls grinned in response as they had managed to get my chair in manual gear without me noticing. They gave me a push toward the library door but didn't go through with their threat.

Y2K

Christmas break came quickly, and everyone said goodbye, adding that they wouldn't return to school until the next century. For several years, news stations and scientists had been talking about the Y2K bug. Since many electronics only used two-digit years, such as 97, 98, 99, it was feared that going to 00 for 2000 would make computers think it was 1900. This would result in massive blackouts and major problems across the world.

I had performed suggested tests on my Windows '95 Gateway and had done updates to prepare, but nobody was sure what would happen. Tom's trusty Apple laptop was designed differently and thought to be immune to such issues, which he made sure I remembered.

On New Year's Eve 1999, Tom came to our annual party with our family and friends. Watching television to see if the world would collapse, Australia and Europe got into the new millennium without trouble. However, it was advised to be off the internet and have computers turned off at midnight, just in case. After too much root beer and sparkling grape juice, the midnight hour approached. I turned my computer off as suggested, but Tom dialed into the Internet just to show off. The clock hit 12:00 and everyone in the house cheered. The electricity stayed on and none of the predicted problems occurred. I turned on my computer again to check, and all was good.

Continuing to work on college plans for the fall, my parents and I took another campus tour of Dordt during the winter to see how well I could get around with the snow. I was thankful to see well cleared sidewalks that were easy to get around on, even in the cold.

In late January, my parents, Voc Rehab counselor, school guidance counselor, and I had a teleconference with Dordt College and the nursing agency. Everything with the school looked like it would work for me to attend in the fall. However, the nursing agency was unable to find enough staff to cover me 24/7 and couldn't guarantee enough nurses would be found in time.

The college was in the small town of Sioux Center and was far from any large populations. Aaron, the quadriplegic I visited in grade school, lived a short distance away from the campus and had some nursing care at home. I would have liked to be near him, but the community couldn't support both of us. Two quadriplegics in a small town both requiring round-the-clock care was too much for available caregivers. After further prayer and discussion, my family decided to stop pursuing Dordt and look at a school closer to Pella. After more than a year of work, we would now have to nearly start over to find a school.

Time also continued to move on with watching my cousins grow. On the third Sunday of every month, Mom's family got together for lunch at her parent's house. February 20, 2000, happened to be the day we headed to Sully for the afternoon. Most of the family lived nearby and came every month, including Levi. With his arrival on my birthday three years earlier, he was now the same age I was when I was injured. As I watched him play, I thought of how our lives would be different from this point in his life forward.

Just like me at that age, the toddler wasn't thinking about his future beyond his current activity. He would not have to learn to watch medical expenses or how to train adults to take care of him. Also, if Levi decided to go to college, he wouldn't need to start planning years in advance to research accessibility and nursing coverage. God had given us very different paths, but I wasn't the only one who realized the anniversary.

A few days earlier, Grandpa let Levi play with his special toy pickup, just as I had years ago. Grandma quickly reminded him of it but still let him have fun. She said receiving the phone call that two of her daughters, son-in-law, and grandson had been in a serious accident was the worst day of her life. However, God had brought us through many challenges since that day.

Closing out the Senior Year

My last half of senior year was moving along quickly. In computer math we had been learning a programming language called Basic. The concept of if/then statements, for loops, and random statements made sense to me, but I struggled writing the programming and remembering all the proper syntax. Accounting class was going pretty well, and I understood the basics. Balancing ledger sheets and getting numbers in their correct columns wasn't too difficult. However, during tests I would try to go too quickly and get everything mixed up. Karen would see me going astray, remind me to focus, and then start again.

Since this was how classes were going in high school, I didn't think I could do computer programming for a career as I had hoped. I decided to apply at AIB and take an accounting major that also included some computer courses. I was starting the process late in the year, but I prayed it would work. A new location for college also meant starting the hunt for nursing agencies again. Kid Care was a care facility in the Des Moines area that served children with significant medical needs. They also provided home care options and said they would be able to help if they found enough nurses. It was an option to try, otherwise I would only be able to attend Central College in Pella and continue to live at home.

Homecoming week was always a fun time at school with each day having a theme. Everyone could dress up according to the theme, and judges would see who did the best. I tried some outfits, like wearing shoes on wrong feet for backwards day, but never too much. When the theme was old person's day, I wasn't the only person in school using a wheelchair, but the other students left skid marks on the cafeteria ramp that could be claimed as mine.

On Friday afternoon, classes were stopped for homecoming games, and competitions were held between the grades to get top bragging rights. One of the challenges was a tug-of-war between upper and lower classman. My fellow seniors pulled valiantly against the freshmen but lost the first round. As he left the rope, one of my classmates said he pulled his back and wouldn't do the second round. Thoughts quickly went through my head that if I was tied to the end of the rope, I could at least act like a large anchor. My thoughts reminded me this would be the only chance I would get to do such an activity. I built up my courage and told the classmates around me, "I'll do it."

They weren't sure I was serious at first, but word quickly filtered through the bleachers behind me, and I was on the crew. A couple of the other pullers, farm boys, started looking over the back of my chair for a good place to tie the rope and discussed different knot options.

The guidance counselor noticed the increased activity around me and came to see if everything was okay. When he learned of our plans, he was unsure of the safety of our thinking. Mr. Van Kooten's wife had become a paraplegic a few years earlier and likely the thoughts of wheelchair expense and repair went through his head. Karen didn't object to me helping my class but did not encourage me either. After further convincing, Mr. Van Kooten allowed our scheme to proceed, but sternly charged the same farm boys with responsibility to keep me from flipping backwards. The time soon came for round two and I rolled out toward the pull line with my support crew. There was a mixture of gasping from teachers and cheers from students as I rolled up and got attached to the rope.

For a moment, I envisioned my backrest being yanked out of place or off my chair. However, I figured it may be a good challenge for Dad to fix, if needed. I faced the gym's wall while the action was behind me. The rope was firmly tied to the back of my seat, with the boys in front of me ready to catch. The first tug yanked my entire chair backwards with my front wheels coming off the ground. I tried to get to my controls to drive forward, but the next yank jerked my head and kept me away from the stick. The match didn't take long and ended with another defeat. My inclusion didn't get the desired result, but at least I gave it a shot.

The journalism teacher snapped a picture showing my shocked face, with wheels in the air, and my support crew looking bewildered. I never saw the photograph but I was told about it by Tom.

By March, most of my classmates knew what they were doing after graduation. Some were going straight into the work force and others to various colleges and academic pursuits.

An award ceremony was held with every student's scholarship or academic success touted. Most of my group of friends were on the honor roll at school, but I wasn't. My GPA was 0.1 points too low to qualify for academic recommendation. A former guidance counselor at Pella Christian sent several students to AIB. I qualified for a small memorial scholarship honoring him, but nothing else.

In early April, the junior/senior banquet came around again. With my group in dresses and me in a tuxedo, we made sure to get a group picture before eating. I again broke Jenny's request not to have special treatment and gladly gave her a corsage to go along with her dress.

As part of supper entertainment, juniors gave predictions about each senior. Their prediction for me was that I would invent a new printer with a stun feature.

A few weeks after the banquet was the annual senior class trip. Like many classes before us, mine voted to go to Chicago. We got to school very early on a Thursday morning and left Pella at 4:00 a.m. so we could get to the city around 9:00. Karen and Rhoda went with me, leaving my parents at home. It was the first time I went on vacation out of Iowa without them.

Two large busses had been chartered for the trip and the planning committee made sure one included a wheelchair lift. My extra vent, battery chargers, and medical supplies for the overnight trip were packed into the vehicle's expansive luggage holder along with my classmate's bags.

After a breakfast stop in eastern Iowa, our tour of the city started with Shedd Aquarium. Then, late in the afternoon, we were dropped off at Wrigley Field to watch a Cubs' game. The travel agency had purchased all the tickets but forgot one for a wheelchair seat. Wrigley refused to exchange my ticket for another one and my teachers and I had to buy additional seats for Karen and me. Our seats were directly behind home plate, and likely a coveted location, but nowhere near my classmates.

The cold April wind froze me as I sat watching a sport I cared nothing about. Around the sixth inning, Karen and I went to the stadium's medical facility to do my afternoon cathing and warm up. Everyone loaded up on the buses before the end of the game, and then headed to supper and the final activity of the day.

My classmates did a riverboat tour of the city, but the boat did not have wheelchair access. Instead, my cousin and his wife met with me, and we visited a coffee shop while waiting.

Strict curfews were in place at the hotel with adult hall monitors ensuring guys and gals stayed in their separate rooms. To save on cost, every room had at least three occupants, except for me. I had a room all to myself with Karen staying up with me. I was also the only male in school history that was officially allowed to have all of my female friends in my room.

With Karen just outside, we simply chatted about the day until midnight when they left to go to their rooms.

The next morning was unstructured time at a large zoo with free entry. Karen and Rhoda stayed at a central dining location while my group toured the animals around the immediate area. It was fun getting time without an adult with us, but easily accessible if needed.

Before heading home, the itinerary had us visiting an arcade type place. Our schedule for the day got delayed, but none of the activities were missed. It was now late and time for my restroom routine, but the arcade didn't have an accessible bathroom for me and a female assistant. Therefore, the tour busses delivered my classmates, and brought Karen and me to an empty parking area. We did my routine in the middle of the empty bus before rejoining the rest of the group.

I drove around looking at the different games, but there wasn't anything I could do without hand control. I got in line to what I thought was a viewing area but it ended up being a queue line for a game. As I approached, I saw it was a virtual reality headset where you had to drive a vehicle through a course. The user's view could also be watched on a television screen by observers to track progress. I figured I could tell Rhoda to turn hand controls left or right while I wore the headset.

Just before getting setup, someone monitoring the game quietly took Rhoda off to the side. He was concerned I couldn't hold the device on my head, and it may hurt me. She told him it was fine, and I could answer any questions on my own. I was soon hooked up and as a team, Rhoda and I did quite well.

On the drive back home through the night on Interstate 80, our bus driver kept falling asleep. After multiple stops for him to rest, I finally got home to Mary, the night nurse. It was nearly 6:00 a.m. by the time I got in bed, and she had been waiting since midnight for my arrival.

Graduation was a few weeks later in late May. After four years of struggling with medical problems and managing school, I received my high school diploma with Pella Christian's class of 2000. Sitting in the congratulatory line with the diploma on my lap, one of my classmates came and grabbed it, saying, "I'll be back." He returned about a minute later and said, "This one is yours." The order was incorrect when the diplomas were handed out and I had received someone else's. Since I couldn't look at it, I wouldn't have known until after everyone left.

At my graduation party the next day, the first guest to arrive was an older man I didn't recognize. Mom knew him immediately, Dr. Kelly. He was the one who warned my parents 15 years earlier that sending me to regular school and living at home would be dangerous for my health. He predicted I would constantly be in and out of the hospital, but I had gone my entire school career with very few illnesses. There had been bumps and twists along the road, but God had brought me safely to this point.

I didn't know what would happen the next few months, but I knew to wait to see God's plan.

13

THE WINNER IS...

Proverbs 27:1 says, "Do not boast about tomorrow, for you do not know what a day may bring forth." After graduating from high school, it's common for people to say what they will be doing. Plans aren't bad, but not everything always goes as expected. Only God knows what He has for a person's future.

Shortly after registering for the draft, I started getting calls from recruiters trying to get me to enlist in various military branches. I didn't want to explain my life history to every one of them, so I just simply said I wasn't interested. A week before another tour at AIB, Mom answered the phone to hear an Army recruiter asking for me. She brought the phone to my room where Karen and I sat, and she held it to my ear.

I wasn't doing anything productive, so I decided to let this recruiter go through his script. He asked what my plans were, and I answered, "My plans are to go to college, likely at AIB." The recruiter acknowledged it was good to go to school but asked if I had considered serving in the military.

Sgt. Hopeful started by saying what I could do after basic training. "Joel, would you like to improve your physical condition and get help paying for college?"

"Yes sir, I would love to improve my physical abilities."

"Well, you'll be able to do at least 35 pushups in less than two minutes and do a two-mile run in under 15 minutes."

With each item, I responded with, "That sounds great, I would love to do that," repeating the ability he listed. As I replied with enthusiasm, Mom and Karen were doing all they could to not burst out with laughter.

"That's just the start Joel, you would build muscle, be trimmer, and ready to serve your country." I agreed I needed to work on my physical condition and everything the sergeant described sounded great.

After finishing his sales pitch, the recruiter asked if I would be interested in talking with him in person. I briefly thought about joining him for lunch somewhere to see the recruiter's reaction. However, the time he suggested to get together was the same day I was scheduled to be at school. I asked him, "This all sounds great, but does it matter if I can't feel or control anything below my neck?" The very chatty sergeant went completely silent.

Several seconds later, he came back with a less enthusiastic voice, "What did you say you were studying at AIB?" I replied with my declared major, "Accounting and PC." Sgt. Hopeful quietly replied that accounting was a good profession, but unfortunately my disability disqualified me from serving in the military. I told him thank you, followed by goodbye and Mom hung up. The stifled laughter now fully exploded in my room and the three of us enjoyed the entertainment.

New Wheels

After leaving the hospital in 1985, Dad purchased a brown '81 Ford club wagon van and added a wheelchair lift to bring me home. It worked well through multiple trips to Ohio, Florida, and many appointments in Des Moines. Now in 2000, it was having more problems with the engine, and I could not sit upright inside. Dad looked at vans that already had lifts installed but couldn't find one that met my needs.

A few months before I graduated, Dad saw an advertisement for someone selling a '94 Ford van with low miles. He set a time to meet with the private owner, and my parents, Mom's parents, and I took a trip through rural Iowa to check the van. We arrived at the address on time and drove into a cattle farm. Nearing the house, nobody came to meet us, and it didn't look like anyone was on the property.

Dad and Grandpa got out of our old van to look around the large farmyard to see if they could find anyone or the vehicle for sale. As the men searched, a farm dog followed along with them. Mom and Grandma stayed in the back seat behind me, unable to get out around me and the lift. Just as the guys returned to our van, a pickup truck pulled up near where we were parked.

The newcomers questioned what we were doing at the farm, and Dad explained the situation. Apparently, the homeowner had left on an emergency and the truck driver was his brother. He told Dad and Grandpa that the dog following them around had attacked the farmer's daughter and severely injured her ear. They were now at the hospital and the brother's assignment was to permanently get rid of the animal. But before carrying out his assignment, the van owner's brother showed Dad and Grandpa where the vehicle was stored. It was in a garage with dark windows and not easily seen, but he let Dad and Grandpa take it for a test drive. I watched the light brown vehicle drive away while Mom and Grandma stayed with me.

Our '81 model van came with dark tinted windows that made it nearly impossible to see anyone seated in the back. As we looked ahead, the pickup truck driver and another man produced a shot gun and started aiming toward the dog as it ran around the vehicle we were sitting in. Grandma grew concerned about stray shots coming our direction. It was unlikely they were even aware of our presence or concern for safety. Grandma couldn't get out from behind me but managed to partially open a door and close it. The sound of the door didn't seem to be noticed and an attempt was made to shoot the canine a few feet away from the van. The shot missed but sent the dog running off with the impromptu hunters in pursuit.

Quite some time later, Dad and Grandpa returned with the potential van. They found the hunting party after the foe had been vanquished and thanked them for the test drive. The vehicle looked good, except that it was again another shade of brown. A few days later, Dad and Grandpa Vander Molen went to get our new, to us, full-size van. Now with summer starting, it was taken to Rollx Vans in Minneapolis to have the floor lowered six inches and get a lift installed.

Summer CHAMP Camp Counselor

It had become summer tradition for me to go to CHAMP Camp, and I didn't see why it had to change after high school. When camp was started in 1991, the founders did not implement a maximum age for campers. The kids that attended had severe medical needs and diagnoses and, unfortunately, often did not live into their late teens or adulthood.

Nearly every year, one camper passed away and they were missed the next summer. Thankfully, with improved care, several of my camp friends and I were now in our late teens, graduating from school, and doing relatively well, so new age limits were added to the rules. If I wanted to return in the summer of 2000, I had to come as a counselor and not rely on any of the volunteers for care. It sounded great to me, so I agreed to come as a counselor and brought three of my own assistants to provide 24-hour care for the week.

When Brian and his wife had come for my birthday celebration, they talked with Jenny about camp and their experiences. She talked with me about it at school and signed up to volunteer as a counselor as well. During senior year, Jenny had become a Certified Nursing Assistant and worked part-time at the Pella hospital.

I was shy about cares such as cathing and never discussed them with my friends. However, Jenny would now be exposed to every part of my daily life. She came to my house a few times before camp so I could give her a warning and brief education on my behind-the-scenes cares, but I couldn't get up the courage to discuss any of it.

June arrived and the caravan of Iowans headed to Ohio. Patty agreed to come and help for the week along with Karen and Leah. Counselors arrived two days before campers to get familiar with each child's needs and how to help them. I was put in the cabin with younger boys and Jenny with younger girls. For the last few years, camper Brenda had called me her boyfriend, at least at camp. Mom was concerned if she was at camp, as well as Jenny, that Brenda may get jealous. However, the graduate camper did not attend that year.

Living in the medical field, I was familiar with some of the boys' needs, but going over their cares and diagnoses still sounded foreign. I recognized some conditions, like MD, MS, CP, and spinal cord injuries, but most were completely new to me. Since I couldn't help with physical cares, I would do more in the way of entertainment and keeping track of ambulatory campers.

Counselors were only assigned to cabins, not certain campers. However, it was common that kids would get to know a few adults well and mainly seek them for help. Two of the boys in my cabin were Keith and Derrick. I saw them the year before as a camper and knew they were great friends, but I didn't get to be around them very much. They both had tracheostomies, but only used mechanical breathing assistance at night. During the day, they walked around under their own power and primarily just needed supervision.

Since their bunks were next to mine, I became one of the main counselors working with them. I directed Patty on how to design a large sign to use for welcoming Keith to camp. Instead of me receiving the cheers and fanfare, I was now helping provide it.

After arrival and getting the first activities, my two boys quickly realized Jenny and I were friends. She became a common target for their squirt guns and various pranks, which of course the boys only thought of on their own.

During down time, while some of the campers had medical treatments, I gladly played Uno and listened to the boys' jokes. Keith asked me,

"How do you make a tissue dance?" The answer to the familiar question instantly popped through my head as I attempted a thinking expression on my face. After a few seconds I replied with, "How do you?" With a grin on his face, I heard the answer I knew, "You put a little boogie in it!" I laughed at the response and loved the gleam of delight in his eyes.

Later in the week Keith found a letter from home on his pillow and tried to hold it for me to read. Derrick noticed it was at an odd angle for me to see. The boy had two prosthetic legs, very short arms, and fused fingers, however, he grabbed the letter from Keith's hand and held it perfectly in place for me to read.

At the end of each day, I made sure the two had brushed their teeth and changed for bed. Before the other volunteers connected the kids to their various machines for the night, I read their favorite bedtime stories. As I recited from a book held by Karen, she would start to doze off while the boys watched me with eyes wide open. I loved helping, but my reading was putting the wrong person asleep.

The end of camp came quickly, and it was soon time to return to the real world. I loved seeing the kids accomplish new goals and being looked up to as someone they could trust. Camp was more fun and energizing than I had experienced before as a camper, and I looked forward to returning even more than before. Jenny got to help with some of the girls' needs and learned new medical procedures but wasn't sure about returning.

College Admission Deadlines

As the weeks passed by, the deadline for new students at AIB came closer. I had declared my major and registered as a student, but not paid any tuition. If I wanted to start class in the fall, I needed to start paying and finish registration. I was hoping I could make it, but the nursing agency wasn't certain. If they were unable to find enough nurses, then I would have to attend Central College in Pella and live at home. I prayed that it may work out for me to go and sent emails to my friends asking for the same.

Kyle completed his freshman year at Central and liked the school. Kyle wasn't sure about praying I wouldn't join him but understood my feelings.

My insurance had increased my lifetime maximum capacity from $1 million to $2 million in response to competition. Mom watched expenses very carefully and, by my 18th birthday, I was still under the original limit. She warned me that the original amount had lasted for over 15 years. However, with using an agency for nearly all my nursing in college, the second half would be gone in a few years. If I didn't find work with good insurance and reached my lifetime cap, then my only choice for living would be a nursing home.

I understood the potential consequences but wanted to attend college and try living on my own. My parents and I had started planning for this transition during my sophomore year of high school. Now, a few months after graduation, we still didn't know what was going to happen. Two weeks before the school's deadline, Kid Care said they had enough staff to cover me. It was a big answer to prayer, and I looked forward to what life would bring in college.

Voc Rehab continued to help with preparing me for school and making sure it would be a successful venture. My counselor said the papers I would write in college were going be too long to type using my mouth stick. Therefore, they would get me a new laptop that could run a program called Dragon Naturally Speaking. With it, I could dictate, and the program would write what I spoke. I protested that it wasn't necessary, but my counselor insisted.

Steve, a technology consultant, was hired to get the software and hardware I needed and teach me how to use it. Tom and I were familiar with current technology, and I knew what options were available. The laptop Steve picked was an off brand that I had never heard of. However, my consultant knew everything about it and what options to include, as it was a brand he just happened to sell.

I again protested that I could get a better machine at the same cost. This time, my counselor listened, and I soon had an IBM ThinkPad with the newest version of Windows 2000. It had a mouse button in the middle of the keyboard I could use with my stick, and I did not have to take an external mouse with me to class. After multiple times replacing or adding components to the Gateway computer, Tom and I happily set up my new laptop.

School didn't start until after Labor Day, but AIB let me move in a couple of weeks early while classes were on break. Most new college students have to learn to adjust to living on their own. However, my transition to independence also included training new nurses to take care of me. I was thankful for the time to get used to life on my own before starting my courses.

Insurance would only pay a maximum amount per day for nurses. The cost varied depending on the nurse's license, but it came out to around 16 hours per day. Voc Rehab agreed to cover the remaining hours so I could live on campus, but only when school was in session. Therefore, I had to go home every weekend and any time school was on break.

Mary, my night nurse, offered to follow me to any nursing agency and help me live on my own. When I was looking at Dordt in northern Iowa, she was even willing to sell her house and relocate with her daughter. Now, Mary would do the weekends while I was in Pella. Insurance still allowed my parents to keep our own caregivers, allowing Karen to help when she was available. This would help cover my hours and decrease some expense for insurance.

As mid-August came, it was time to leave the only town I had known and start a new chapter in Des Moines. My parents and I said goodbye to Leah and most of my nurses who had helped me for many years through every situation. I also wished Jenny well as she moved to another school east of Pella to study physical therapy.

My parents and I made the familiar trip west to Des Moines with the new van packed with my belongings. The dorms at AIB were not typical college lodging but were all small apartments. My room was a one-bedroom dorm with its own kitchen, bathroom, and living area. Since I had enrolled late in the year, most of the dorms had already been taken. The one I was given had been used for storage but was made available for my housing. It was at the end of long hallway that had an auxiliary classroom, but no other dorms. Therefore, I had a quiet place all to myself that was directly across from the laundry room.

The first trip up was to bring my tables, clothes, and some medical supplies. Another trip would be required to bring my hospital bed and air mattress. After unloading the van, Dad and I left to go to the nearby Hy-Vee grocery store. I had a completely empty refrigerator and needed to be responsible for my own meals. While we found food essentials, Mom met with the nursing supervisor to go over last-minute items and meet my new nurses.

Dad and I soon returned with a supply of milk, eggs, bread, and other items to cook. As I bumped through the outside entrance into my open living area, I saw Mom crying and looking overwhelmed. The night nurse that had been hired to cover most of my hours decided that morning she didn't want to work with a vent dependent person. She was now signing her resignation papers and Kid Care was no longer sure if they could provide the nursing I needed.

This was not the start to a new chapter in life we had planned. After more than two years of preparing for college, the next few hours would determine the course of my future.

14

HIGHER EDUCATION

Proverbs 9:9 says, "Give *instruction* to a wise *man,* and he will be still wiser; teach a just *man,* and he will increase in learning." No matter what stage of life we are in, learning never stops. Working toward a college degree is a challenge for most people, without worrying about nursing care. I didn't know where life would lead but trusted in God through it all.

Even though night hours were uncertain, Mom and I started training the new day nurse while the supervisor made phone calls. The daily routine consisted of cathing three times a day, meds at various times, and constant monitoring of the vent and suctioning as needed. My vent tubes and trach were reusable and had a schedule for changing and cleaning. It all took time to show and was a lot for anyone to learn at once.

After several phone calls and waiting for messages to be returned, Mary agreed to do more nights and come to Des Moines to help me. Kid Care could also subcontract through other agencies and believed everything would be covered.

The next day, we moved more of my belongings and Tom came along to see my apartment. He and I took the trek from my dorm up to the main classroom building. The campus was near the Des Moines River and was built into a hillside. Steps went off in all directions, but there wasn't a ramp in sight. As the crow flies, my dorm was the closest to the main building as possible, but wheelchairs take different paths.

After traveling half the length of the large dormitory, we exited the main doors. Then our journey took us all the way to the opposite end of the building, past the gymnasium, and onto the parking lot. We then went past four rows of parking before turning again, back the opposite way we started. Then going up the hill, through the parking lot, past one classroom building, onto the sidewalk, and another couple hundred feet to the top of the hill. The entire journey took about ten minutes through the hot August sun. I had only taken the route once before when exploring campus and hoped Tom didn't notice I was somewhat guessing what path to take.

At our destination, we hoped to find an ethernet card to help connect my laptop to the campus network. The bookstore was in the main building, and we presumed they would have the required hardware. However, nobody was anywhere to be seen and we only found locked doors.

Tom sat on a picnic table for a few minutes as we looked at my van parked by my door just down the hill. If Tom had a rock and a strong arm, he could have hit the vehicle. Even though it was close, we would need to reverse our journey without fulfilling our goal.

The school designated three parking spots for my use. One was for the van and two for the nurses, the one on duty and the next one coming in. It was part of our discussions with AIB and Voc Rehab. Instead of having my caregivers try to find parking, they could easily have a spot near my dorm.

A few days later, my county DHS supervisor came for a visit and wanted to see how I got to class. It was one of my first full days living on my own and I was with one of my new nurses. I had yet to take the journey with her and agreed it would be good to go over the route. When we exited the dorm, I noticed a few recent changes to the parking lot. A ramp had been added to one of the high curbs and a cement cut-through placed between two of the lots. I still had a long journey, but it was now cut down to just over five minutes each way.

Since I had been to Des Moines countless times for medical appointments, I only knew the area by the hospital. Classes hadn't started yet, so my new day helpers and I toured the area around campus to find points of interest. A new bike path around Gray's Lake had opened a few days earlier. It was a very warm day, just as I liked, and thought it would be fun to roll down the new path around the lake.

Not knowing my nurse, I didn't want her to get too hot and possibly not want to work with me. Every few minutes, I asked if she was getting too warm, and let her know we could head back at any time. Partway around the lake, she asked to stop by a picnic bench for a rest. I parked beside her and, as we rested in the sun, a reporter approached us. The journalist was from a small, free newspaper in Des Moines that I didn't know existed. Since the trail had just opened, she asked to take our picture and get our thoughts about the park. After living in Des Moines a few days, I was already in the paper.

The new van was an added blessing and convenience for me and my caregivers. With my first vehicle, I sat in the middle of the van behind the front seats. It worked, but it wasn't easy for the driver to reach behind them and help me. My new van had a lowered floor from the front seats all the way to the rear axle, which allowed me to park where the front passenger seat would normally go, right beside the driver. With just a caregiver and me, it was easier for them to help if I needed anything, or for eating in the van.

After a few days of living on my own, the first weekend came, and I was back in Pella. In preparation for my move, Mom had ordered a new hospital bed and an electric Hoyer lift to get me in and out of my chair. The bed included wooden head and foot boards so it looked closer to a regular piece of furniture. The lift came and worked well, but the bed still hadn't arrived so, not only did I need to be picked up to go home, so did my entire bed.

Going home every weekend required me to pack extra supplies, but moving furniture each time wasn't something we wanted to continue. Thankfully, the bed arrived within the week, and we only had to move furniture once.

Labor Day weekend came, and the other first-year students moved to campus. Just as school started, Steve, the tech consultant, came to train me on the voice dictation system. He and his wife showed me what the Dragon speaking system could do. They emphasized that I needed to speak clearly for it to learn my voice. Instead of saying, "Whad je'eet last night?" I had to say, "What did you eat last night?" As I used my stick to click the mouse and do some typing, they also showed me a grid system that could be used for mouse commands.

I knew my class schedule included more computer programming, and I wondered if it would help with remembering proper syntax. Unfortunately, it couldn't, and programming would need to be done by stick. As I typed over 30 words per minute, they commented this would be a great second tool.

After they left, I attempted using my voice to write a test document and quickly got frustrated. After a few days of attempting to dictate notes, I quickly gave up on the system. I had to constantly go back and correct words, and I couldn't use it daily and keep up with my homework. I needed my mouth stick to turn pages in books and notebooks, but it hardly understood anything I said with the stick in my mouth. I tried coming back to it a few weeks later and found that the little progress I had made earlier was gone. I soon fired the dragon and banished it from my computer.

College Courses

My first college courses were Principals of Accounting 1, Introduction to Composition, and a few general education classes. Within the first few days of Composition, everyone was tested on their knowledge of basic grammar. If you received a high enough score, you didn't need to take the course and could go on to advanced English. I felt I knew grammar well and was confident about the test and hardly looked at my book.

As part of my admission process, I arranged with my instructors to take written tests in another room so I could tell my caregiver what to write. I could have written out answers on my own, but it would take much longer than just dictating. When the 50-minute period was complete, I didn't feel as confident as when I had started. By the next class, our teacher announced that nobody had tested out. I figured it would be nice to have an easy class anyway.

By October, classes were going okay, but accounting had already covered everything we did in one year of high school. It was getting more complicated and my grades in the class were going down. I tried to remind myself to go slowly and not rush, but it didn't help much. College life wasn't only about studying and taking tests though.

I heard that one of the CHAMP camp volunteers was having a get-together at his acreage near Indianapolis. It was an open invitation for any counselors from that summer. Patty, her husband, and their son were going and offered to take Jenny and me. I hadn't seen Jenny since August and I was excited to see her and catch up.

Classes were done by noon every Friday, so my nurse and I quickly packed for the weekend and Dad picked me up and took me to Pella. Once there, the rest of the group joined me, and we made the eight-hour drive to central Indiana.

The counselor I helped mentor as a camper, Pastor Dave, offered his home for lodging and we arrived late in the evening. He set up a ramp for me to get in the house and I carefully navigated around the walls and furniture. This was the second time in my life I traveled out of Iowa without my parents, and my second time staying in someone's house.

On Saturday, Dave showed us around the city, and we took a guided tour of the Indianapolis Speedway. As evening approached, we joined several counselors for dinner in a grassy lot. Dave used my computer to show pictures from the summer and gave everyone a chance to catch up on the previous few months. Overnight, I slept on the floor in a sleeping bag with Patty and her family nearby, in case I needed anything. She also got up regularly to move me and do some of my night cares.

Sunday morning, our small group joined Pastor Dave at his church. I hadn't attended a Methodist church before but didn't notice many differences in the service. Before heading home, Brian, his wife, and infant son joined us for lunch. They had been in Iowa for my birthday less than a year earlier and it felt like we were getting regular visits.

Partway through rural Illinois, Patty started falling asleep and I noticed the van heading toward the median. She woke up when the wheels hit the rumble strips and quickly got us pointed in the right direction. She changed seats with her husband and napped a few hours. Jenny also traded seats so she could sit beside me, help feed me a snack, and catch up on the weekend and the last few months. I enjoyed being with her again, but the time soon ended.

Arriving in Pella, Dad took the extra seat out of the van, and I returned to my position up front. I got back to my dorm just in time for the 10:00 night nurse to take over. It was a busy weekend, but this time, going out on my own went without trouble. I had learned from my previous trip and knew better how to handle my care.

Every weekend I was home, Tom came to see me. He said he was enjoying his senior year of high school, but it was boring without me. During down time, Tom built a website for the church and started to put up the weekly bulletin and other information. He explained that he was going to be attending college in Michigan and likely wouldn't be back in Iowa and, if the site was to continue, someone would need to take responsibility for it. Church was okay with the site existing, as long as it didn't cost any money. Tom used a program called Adobe GoLive and his dad, the pastor, agreed to get me a copy. Once I had it installed, Tom showed me how he did the weekly updates. I thought doing web updates was fun and by November, I had taken the site over. GoLive completely took care of the programming in the background, but I started to learn web coding as well.

Oops, My Faux Pas

By the time Thanksgiving break came, I was getting used to living on my own five days at a time. I knew I had to be careful about pressure sores if I was to keep up with school. I had heard about doing regular skin checks, but had not done this before. Shortly after moving in, I got a full-length mirror that could be propped against my bedroom wall. It was great for checking my appearance prior to heading out, but it served more purposes.

Before getting in bed for my afternoon cares, I had the nurse get me undressed in my chair. It was a challenge getting my pants off, but we figured out the process by tilting and pulling. When everything was exposed, I could check my skin from head to foot. Spreading my legs apart let me see between them and crossing them allowed me to check my hips. I didn't know how other quads monitored their skin, but I could at least keep track of my front half. Without being able to feel anything below my shoulders, I also liked being able to see that I had a body underneath my clothes.

After finishing one of my visual examinations, it was time for my nurse, Erin, to get me in bed for my afternoon routine and to get dressed again. I parked in the corner of my bedroom, hit the switch to turn off my chair, and moved the controls to the side. Erin started putting the lift's sling in position so it could be attached to the Hoyer and hoist me out of my chair. She leaned me forward to slide the device behind my back. To free her hands, Erin rested my head on her well-padded upper chest. As she started moving the sling, I heard my chair give two beeps, indicating the power switch had been hit. I knew that if my controls were bumped again, the chair would move and potentially injure one or both of us.

With my head on Erin's chest, I said, "Be careful, you turned me on." As I felt the sling get in place behind me, I didn't hear a response. When I was pushed upright again, I explained to my new caregiver how to turn off my chair and why I said to be careful. Erin acknowledged my instructions but had initially thought my warning had a completely different meaning.

On My Own

AIB had a cafeteria, but it closed at 1:00 every day when classes were complete. The school encouraged students to work part-time and, to help students with this, only held class the first half the day. Evening courses were also part of the curriculum but didn't start until 7 p.m. Any student would have at least six hours a day available to work, study, or take care of any other needs.

I got used to grocery shopping and preparing my own meals. I would sometimes get lunch from the cafeteria or local fast-food restaurants, but often had to prepare at least one meal a day. Sometimes I made a menu plan, but often picked up common ingredients at the store and ate what I had available.

After collecting my items in the grocery store, my nurse and I would head to the checkout lane. She filled in what I owed on my check, then I signed it. Some of the cashiers were quite impressed after seeing my mouth signature, but they got used to seeing me on a regular basis.

Trying new recipes was fun, but tricky, as not all my nurses were experienced cooks. As one younger caregiver cooked a chicken breast with a recipe I found, she talked with her boyfriend on a cell phone. He was surprised to hear she was making something, and I heard her respond, "I can cook if I have a recipe." However, when the cookie sheet came out of the oven, a large piece of charcoal that had once been meat emerged. The cracker-crumb topping that I hoped would be tasty was now beyond recognition. I thought it was likely a good thing her boyfriend was a fire fighter.

The next day, one of my older nurses with much culinary experience tried to clean the once spotless baking pan. Several attempts of scrubbing couldn't remove the petrified topping. Mary tried at night, but the blackened pieces became a permanent reminder to be more careful with meal planning and my caregiver schedule.

The Challenge of Social Life

Similar to high school, I didn't make many friends on campus. I didn't try to avoid people, but I primarily stayed in my dorm after classes. Most social activities were either on the weekend, while I was at home, or late in the evening. However, I did get to know a few students that I frequently saw in class.

Rich was an outgoing, tall guy who was also taking computer courses. He lived in one of the fraternity houses and spent time with his girlfriend when he wasn't serving his weekend in the Army Reserve. Rich was curious but wasn't as concerned with my medical equipment as some others. When our schedules allowed, he was fun to talk with and get to know.

I noticed another student who used a wheelchair but had full use of her arms. She was often waiting to be picked up when I headed to my dorm, and I wondered about her story. We eventually had class together and Jayde was a friendly face who knew some of the challenges of wheelchair life.

After two quarters of taking accounting classes, I knew I wasn't doing well enough to continue, so I changed my major to Information Technology (IT) and dropped the accounting portion. Since I had already taken the basic computer classes, I hoped it wouldn't add much time to my eventual graduation. Now when anyone asked what I was studying, I could say I was taking "it."

Winter 2001 came with a lot of snow and cold weather. Getting bundled up for my trek around campus was a challenge I dreaded every day. I would give in some days and opt to get in the van and drive to the top of the hill, but the process of loading and unloading me took as long, if not longer, than walking. AIB liberally salted the sidewalks and parking lots, and my chair and van lift started showing rust. Dad carefully washed the van every weekend to remove the metal eating rock, but it only helped so much.

There were two primary classroom buildings, each with multiple floors, however, only one had an elevator for easy access. The other building only had outdoor access that would require me to go around and through the parking lot to access either level. To help out, the school had some of the professors move a session so I didn't need to change buildings.

Winter weather was also a challenge for my caregivers. Over the years, my parents and I were familiar with nurses calling in due to illness or bad weather. Some would give notice long ahead of their shift, but others waited until they should have already arrived. In either case, Mom, Dad, or sometimes my grandparents would cover the shift. Now that I lived an hour away from Pella, it wasn't so easy. As winter dragged on, nurses who lived in Des Moines or the suburbs would call saying they couldn't come due to bad roads. My parents were then expected to drive more than 40 miles through open country to cover the shift. If a storm was predicted on a Thursday or Friday, I would sometimes return to Pella early, but that didn't always help.

On one snowy Friday in January 2001, classes had been cancelled and my nurses didn't know if they could make it. Mom and Dad headed to Des Moines early and got there just before the worst of the storm hit. Packing up my battery chargers, vents, and portable suction like we did every weekend, the three of us ventured toward home. A few miles east of Des Moines, in near white-out conditions, a semi we were following quickly changed lanes. Dad thought he better do the same and a few seconds later we passed a car spinning its tires on a hill. We didn't see it until it was a few feet away. As conditions worsened, we wanted to stop in one of the towns between Des Moines and Pella but couldn't see the exits. Eventually, three hours after leaving my dorm, we were safely home and questioning if college was worth the effort.

Thankfully, spring soon came with better weather, and I began taking classes in my new major. One of my courses was Multimedia Applications and covered website programming languages. After working on the church's site for a few months, I was familiar with HTML and making web pages. Building pages and coding them manually was slow and much more labor intensive than the program I used, but it did help me learn the code better and understand how to add different elements. An older student was having a hard time understanding the work, so I gladly helped her find bugs and areas to watch.

I was glad when we moved on to using a web development program for coding, but I quickly learned I liked my software better. While working on our final project, I saved two versions so I could test different designs, however, the school's database didn't like it and, before I could blink, both were deleted. I didn't have enough time to build one again and had nothing to show at the end of the class. So, I watched my classmates present their work, and receive stark criticism from the professor for every error. Since the instructor had seen my work earlier, I didn't fail the assignment, but ended up with a C.

Commuting to and from Des Moines every weekend, the trip became monotonous, and Dad found different routes to break up the drive. We would sometimes take country roads through small towns; other times we would meander through downtown Des Moines instead of taking the four-lane roads. We also got familiar with listening to an evening radio host who played songs for people calling in with various challenges in life. Delilah always had a great song for each situation and helped provide a little entertainment.

Summer 2001 had the start of another semester at my year-round school. I tried to convince my parents to let me take a week off for camp, but they wouldn't hear it. If they had, it would have been one of the lesser concerns for the year.

Just when things are going relatively well, that's when accidents happen.

15

TAKING A BREAK

In Luke 13:1-5, Jesus was told about some Jews who had been killed by Pilate in a tower collapse. He answered that the ones killed weren't worse sinners than anyone else, and He went on to tell His listeners that they needed to repent.

Tragedy happens to both Christians and non-Christians alike. For those who have truly repented of their sins and trust solely in Jesus for salvation, they will live forever in heaven. We need to always be prepared, for we don't know when our end will come.

The summer of 2001 was a lonely one. A few days after graduating high school, Tom left for college in Michigan. I talked with Jenny on the phone a few times, but she was now dating a man she met at school. I was used to having few friends and being on my own, but this summer seemed particularly lonely. It was also the first year I had missed camp since 1993.

No matter to my social life, I enjoyed warm months and getting out in the sun as much as possible. After class, my nurse and I picked up lunch from Long John Silvers and sat in the van by a pond at Water Works Park. Eating our fried fish, we chatted about whatever came to mind. She said when Kid Care agreed to take my case a year earlier, they knew there weren't enough people to cover me; however, they saw the potential to make a lot of money so they agreed to take me as a patient. Normally, when one of their clients turned 18, they would be sent to other care providers. At 19, I was now considered an adult, but they still kept me as a patient.

Shortly after starting with the nursing agency, Mom made sure I kept track of hours and expenses. I set up a worksheet on my computer and recorded who worked, how long, and if they were an RN or LPN. It automatically calculated what the day's charges should be and what part went to insurance and what part went to Voc Rehab.

When insurance was billed, I received a detailed sheet going over daily charges. I looked over the numbers carefully and regularly had to contact the nursing agency's billing department with corrections. Some days had charges totaling 25 hours and billing rates were frequently off. The adjustments had to be resubmitted to insurance and hopefully billed correctly. It became a routine for me, one that Mom had done for over a decade.

Kid Care could barely keep my hours staffed and had time slots they couldn't fill. To help, Karen came to Des Moines and worked from 5:00 p.m. to 7:00 a.m. once a week. Before heading home, she would sleep on my dorm's couch for a few hours while I was in class.

If nobody was available to cover a shift, Mom would make the 40-mile drive and help for a few hours. While heading home once, she had to pull over and stop as tears filled her eyes. Every other 19-year-old college student could easily attend class without needing monitoring every hour. They didn't need to plan caregiver schedules and rely on parents to provide physical help. She knew God is in control of everything, but some days were difficult to cope.

The agency was always trying to hire new caregivers and train them to help take care of me. During one of her mandatory recertification visits, my nursing supervisor, Jesse, joined Sandy and me after class for our long stroll back to my dorm. She told me about a nurse who had recently become available and could help fill my day shift for either eight- or twelve-hour periods. She said this nurse could come to be trained within the week, but the caregiver would need to have regular smoke breaks while working with me; at least every two hours.

I initially said I was willing to accommodate her and let the potential nurse come to train. However, Mom called that evening, as she regularly did, and we thought it over more carefully. The school did not allow smoking in the dorms or inside any building. Therefore, if I was in bed, she would have to go outside to have her break and I wouldn't be able to see where she was or likely get help if needed. I couldn't smell very well, but cigarette smoke was something I did notice, and the odor would likely get on me and my clothes. After further consideration, I contacted Jesse and told her not to send the nurse. She was sorry to hear my decision but understood my reasoning.

Shortly after, another day shift couldn't be filled by the regular caregivers. Instead of asking my parents to cover, Jesse came to fill the time. As she was helping me get out of my chair after class, I explained how to get the sling behind my back, under my legs, and then hook it to the lift. I parked so I could be connected to my bed vent and start the transfer process. As my weight shifted from chair to sling, I noticed I was hanging a little different than normal, but I trusted Jesse knew what she was doing. As the machine lifted me up, my back was sitting straight. The strap that normally came up between my legs and sat in-front of me also wasn't there.

When my body cleared the chair, I could feel I was teetering on the verge of falling forward. If I tried to speak, it felt like the movement would get me off balance and I would fall forward. Jesse pulled the lift away from my chair watching the vent circuit and how much leash I had. As she pushed the lift forward, my body backed toward the bed and the precarious balance was tipped. I felt my head and upper body start to fall forward and saw the arm of the lift come closer. I quickly imagined my head hitting part of the lift before I completely fell to the floor.

Jesse saw me start to fall forward and caught me with my chin landing on her shoulder. She then carefully shuffled forward with my butt barely staying in the sling. After doing an odd sort of dance, I was soon safely in bed again. I learned not to trust supervisors completely and to be more careful in strap positioning.

Three to four times a day, I did a regular exercise routine. The nurse would stretch my arms and legs to different positions, hold it for a few seconds, then go to another position. My nurse, Shelly, had been with me a few months and knew my routine well. However, as she stretched my right leg, she felt it give and we both heard what sounded like the breaking of a wet tree branch. Shelly quickly put my leg down and carefully felt it.

Near the hip, it felt like there was a protrusion, like the joint had popped out. Shelly called the Iowa Methodist Emergency Room and spoke with a nurse about what to do. She recommended bringing me to the hospital to get checked and gave the phone number for non-emergency ambulance service. They arrived not long afterward and came through the main entrance of the dorm. As the paramedics slid me from my bed to the stretcher, they agreed it felt like my hip was out.

Since I was familiar with Iowa Methodist Hospital, I decided to go there for treatment. In the ER, Shelly stayed with me and made sure the vent and everything remained connected. An x-ray revealed my hip was fine, but my femur had broken just below the socket and needed attention. At 10 p.m., we called my parents from the ER. Long distance calls weren't allowed, but I remembered the number from my prepaid phone card I used to call home.

Mom and Dad were already in bed, but Dad was quick to get up, as he had a feeling earlier in the night something was wrong. Shelly was scared to meet with my parents, but they arrived a little over an hour later and let her know it was only an accident. I knew broken bones were usually very painful, but I didn't feel anything. However, I noticed the stiffness and muscle spasms I always had were non-existent and my body was completely limp.

I was given an orthopedist, Dr. Gunke, to decide a course of action. He picked up my leg and moved it around like some sort of toy. Not being able to feel can sometimes have advantages, as I guessed this would have hurt badly. The doctor didn't see a point in doing surgery to fix the break since I couldn't walk anyway. He said if he did a plate or rod, he was certain it wouldn't stay and would cause more problems since I must obviously have weak bones. I pointed out that rods were holding fine in my back, but it didn't matter to him.

After 36 hours in the hospital, I was released. My leg was surrounded by a foam cushion and bandage wrap, but Dr. Gunke refused to do anything more. I tried to get transferred to another physician who would treat the bone but was told I couldn't switch. My parents' protests also fell on deaf ears. To get back to my apartment, Dad carefully picked me up from the hospital bed and put me in my chair. He usually tossed me around like a sack of potatoes without any trouble, but we knew any movement had to be made with caution.

Back at my dorm, the nurses and I came up with a plan to further support my leg when transferring with the lift. Having directed the ambulance crew, the dorm administrators had been concerned and were glad to see me back. AIB had a policy that if you missed more than eight classes, or two weeks, in a quarter, the class had to be taken again. Fortunately, I only missed three days and could easily catch up.

With my oversized upper right leg, getting dressed was challenging. Thankfully, summer meant I could wear shorts and Grandma Vander Molen modified a pair so that one leg could be opened with Velcro. It wasn't a great fashion statement, but I needed function over form.

About a week after the incident, as Erin got me in the sling to put me in bed, I noticed the straps weren't supporting my leg as planned. She responded by saying the way the other nurses and I were doing the sling didn't support it any better and her way was fine. As my lower body elevated, I saw my right leg jerk in a position I hadn't seen before. Not long after getting me down, Erin's shift was over and my primary day nurse, Sandy, started her shift. As soon as it was just us in my apartment, I explained what happened and told her I wanted to check my legs.

Laying them out straight in bed, my right foot didn't extend as far down as the left. Sandy called the ER and was told we could come and get checked, but the change was likely just part of healing. After carefully getting me up and driving to the hospital, I was again in a bed in the emergency room.

As Sandy sat beside me, an immense pain raced up the left side of my neck and through my head. I screamed as extreme pain shot through my head, then disappeared. I wondered if my leg's movement released a blood clot that traveled through my brain. The ER nurses didn't seem concerned with my fear and pointed out the monitors I was attached to. They said if something happened, the electronics would inform them. A couple of hours after arriving and getting more x-rays, the two of us were sent back to my dorm.

Nurse Erin seemed to have a legal solution for every malady. Along with a door to the hallway, my apartment had an outdoor entrance that went to the parking lot. It had about a six-inch step to get over, so I didn't normally use it. I could manage the step if I really needed to, but I didn't care to make the effort on a regular basis. Erin wanted the door to be made more easily accessible for me for two reasons. First, to shorten our trips outside by 50 feet and, second, she said it was a fire hazard.

Despite my requests that she not say anything, Erin regularly complained to the dorm staff. She said a ramp had to be installed at my door or I could sue the school. As a result, AIB took out some landscaping and a large section of wall near my dorm to construct an over-sized ramp.

Erin had come to Iowa a few years earlier from her native New Jersey. A frequent conversation on her shift was how I should take my parents and trucking company to court and sue them for my injury. She also told my other nurses how they should be caring for me and that she would be monitoring what they did. After putting up with Erin for nearly a year, I was tired of her attitude. Ignoring my requests to adjust the sling's straps for better support was all my parents and I would tolerate. Erin was knowledgeable about medical needs, but she did not have a good temperament.

Nurses were hard to find, and I didn't like to complain, but Mom was willing to come to Des Moines more often, if needed. Erin came on Sunday evening as scheduled, but that was her final shift with me.

September 2001

September 2001 marked the completion of one year in school and started my second. I had changed majors, learned to live on my own, and managed training caregivers without my parents. With the new quarter, I had two classes during the day and a night class. Each 50-minute daytime class period only met four days a week. The class schedule made it so that I had only one class for less than an hour some days.

The evening course, MCSE, met for two hours, twice a week. It covered Microsoft computer systems and networks and could lead to a certification, if desired. On the first night, as everyone sat by our desktop computers, the instructor had each student stand, state their name, and give a brief introduction. After a few students did the requested steps, one man stated he was too lazy to stand and just sat to report his information. The following three classmates followed his lead and remained seated. I was next in line for the informal greeting session.

Getting my chin controls, I backed away from my desk several inches. Then I started, "I'm Joel Vander Molen. I would love to stand no matter how lazy, but don't have the ability." My fellow classmates halfway looked at me, glared at Mr. Lazy, and back to me. He briefly stood from his chair for about a second before plopping back down. Remaining introductions went about half and half, with some stating they didn't stand so I wouldn't feel left out.

About two weeks into the quarter, on September 11, it was a beautiful sunny Tuesday morning as Sandy and I did the morning routine. With my bed lined up with the bedroom door, I could watch the television on the opposite wall in my living area. I usually had the TV on while halfway listening to the morning news. As my legs were being stretched, I looked around the hair on my calf to see an image of one of the World Trade Towers on fire. I commented that they must be advertising a new movie and continued to talk with Sandy.

A few minutes passed and the same scene was still on the television. I refocused my attention to listen and heard the CBS reporters talking about how a possible plane had hit the tower. Just then, I saw a brief blur of an aircraft and the second tower blew up in a cloud of flame and black smoke. Cameras were adjusted and refocused to confirm the second tower had been hit.

Our attention was now fully focused on the news as I got dressed and in my chair. I had a quick breakfast and sat glued to the screen. My 9:00 class on Principles of Marketing was about to start, and we left as late as possible to make the commute up the hill. Passing the City View Café, I could see everyone fixated on the events on the suspended televisions.

Sitting in class, the students were quieter than usual with some not aware of the morning's events. Mr. Clark arrived a few minutes late and told us one of the towers had just collapsed. He commented that this felt like a book from someone named Tom Clancy. Since the events of the morning would likely be popular topics for several days, he wanted to hold class as usual.

The marketing class proceeded as any other day, but everyone wondered what was happening outside our classroom walls. My next class was in the same room and most of the students filed out as the next group trickled in. Composition II always started with journaling. Sandy set up my laptop in front of me to get prepared, and I considered a multitude of thoughts to record.

When Mrs. Smith arrived, she had us write for a few minutes, then stop. One of the students commented that we could probably write the entire period. The professor talked with us about our thoughts for the day. One woman said she had family in New York City but hadn't heard from them. Mrs. Smith said she didn't feel right keeping us stuck in the room while events unfolded. She dismissed everyone 15 minutes after arriving.

Since it was my last class for the day, Sandy packed everything up and we headed to the bookstore. The AIB bookstore was small and busy selling schoolbooks at the start of each quarter. The rest of the time, it was quiet except for a few students buying AIB apparel, notebooks, or writing utensils. I was friends with a few students, but also with Becky, the lady who ran the store. She was probably close to mom's age, but I connected more easily with older adults.

As Sandy and I entered, Becky was glad to see us and had a radio tuned to a news station. Since I left for class, a plane hit the Pentagon and another suspected hijacked plane crashed in Pennsylvania. As a response, all aircraft in the country had been grounded. Becky said she heard reports of people dancing in Afghanistan over the apparent terrorist attacks. As we talked, a student entered, and I moved away from the counter to give room.

Becky quickly responded in a frightened tone, "You aren't leaving, are you?" I assured her I was just making room. I stayed for about half an hour as we listened to the radio and discussed possible future military responses and the world ahead. Eventually, Sandy and I made the journey through campus back to my dorm. AIB was about two miles from the Des Moines International Airport and aircraft sounds were quite frequent. During this commute, the bright blue sky was clear without a hint of airplane noise. The silence was a very loud reminder of what was happening in the country. The sun eventually set on September 11, and I finally turned off the television around 10:15.

Shortly after starting school, I had increased my nightly Bible reading from one chapter to three. My mind was easily distracted as I poured through Scripture but was thankful to be safe in my apartment.

With the large foam cushion on my leg acting as a cast, it caused me to sit differently. As expected, I started getting another pressure sore on my butt. After four years without problems, I returned to my plastic surgeon, Dr. Rouce. On days with night classes, I had been staying in my chair all day and tilting. To help decrease pressure, I started getting back in bed after my final day course and stayed down until the evening session started. It was more work for my caregivers, but I hoped it would help.

Unfortunately, decreasing the amount of time in my wheelchair didn't improve the area. By October, the doctor said I would need to have another muscle flap surgery and would need complete bed rest for six weeks before starting the slow routine of increasing time in my chair again.

My parents and I didn't want to waste the progress I had made in school for the quarter so I worked on arrangements to finish both of my day courses through email. MCSE required specific software and computers to complete the assignments, which meant I had to drop the class.

AIB allowed me to keep my dorm as long as I wasn't gone too long. That meant I could at least keep my bed, television, and other belongings in Des Moines for an easier return. I was scheduled to have the procedure on December 1, with six weeks of bed rest following.

December started off with surgery and recovery at Iowa Methodist Medical Center. I had to stay at the hospital for several days to monitor initial healing. Once the anesthesia wore off, I was able to run my laptop from the hospital bed and do schoolwork. From my bed in Des Moines, I emailed Mom my final papers to print. She brought them to me during a visit and I had everything ready when my professors, Mr. Clark and Mrs. Smith, were scheduled to visit me in the hospital.

Sitting in a hospital with a sitter monitoring me was now very familiar. Anticipating my professors' visit, I planned on talking with them for a while, but they were not as comfortable in the medical setting as I was and conducted the briefest possible conversation. I gave them my paper, showed I kept up on daily journaling, and they were satisfied. Even with the hospital interruption, I finished my two classes with excellent grades. For the first time in my academic career, I made the Dean's list.

Recovery continued at home in Pella over Christmas and New Year's. I didn't mind staying inside from the cold but wondered about finishing my degree. The next few weeks would again determine how the future would turn out.

16

RETURNING AGAIN

In Jeremiah 29, God spoke through the prophet to the Israelites who had been taken by Babylon into captivity. He assured them that they would return to their land and again worship the Lord. Sometimes, even when we are doing God's will, trials come that require us to pause. However, if it is God's will, we will once again return to serving Him.

With my nursing agency based near Des Moines, most of my caregivers would need to commute quite a distance to continue to help me. Thankfully, most were okay with the travel time and drove the extra 40 miles each way. My parents had become familiar with me living on my own during the week, and we had to adjust to me living at home again.

Mom showed everyone around the house and where to find supplies. For the most part, I had already directed them where to find everything, but my nurses just smiled and went with the tour. Without school work, I spent a lot of time playing games on my laptop. Thankfully, I had two websites I could work on, but they didn't fill many hours.

My caregivers reported my healing progress to the doctor and they were able to remove the staples that had been holding my skin together. Mom pointed out that if I was going to be able to tolerate enough sitting hours to return to classes in March, I needed to start the routine early. By mid-January, I was cleared to sit for 30 minutes a day for seven days and then increase by half-an-hour each week. When the next school quarter started, I could sit just long enough to attend classes. I was very thankful to return to school and live on my own.

Making the Dean's list in December included receiving recognition. Rolling up to President Sandy Williams in the school gymnasium to receive my award was a new experience. I had never achieved anything above my classmates, but I hoped to be able to do it again.

My new daytime courses were Principles of Management, Technical Writing, and Microsoft Access and I had one evening class a week, Business Law. With only two to three classes per session, I started the quarter with barely enough time allowed in my chair to attend. Four hours straight for my evening class was a little much at the beginning, but it soon worked better as time in my chair increased every week.

Sitting through multiple hours of law education, I frequently dozed off as the sun dipped below the horizon. My classmates and I would regularly find the instructor holding his hand like a gun and pointing it to our heads. They were then asked if a contract signed under these circumstances would be legally binding. The demonstration was a vivid reminder to stay alert, but nodding off in class kept me from making the Dean's list again.

Warmer Weather and Summer Classes

One of my routines after class was to get my shoes off as soon as I got back to the dorm. I preferred to be barefoot, but I also started noticing I had fewer muscle spasms when my feet were free, so I started wearing the absolute minimum on my feet and only wore footwear when required. As my allowed sitting time increased, I also enjoyed getting on the bike trails at nearby Water Works Park. After lunch, my nurse and I headed to the park for a walk, or roll, before errands. I loved the feel of the sun on my face and attempted to get a tan on as much skin as possible.

It didn't take long to learn that a new day assistant, Mark, enjoyed the outdoors as much as I did, so we were frequent visitors to the park. After our stroll, we headed to the Hy-Vee grocery store. On one occasion, as he started to get me out of the van, Mark realized we left my flip-flops at the dorm and forgot to take any footwear. I thought we had to go back, but he was sure nobody would say anything. Going through the aisles of Hy-Vee, I drove behind Mark trying to hide my feet from anyone. At the end of the trip, we got back to the van without anyone appearing to notice my forgotten footwear. Going through the store, I liked having fewer spasms, but I wasn't quite comfortable with always staying barefoot.

Warmer temperatures were great for getting out, plus there was no additional salt on the sidewalks and parking lots at school, but the corrosive substance left its mark on my equipment. Even though I missed winter classes, I had still driven through some remaining salt in early spring. Some of it had worked up into the wiring of my wheelchair and corroded electrical connections. I tried getting help from a wheelchair maintenance company in Des Moines, but they couldn't solve the problem. The company guessed one of the motors on my wheels was going bad and wanted to order a new one.

I frequently could only turn one direction, and my chair's motors wouldn't respond to any input. In order to turn left, I had to turn nearly a full circle to my right. Dad looked at my chair and switched a few wires around. The adjustment allowed me to turn both directions again but reversed my controls. Instead of pushing my chin to the left to go the same direction, I turned right. It was nice to be able to turn either way, but I had to stop and think so I didn't go the wrong way and hit someone or hurt myself. Dad came to Des Moines to help and set up a makeshift repair shop in my dorm. Tilting back in my chair, he soldered a few new connections together. As I heard a few sparks pop, he said it wasn't ideal to work on a battery that was connected to something. After a few more sparks and singed spots on the carpet, everything was working properly again.

Summer came with another year of attending class and missing camp. The classes this quarter consisted of Advertising, Speech, Pagemaker, and the programming language Visual Basic.

In advertising class, I was placed in a group with five ladies. Mr. Clark explained that the entire class was to do a marketing campaign for a car dealership in Ames, Iowa. Everyone was divided into separate groups and the winning team would receive a monetary prize. To help my group, I volunteered to get advertising rates from the radio stations in Des Moines. Some of them were familiar to me as Dad sometimes listened to oldies music as we sat by the train tracks. As I found each station's physical location, my caregiver and I drove to each one to get rate cards. I was pleased to find all of them accessible and nobody seemed to mind the AIB student rolling in for quick visits.

For speech, we did different types of presentation: persuasive, impromptu, informational, and demonstration. I didn't mind going to the front of class and speaking because I was used to people looking at me. When the time came for my demonstration speech, I wasn't sure what to do. My classmates showed juggling, cooking, how to strap a baby in a harness, and other advice. Everything they did required the use of hands to show a topic.

I thought about things I could do that were unique and came up with mouth writing. Mrs. Smith approved the topic, and my ten-minute time slot was a few days later. I started by having the class write their name in a notebook. To fill time, I talked a little about different forms of writing and using various instruments. With Sandy holding a notebook, I showed how I wrote with my mouth, then I had the students do the same. Everyone, including the professor, attempted to duplicate what they had seen. I tried not to laugh at the results, but we could hardly read anything. I offered a tip about holding the pen with their side teeth, on the same side as their dominant hand, and had them try again. The demonstration worked and I was able to fill the assignment primarily on my own.

Near the end of the quarter, Mr. Clark had every group present their final marketing campaign. He requested that men wear a tie with a dress shirt for the final presentation. Looking down at my ventilator tubing, I told him, “I don’t know if I can fill that part of the assignment.” He said that was fine and the request was mainly for the fraternity men who liked to party. On presentation day though, Sandy managed to get a tie over my trach and vent tube. My group won the $100 prize, and we were glad our hard work paid off.

With that project complete, I could give more attention to another. Earlier in the summer, my friend Rich said the student government association needed a website, so he convinced me to join the governing body and see what I could do. The two sites I was already working on had been designed and constructed before I started. It was a fun challenge to consider starting one from scratch, but I wasn’t sure where to begin. Near the end of the quarter, I completed building the website for the student government association and presented it to the president. She was initially surprised to see the design featuring her picture on the front page but liked it overall. The site was accepted with few changes, and I gained another client to increase my web building experience.

Even with the busy summer semester, I again got on the Dean’s list for another quarter.

A Surprise for Dad

That summer, the Union Pacific Railroad would be running steam excursions through the Midwest. Their largest operating steam engine, Challenger 3985, would be going through Iowa as they traveled from Des Moines to Kansas City. The excursion run was open to the public, but none of the cars were wheelchair accessible. Even though I couldn’t go, I got tickets for my parents to ride the train.

Near Dad’s birthday, I was home for the weekend, as usual, with the gift sitting on my dresser. I had yet to receive the actual tickets but made up same fake ones to use as an announcement. The excitement got to me and, while Dad did my afternoon cathing and exercises, I had him open the card.

June 23 was a warm and sunny Sunday. No matter what was happening, Voc Rehab wouldn't cover nursing when classes weren't scheduled. However, I could have nursing all day if it wasn't going through the agency. Karen and I didn't like missing church, but she agreed to come for the day so my parents could have fun. We took the van just south of Des Moines to Carlisle to watch the big engine steam through town.

We took pictures as it whistled through the small town, then Karen and I ventured further south to continue watching trains. After several hours on our adventure, we returned to my dorm. Late that evening, a bus returned my parents to Des Moines after their trip, and they stopped in to give me a full report. It was a rare opportunity I was happy to witness and let them enjoy.

Summer finished without any new open areas on my skin, but I stayed in bed on my air mattress most of the time. As I sat in bed with my computer in front of me, the air pump would frequently stop working. As soon as it turned off, the bed deflated, and I sank down to the bed springs. Turning the mattress on and off didn't help. It would regularly stop working and then restart a few minutes later. I didn't think sitting on springs would be helpful to my skin, so I called my equipment supply company. The next day, a new mattress was delivered, and the technicians set it up on my bed. Exchanging the equipment appeared to fix the problem, and I thanked the technicians for their help as they left.

A few minutes after their departure, the same issue started again. Nothing else was running in the room, so it couldn't be related to a power issue. I called again and explained what was going on and the next day another mattress pump was brought for my KCI tri-cell bed. Everything worked perfectly again, until they left.

By the third time, my equipment supplier was getting frustrated and started to wonder if I was making things up. However, they said they would try one more time with another mattress pump. I was getting tired of the problem as well and didn't like staying in my wheelchair longer than needed.

My bedroom had one door into it with a window for emergency access. The previous deliveries were done quickly, without enough time given for the pump to completely fill the mattress. I thought if I parked my wheelchair in the bedroom door and had the technicians stay longer, they would at least observe the issue.

Yet again, two technicians came with another air pump for the bed. As they unhooked the old one and set up the new, I casually parked in the only entrance to the room. They quickly had the new pump running again and I conversed with them about the previous problems and possible causes. I continued chatting as I hoped the technicians wouldn't notice they were stuck in my bedroom and being detained. Sandy sat on the couch near me, outside my bedroom, and grinned as she knew what I was doing.

After five minutes of small talk, the bed sputtered, just like the two previous times, stopped, and started again. This time, my nurse and I were not the only people to witness the act and the unknowing hostages suddenly became convinced of the issue. They investigated the room further and I discreetly backed out of the doorway, having proved my point. Another exchange solved the unknown issue, and everything worked well again.

My Final College Days

Between quarters, the school had a three-week break. Some of the dorms were being refreshed with new paint and improved heating and air conditioning units. Mine was due, so my bed and everything else had to be removed before going to Pella for the break. It was a lot of work for Dad to move furniture, but I looked forward to better heating before winter.

September 2002 came with another year of school complete. My apartment looked much better, and I was glad to be back. If I had stayed with my original major and not missed any classes, I would have been graduating. However, that was still several months away with a career to follow.

It didn't matter to the insurance company what I was doing in school. Funds continued to pour out for nursing and drain my lifetime limit. It would not be long until I was out of funding and would have no choice except to go into a nursing home. Mom had warned me this was a possibility, and now it would come true. Instead of being independent and on my own, I could only be in a small room in a care facility and not a productive citizen. I prayed that God would allow me to continue to be free of a nursing home, but His will be done.

One of my fall classes was investing, led by one of my former accounting professors who taught about the stock market as well as good and bad debt. The class was separated into several groups of 4-5 students with most people choosing to partner with friends.

This time, I was placed with a few other guys. The assignment of each group was to be an investing firm with a seed of $5,000 to invest in the market. Every investor in a firm could select the same stock as the other people in the firm or select individually. Every Friday, we had to sell all shares of stock and reinvest it in something else. The firm with the highest amount of funds at the end of class would win.

Since we only had numbers on paper and no actual cash, I thought it sounded fun. With fall approaching, I knew farmers were starting to harvest and crops were often transported by rail. Within the first few weeks, I invested in the Union Pacific Railroad, then GATX. Grain cars were leased by GATX to railroads and I encouraged my group members to follow my lead. They decided not to, but by the following week I was the only one who had earned an income. It wasn't long before I was making suggestions that received attention. Some weeks I didn't want to sell the stock I already had but it was part of the rules.

Rich and I had an evening class covering the computer programming language C++. The only desktop I could drive up to was in the back of the room with Rich on the machine beside me. It felt like high school again with Tom and me as computer neighbors working on assignments.

From my position, I had a full view of most of the other students' screens. I learned not to look around before class as some people checked email with pictures of what they did over the weekend. Several images would have resulted in expulsion from Pella Christian, and I saw a completely different side of my classmates.

From my seat, I could barely read what was written on the white board in the front of the class and had to carefully concentrate before it was erased. As with previous programming courses, I struggled as the class advanced and Rich and I would immediately raise our hands, or stick, when time was given to work on building our assignments. We noticed the professor would briefly answer our question but then quickly move on. If the student was female, and especially blonde, they received his full attention as long as desired.

Dad came with me during one class when the agency couldn't cover the evening. He noticed the same thing I did with the instructor, so Rich and I tried to help each other muddle through as best we could. He had me print out some of my coding so we could both look at it and find errors. I suggested it would be easier to email it but he insisted on printing. Two students were later removed from the class as the IT department noticed they were emailing assignments to each other and copying them. We weren't doing anything of that sort, but I understood the need to use paper.

Evaluating Career and Housing Options

Before finishing my college courses, Vocational Rehabilitation started looking at what I would be doing after school and where I would be living. If I was going to look for work in the Des Moines area, then I needed to have a place to live that was more permanent than a college dorm. However, being able to afford an apartment somewhere without a job would be difficult. The director of housing at AIB said I had been a good student and they would be willing to let me stay on campus for one quarter after finishing classes, but not in a long-term apartment.

Even though I lived in Des Moines in Polk County for school, my official address stayed in Pella in Marion County. My DHS case worker from Marion County was able to find a program that would cover my monthly rent until I found work. It would not always be available though and would only be a temporary option.

Housing wasn't the only problem. I was nearing my lifetime cap on insurance after two years of nearly daily nursing through an agency. With Dad being an integral part of the Town Crier, they were willing to work toward a new plan to keep him on staff. My parents, county supervisor, insurance case manager, nursing agency, and I all met together on what I needed for coverage.

The time it took to search meant another day closer to reaching my limit. At home, Mom had a tearful meeting with some of the church council members explaining our situation. The elders came for another visit on a Saturday evening when I was home. Mom asked me to talk as she couldn't explain without getting choked up. I told the men that I was nearing the end of my $2 million lifetime spending limit. If that happened, I would go completely on state funding, which would only cover my needs if I was in a nursing home. I also would no longer be eligible for a different insurance plan because the rules made it so that I couldn't get a new limit. I also reminded all of us, "God had brought us safe this far, and I trust He would continue to do so."

After a few months of a lot of work, a new plan was found for the Town Crier, and therefore, for me. Monthly premiums would increase as well as annual deductibles, but it was still funding. The coverage for equipment, like wheelchairs, wasn't as good, but it allowed for the nursing care I needed and a new $2 million policy. The approximately $100,000 left from my original cap would be deducted from the new policy. We were surprised but thankful that it came through and would start on April 1, 2003. The plan also continued to allow my parents to hire our own caregivers, pay them, and get reimbursed through insurance. No other insurance plans had this allowance, and we were thankful to see it continue, and to see God's provision once again.

With medical funding secured, I contacted apartment complexes around Des Moines to try to find places that were wheelchair accessible. Very few were available, and others had a requirement that the resident be over 50 years old. Mom helped look at one apartment that the landlord said had wheelchair access, but when she toured the property, corners and hallways were too tight for me to negotiate. The property manager was certain it was enough space, but Mom knew better.

Weeks of calling and looking for living quarters turned into months. Voc Rehab added pressure saying I couldn't look for work if I didn't have a permanent residence. I countered that I could commute from Pella to Des Moines, as many people did, for a temporary solution. The idea wasn't acceptable as I still had the possibility of not having housing for an indefinite period of time.

As fall quarter neared completion, my DHS supervisor heard about an accessible apartment that had become available near campus. My parents initially toured the residence and it was large enough for me to get into. I visited the two-bedroom home and was able to get down the hallway to the bedrooms and mostly everywhere else. The bathroom door was tight, but I didn't really need to get in it much anyway.

In November, I finished the quarter with a GPA high enough to make the Dean's list. I signed a six-month lease on the apartment and planned on moving in December. Marion County would pay for part of the rent, and I was responsible for the rest.

Most of my income was through Supplemental Security Income, or SSI, which I started receiving in high school. It was a social security program that provided monthly income for people with severe disabilities that make working difficult. My SSI got me through two years in school, paying for groceries and helping my parents with tuition whenever possible. Now I would need to carefully balance rent, utilities, groceries, and any other expenses.

My last quarter at AIB started in December with three classes during the day and one evening computer class. As I continued the routine of studying and commuting through campus from my dorm, my parents and I started accumulating furniture. All I owned was a television stand, dresser, and hospital bed. Everything else in my dorm was provided by the college.

Mom's parents had an old chair and couch in their basement I could use in my living area. They also had a small table with a few chairs that would work in the kitchen as a dining area. My parents purchased a roll-away cot for my second bedroom that Karen could sleep on when she worked overnight.

Moving to Sunburst Apartments

Over the two-week Christmas break, I left my dorm and everything was moved to my new place. The commute from Bell Ave. to Sunburst Apartments on SW 9th was only about 2.5 miles. I was still near the airport, just a different side, and near the same grocery store and pharmacy I had been using, but it felt like a big step toward my future. It increased my responsibility of living independently and potentially a long future on my own.

After school resumed, I took Rich to see my new residence. He rode with me in the van as Sandy drove. When we arrived, I saw Mom's car parked in the only handicapped spot I could use. Grandpa was taking in a box of stuff and waved when he saw the van. I commented on Mom's parking and Rich responded, "Your mom has a disability too?" Rich had met Dad when he covered for nurses that couldn't come, but he hadn't met the rest of my family. Living in Pella, most people knew my family's history due to small town relationships. However, that wasn't the case in Des Moines, and I had never fully explained my history. I told him a brief synopsis about our accident, who was involved, and the injuries received by me and Mom.

Furniture was moved during the break, but not much had been put away. Since I wasn't in class, I couldn't stay in Des Moines until January when Christmas break was over. Grandpa was helping vacuum and do final cleaning as Mom put away dishes and organized the kitchen. Rich liked the layout of the apartment and helped nail a loose floor molding in place.

My bed was in the back room, and my television, along with the borrowed furniture, was in the living area on the opposite side of the apartment. It meant I could no longer watch the news or any TV from bed, but I figured I could try to get current events online. For finishing touches, I put a few railroad themed posters on the walls to make it feel like my own place. I also invited Rich and his family to visit any time.

With housing established and college completion looming, it was time to think about employment. I used a template in Microsoft Word to build my résumé, but it was frowned upon by job services at AIB. They helped me build one from scratch, listing the computer software and programming I knew, as well as my work and volunteer history. With a customized document complete, AIB said I had the best résumé they had seen in years. No other students had done volunteer camp counseling, worked for a newsletter in high school, or done volunteer web development.

I felt confident in looking for work on my own, but Voc Rehab required me to hire a job developer. The developer would help with the job search as well as talk with potential employers about possible concerns in hiring me. I interviewed candidates from Goodwill, Easter Seals, and a developer who worked independently. Two of them said they mainly looked in the newspaper for openings and would pass them along to me. Guy, from Easter Seals, appeared to be the best choice. I agreed to work with him and see what he could do to help.

Disability Awareness Presentation

A few months before my senior year of high school, I had been a delegate with the Youth Leadership Forum. During college, I somewhat kept in contact with the organizers of the forum. The head of YLF contacted me to see if I would help with a group of speakers at Southeast Polk Junior High. The seventh grade class was having a section on disability awareness and had asked if anyone from YLF could help. It was in late February during my final week of school, but I agreed to join a few other former delegates after my class was out for the day.

On Monday, I arrived at the school in early afternoon just as a class period was about to close. I tried to hide in a corner to see what was going on but was immediately brought up front and asked for some input in the last five minutes before the bell. I had no idea what had been discussed or what to say, so I thought back to speech class and had the students get out a pen and notebook. I quickly showed them how I sign my name with my mouth and had them do the same.

The students attempted to repeat the action, but with very little success. In the few remaining seconds, I quickly added, "Someone with a disability may do things a little differently, but we still get the same things accomplished." My improvised quick response went well, and it unexpectedly became part of my demonstration for the remaining classes.

Tuesday had the same routine but this time I was more prepared. Our panel of four finished the presentation early, so we opened the floor for questions. The teacher asked, "Joel, what are your plans for the future?" It wasn't something I was prepared to answer. However, with two days left in my college career, I at least knew school plans. I responded, "For the immediate future, I look forward to finishing my degree and finding work in the Des Moines area. Beyond that, I suppose I am the same as most people and hope to get married and have a family."

It had been a good two-and-a-half years, but completion was now in sight. Just as with starting college, I didn't know what was around the corner, but looked forward to life ahead. I would quickly learn new lessons about working with people and how expectations could change.

17

OFF TO WORK

Second Thessalonians 3:10-12 gives a command that if someone is not willing to work, they shouldn't eat. There are some legitimate circumstances that make it so a person is unable to work. However, I had just been through many years of school and didn't see any reason not to earn a living. Just because I can't move or breathe wasn't an excuse to not be productive.

February 27, 2003 was my last day of class. I had one test to pass in Project Management in the evening, and I would then be a college graduate. Before the final exam, I met with Guy from Easter Seals to go over my school history and discuss how to look for employment.

Mom came up for the meeting as well and we started to discuss strategy. Guy started by looking at job offers he had found for Information Technology graduates. He listed a job doing computer repair but said I couldn't take apart or put computers together, so that was not for me. He continued to list more openings and immediately struck them down as tasks I couldn't perform. After a few minutes, Guy asked why I decided on an IT degree.

I started to regret hiring him until Mom spoke up and asked Sandy, "Aren't you able to help with some of this?" "Yes," she answered. With my knowledge and directing, my caregivers should be able to help with some of the physical requirements. Guy looked surprised by this revelation, but we went on to my education background. He wondered if I had made any academic achievements. I told about making the Dean's list twice and receiving an award from student government for web development. Guy said he would mark me as being on the list multiple times and doing extra work. I didn't think that saying twice was enough to earn the label multiple times, but I agreed.

When Guy's paperwork was complete, it needed to be signed. Sandy got a pen for me, but he hesitated and didn't think I should do it myself. Guy said, "I don't know you, but this signature needs to look neat, and I should probably do it." I sternly responded, "I sign all my own paperwork and it will be fine." After signing my name, he was surprised to see the results and considered noting it was my actual writing.

When evening came, I quietly completed my last exam for class and for my degree. Project management tests were done on the computer, and it was a nice change to answer the questions without writing assistance. As I rolled off campus in the chilly night air, I was glad to be finished. However, AIB graduation wasn't until September. Even though I had completed my courses, I wouldn't have a diploma to show for nearly seven months.

Even before working with Guy, I applied for a few job openings I found on my own. I didn't hide that I used a wheelchair and needed caregivers, but my résumé didn't say anything about it either. I got a call from a web development firm that liked my qualifications and wanted to interview me. They knew one of the instructors at AIB and liked that I had some experience in the field. We agreed on a time to meet the day after my final exam.

The potential employer was just a few blocks from my apartment and would easily be within rolling distance during nice weather. On the phone, the head developer told me, "Just come in the front door, go up the stairs, and my office is at the top." I knew this wouldn't work so I let him know I use a wheelchair and asked if they had a level entrance. After some thought, he was pretty sure one door on the lower level was flat but could be tight navigating inside.

Before leaving school, I talked with Mr. Clark about my upcoming interview and he said the interviewer was a good man, had been in politics for a few years, and advised me to get everything in writing. I dressed in my Sunday best and Sandy drove us the three blocks to a plain, square, gray building. We found the lower door and, upon entering, were greeted with two small printing presses. The sound of the machines was just like what I knew when visiting Dad at the Town Crier.

Bill found us and escorted Sandy and me to an area where we could talk. I answered questions and talked about how I started working with websites. He wanted to see my work, so I gave him the addresses of my sites, all three of them. His company's primary work was web development, but they did a few small printing jobs as well. About half an hour later, I left and thought it went pretty well. Before heading home, Sandy and I went to get groceries.

When we got back to my apartment, the answering machine was blinking with a new message. Bill called in the short time while I was out and wanted to set up a second interview. Returning his message, we agreed to meet again on Tuesday morning. Guy also wanted to meet with me, so I scheduled him for Tuesday afternoon.

While looking for a job, I was also trying to learn to manage my budget. February had been cold, so I ran my apartment's heat a lot in the month. All utilities, other than gas and water, were my responsibility. However, everything, including heat, was electric and nothing used gas. In addition to utilities, I also had to pay for my landline phone and dial-up internet access. My electric bill came and I was shocked at how much I owed for staying warm. December and January weren't bad, but this was a surprise.

In the third quarter of my first year at school, one of my classes was College Math. The name scared me, but it was a practical course on real-life financial decisions with things to do and avoid. A few of the topics were budget billing for utilities and rental insurance. The insurance was usually very inexpensive, but not many people got it. After calling different companies for rates, I got a policy a few weeks after getting my apartment.

For less than $3.00 per month, I received $25,000 in coverage if needed. As I signed the insurance contract, I thought it was a little low. I was sitting in a wheelchair and attached to a ventilator with combined value more than my plan covered. However, I figured if I wasn't already in my chair and my apartment caught fire, I likely wouldn't need the chair or vent any longer.

I was just able to cover the electric bill but decided to register for budget billing instead. This change would make my monthly cost about the same. In the winter, I would pay less than what I used, but it would even out in the warmer months when I didn't use much air conditioning.

After a weekend in Pella, my second interview with the web developer came as scheduled on Tuesday morning. Once I got into the building, Bill took me to the same location as a few days earlier. He liked what I did, even though one site didn't come up for him. Pointing toward Sandy, Bill asked, "Is this your sister?" Since she was close to my mom's age, I thought it was an odd assumption. However, I explained a little about why I had nurses and some of the hardware I used.

Bill then asked, "How much would you like to earn per hour?" I had no idea what a web developer made or what to say. It briefly ran through my head that my Medicare had very strict limits on what I could have for income. I primarily used the Town Crier's insurance for medical needs, but still had to keep on the program. I answered, "I have a cap of $2,000 per month for some of my funding but would like to earn near that if possible."

The proposed amount didn't seem to be a surprise, and I was asked how long I could stay while Bill made some phone calls. My meeting with Guy was in two hours and required about 30 minutes of travel through the city. I considered saying I had another interview, but as that wasn't accurate, I just gave a time limit.

Another developer showed me an office area that I could access with a few computers. He said a lot of people work from home doing web work, but they could also come in if they needed more tools or to get out of their house. Going to his computer, I helped him find my site they couldn't access earlier, and he went through areas that I could adjust.

Not long before I had to leave, Bill returned from his office upstairs. They wanted to offer me the position but needed to hear back from some people first. He said that he looked forward to working with me and would contact me soon.

With the second interview complete, Sandy and I talked about how it went as we drove to Easter Seals to meet with Guy. After finding our way in, Guy said he had talked with a company in downtown Des Moines and gone over what accommodations I would need if I worked for them. The company was interested and would possibly like to meet me. I told him about the interview I had come from and that I expected to be offered the position. Guy was surprised and said he would inform the company I was no longer available.

> *Memories of interviewing at the Diamond Trail News were going through my mind and how I was quickly hired on. I hoped I would have the same experience now in Des Moines.*

Memories of interviewing at the Diamond Trail News and how quickly I was hired were going through my mind. I hoped I would have the same experience now in Des Moines. A few days passed and I didn't hear anything from the web developer. However, I had applied for more positions at other companies and started getting calls for interviews.

Even though I was finished with school, Voc Rehab continued to help cover part of my nursing hours so I could stay in Des Moines. Days would be covered as long as I was actively applying for jobs, interviewing, or working. It still meant going home every weekend, but I could continue to live on my own.

A week passed after my second interview, and I still hadn't heard anything. I called Bill to ask how it was going and received a brief, "We're working on it." I contacted Guy to update him, but the company he contacted was no longer interested. Throughout March, I interviewed at different locations around Des Moines with Wells Fargo, government positions, and a real estate company. They were general help desk and IT positions, but jobs that seemed accessible to me and good for just starting my career.

The realtor had two offices in Des Moines and was looking to hire a web developer. The person interviewing me said they were just starting to advertise real estate online, but already had a large market in the area. He was particularly glad to see I worked with a church site as they also regularly worked with churches. After the initial interview, I didn't hear back. However, they were on the local news a few months later as being investigated for fraudulent spending and were subsequently closed.

April came with more job interviews, but no offers for employment. I got into a routine of working on websites on Monday with an interview or two during the week. Every place that contacted me was through my own initiative, with nothing coming from Guy. Sandy told me about an agency called Adecco that filled part-time positions for businesses. It sounded like a place to get some experience and it was worth giving it a try. I hadn't heard of such a place before and thought they would hire anyone. I came to the office in Des Moines, rolled in with Sandy behind me, and asked about getting placed for temporary IT jobs. The lady at the desk looked a little surprised but asked about my qualifications. I gave her a résumé and told her about recently graduating from AIB. I would need to take a test and watch a video, but she said they may be interested.

A few days later, I returned to watch a job safety video. It went over proper use of ladders, forklifts, and other basic industrial tools. Looking down at my arms strapped to my wheelchair's armrests, I didn't think the instructions pertained to me very well. I managed to stay awake through it and did at least learn how to report my hours if I was assigned to work somewhere on my own.

After the video was the technology test. I brought one of my bedside tables and Sandy put the keyboard and mouse on it so I could reach with my mouth stick. The lady evaluating me didn't say anything but was watching closely. The test started with different functions of Microsoft Office. I had taken four classes in school covering everything in these programs, or so I thought. The evaluation used an older version of Office than I was familiar with, requiring me to do some searching, and guessing to find some items. Each question only allowed a certain number of clicks and time limit before moving on. One problem was how to open a corrupted file with Microsoft Access in one click. I hadn't heard of such a thing before but tried clicking on the open file button. My guess was incorrect, and I was moved on to the next question.

I completed the evaluation in about 20 minutes, feeling like a fool, receiving what I thought was a low score. I wondered if I had just wasted over two years and much of my parents' funds for school. However, I was told I scored higher than most applicants and would get a call if an appropriate position was available.

Interviews through Guy were still non-existent, but he let me know about a job fair in Des Moines I had already planned to attend. The day came, and I printed out several copies of my résumé and went to meet Guy at the job fair. He said he would tell potential employers the benefits of hiring someone like me and cover any disability related questions.

Upon entering, the independent job coach I had interviewed a few months earlier was standing by the door giving out maps of where employers were located. It felt awkward saying hi with Guy behind me, but I entered the large room at the Civic Center to see tables set up everywhere with all the major companies in Des Moines represented.

Rolling down the rows, I approached each booth and asked about IT openings for entry level jobs. If they had any, Sandy handed them my information as I talked with the recruiter. As I moved on, I could hear Guy come up behind me to the same person and talk more about me and working with someone with a disability. I wasn't sure if he was helping or hindering prospects, but hoped he knew what was best.

Guy told me about a business called Criteria 508. It was run by a person in Des Moines and tested websites for accessibility. A government regulation called Section 508 required some sites to meet certain requirements so that everyone could use them, regardless of physical abilities. I met with Anna, and her company seemed like a good fit for me. However, it was only occasional, short jobs, not anything full time. I agreed to help and was told to buy a few books to help get me acquainted with what to test. One book covered disabilities in general and said that young children in wheelchairs often spin in circles. It said the behavior helps them learn what size they are and general spatial recognition. My thoughts returned to grade school and waiting for the bus to pick me up after school. I would spin circles endlessly, never getting dizzy, and drove my nurses crazy. I wondered if it may have contributed to my good driving award at VACC Camp so many years earlier.

Adecco called late in April. They had an upcoming customer service job that I could do, but they were concerned about whether I could be understood on the phone with my mouth stick while typing. I tested it while the Adecco representative was on the phone with me. I typed on my laptop while speaking to her and tried to record what was said. I passed the test and was told that I would be given further information soon.

The job hunt wasn't progressing any further. I continued to get interviews, but never any return visits. Guy had me come in for a typing test to show I could run a computer at a decent speed. I had typed around 40 words per minute in high school but hadn't been evaluated since. I was brought to an office with a desktop computer. It had words on the screen for me to copy for one minute and time my speed. The tester put a sticky pad under the keyboard so it wouldn't move as I typed. Looking at the screen and down to my stick on the keyboard wasn't ideal, but I timed at 29 words per minute.

With the keyboard stationary, it felt like I was jabbing my stick into my teeth. I tried the test again without the pad but got the same results as the keyboard slid around like it was on ice. I had been using my laptop with a smaller keyboard for a few years and was used to it. Therefore, she let me try again with a laptop. It looked like I was typing faster, but the time was still close to 30 WPM.

Guy came to my apartment the next day and wanted to take pictures of me getting in the van to show I had reliable transportation. Finishing something on my computer first, he said, "You *can* type fast." I told him it depended on what I was doing and that I could go faster if I was going by my own thoughts. Sandy and I went out to the van, put the lift down, and I sat on the platform as he took pictures.

I soon found myself back at Easter Seals with Anna from the web checking agency. There were three other people and me in a computer room. We would be testing websites for a few clients while they watched us. One tester had trouble with seizures and the other two had some mobility impairments, but I was the only one using a wheelchair, ventilator, and mouth stick.

Each person showed how they navigated the site and what worked best for them. Then the attention turned back to me. I resized the browser to demonstrate how the site would look on different computer screens and how I use my stick to operate the keyboard and mouse. I somewhat felt guilty as I looked to have the most significant physical challenges in the room but had the easiest time of anyone running the tests. Having the clients watch us work showed a sample of what we could do, but also advertised who was doing the work. Three different site owners came, one at a time, as we tested, and I hoped we were able to improve the finished product.

Some job applications I submitted were in the financial industry. I didn't really expect a response, but they still asked for interviews. Sitting in a small building directly across from my favorite model train store, Sandy helped me fill out one company's required information. Along with listing references and work history, it asked if I looked at my hands when I type. I hadn't considered the question but could honestly answer no. I concluded my hands just sit under my table where I can't see them, so I don't look at them when I type.

When the interviewer first saw me, he didn't seem surprised to see all my hardware. During the question session, he said they had another quadriplegic who worked for them part-time. His company didn't provide insurance, but the other man also worked at a hospital that covered medical expenses. To approve loans for his agency, all I needed to do was watch a video and answer questions at the same time. He called me back a few days later to see if I was interested, but I declined. Having a job with an income would be nice, but I wouldn't be able to stay without insurance coverage.

A Temporary Position

The temporary job with Adecco started in early May and would end in June, the week before camp. I was glad to finally return as a camp counselor again and show Sandy what I had come to love. Before fun though, it was time to finally get to work.

My assignment was in West Des Moines at a place called ADP, about 30 minutes away from my apartment. I found myself in a room with 90 other temporary staff members for a week of training. A large airline had recently declared bankruptcy, and as part of their restructuring, every employee had to re-enroll with their medical and dental insurance. My hours would be 8:00-4:30, Monday through Friday, with a 30-minute lunch break at the on-site cafeteria.

This was my first experience working full-time, and I wanted to do well. However, my hours were too long to go between my regular cathing times. I didn't like to discuss bathroom issues with my temporary employer, but I didn't have a choice.

Sandy and I met with the human relations person we had been introduced to in the initial orientation meeting. I explained that I would need a restroom break during the day but would always have a female assistant. Therefore, I wouldn't be able to use the designated male or female bathrooms. She thought of a few ideas but decided on posting a sign. When I arrived at work the next day, I was given a laminated sign saying, "Out of Order," with a Velcro pad on the back. A corresponding strip had been glued on the wall by the women's restroom and I could use it whenever needed.

As training continued, the influx of staff was shown how to work the computer system, phone system, and how to answer airline employees. ADP also worked with a major railroad, and we were told the most difficult people to work with are pilots and train engineers, who thought the company would be nothing without them and they deserved the best treatment. I wondered how I could get transferred to the railroad account but didn't see any options.

Since starting pre-school, I had been in class all my life. This week didn't feel any different until late in the training. The realization came to me that this wasn't another instructor giving information to pass the next test. It was for work. There wouldn't be any grades or further courses, this was to earn a living or lose my job. With this realization, I started paying closer attention to everything I was being shown.

On Friday, the week of orientation was complete, and everybody was shown to their cubicle. My supervisor said mine was made a little larger than the others so I had room to get in. Sandy rolled my bedside table in and put the keyboard, mouse, and telephone on it. I parked in my desk just as I had in school and checked the placement of everything and saw if I could reach with my stick. I could just see my computer screen over the table and access all the equipment I would be using. Beyond that, all I could see were three gray walls on each side of me that funneled my vision to the ceiling.

My computer screen had a small script taped to it, "Hello, my name is. Thank you for calling the airline service center, may I please have your employee ID?" Sandy picked up a small book that was in my cubicle with questions that I needed to answer through the computer system. With my phone headset on, I could hear her behind me as she asked each item. I struggled to find the first answers, but I soon became familiarized with where to look and remembered the training. I was able to complete the practice test, but Monday would be real employees relying on me to get their correct information.

After my regular weekend in Pella, my first day of actual work came. Even though the people I interacted with would never see me, there were strict rules on what I could wear from head to foot. I dressed as required, and logged into my computer just barely before I was to start my shift. After a couple minutes of staring at the computer screen, my phone headset buzzed, and the display showed the pre-entered employee ID. I read my script and entered the number in the correct spot. As the person on the other end spoke, I could hear what sounded like my computer's flight simulator in the background. My first call was from a pilot in the air, and he wasn't happy.

I attempted to answer his concerns but didn't make progress as the pilot just wanted a supervisor. Sandy listened behind me and when I said, "I'll get my supervisor," she raised her hand to get his attention. He responded promptly, but I had to be told of his arrival as I couldn't see behind me. I muted my phone, explained the situation, and the supervisor took over the conversation with the pilot on another headset.

It only took a few minutes to complete the application, so I entered everything into the computer as it was coaxed out of the disgruntled pilot. When we were finished, I was thankful for my phone going silent again. From somewhere behind me, my supervisor asked, "Was that your first one?" I confirmed it was and heard a slight chuckle and assurance that it would get better.

By the time lunch break came, I had successfully handled more calls from much easier employees. I got into a routine that my assistant would write down the employee ID if it came up on the phone where she could see it. If it came up incorrectly, then I would get it from the caller and repeat it out loud to be recorded. That way I could track how many people I helped, and it gave my caregiver something to do.

With my wheelchair's chin control off to the side, I couldn't reach it. I showed my assistants how to tilt my chair so I could have some adjustment throughout the day. I could only move a few inches with my lap under the table, but I thought it was better than nothing.

Every person that I talked to had to say what option they wanted to choose. They could have no benefits package with no fees or continue with insurance through the airline. If they chose the second, the employee would get health coverage with an unlimited lifetime capacity for $50 per month for an individual or $200 per month for a family of any size. Each employee that opted to keep medical insurance was receiving what I was dreaming and praying about. For my insurance, my parents were paying more than five times what a family plan costs for airline employees with a constant lifetime cap looming over me.

Several of the employees I talked to lamented how terrible the airline was and that they now had to pay for what had formerly been free. I was told I should be thankful that I worked for someone else. With every comment, I wanted to educate them on how good these benefits were and that I would love to receive a similar package. Sometimes I responded that everything looked good from where I sat, but I mainly kept quiet and just worked as required.

After I responded to questions, I entered in every family member's social security number and primary doctor. When all the boxes were checked and spaces filled, I read a short disclaimer paragraph before clicking submit. I didn't remember being told to read it and I normally would skip it myself, but I thought I should in order to cover potential problems.

All my fellow temporary employees were allowed to take a short break two hours after starting our staggered shifts. I knew my afternoon bathroom break took longer than everyone else, so I worked through the break and didn't pause until lunch. With my caregiver feeding me and herself, it was sometimes hard to get lunch complete in 30 minutes.

There was a cafeteria in the building we could use, so I generally just ordered a sandwich for quick consumption. My normal order was pepper turkey lunch meat with some type of cheese and bread. I wasn't familiar with some of the options, so I tried a different cheese each day for some variety. One of the options was called pepper jack, something I hadn't seen before, so I added it to my pepper turkey. Sandy warned me it was a little spicy, but I thought it sounded interesting. Less than an hour later, I was back in my position inside my gray walls. With my nose running and eyes watering from lunch, I attempted to sound competent on the phone while Sandy reached from behind me to wipe my nose. I learned to never touch that cheese again and to listen when I was warned about spicy food.

Memorial Day weekend came, and it was nice to have three days off from my cubicle. In the month I had been working, the wall to my left had become mostly filled with notes handed down from management with adjustments in what we could or could not say. One list had names of airline staff who had been killed in the terrorist attacks nearly two years earlier. The surviving family members could still get full benefits if they wished.

Someone had very good negotiating skills when the airline contract was established. Since we missed one day for the holiday, everyone had to work two extra days over the following weekend. I absolutely did not like the idea of missing church and working on Sunday, but I got it arranged that Karen would help me over the weekend so I could stay in Des Moines and work. On Friday, a paper went around to see who wanted to take Sunday off. I wanted to take the day off, but I didn't feel I could cancel since I had nursing arranged.

On Saturday morning, the usual main door we entered was locked. I tried checking other entrances, but they didn't all have curb cuts or recognize my ID badge. After several minutes of trying to enter the building, another worker let me in a side door. It was then a challenge to navigate through the building to the elevator to get to my desk. I had a badge that could be swiped at doors to allow entry. However, I was in a different section of the building and couldn't get through. With help from other weekend staff, I finally got to my workstation a few minutes late.

The cafeteria was also closed, unknown to me. The other temporary staff took off for fast food, but I didn't have enough time to leave, eat, and return in my lunch break. Food wasn't allowed in cubicles either, so Sandy and I dined on vending machine snacks in a corner room and looked forward to getting home.

I learned from my experience, and I came better prepared on Sunday with a sack lunch. With the top supervisors not around on the weekend, several of my fellow workers disregarded clothing rules and wore shorts and regular t-shirts. Even though I didn't agree with the garment stipulations, I tried to set an example and still followed them.

Monday, June 2, was the last day for enrollment with the deadline at midnight. As I got settled into my familiar gray walls, my computer slowly started up. I quickly checked the phone system and saw a queue of people waiting, even with 90 of us taking enrollment calls. As soon as everything booted up, I hit the button to say I was available and immediately had a caller. The busy morning went by quickly with people who had waited until the last day. One caller wanted to know if enrollment was available until 4:00 A.M. eastern time, which would be midnight in Hawaii. I explained he had until midnight in the time zone he lived in and offered to get him enrolled, but he wanted to wait.

Calls slowed down in the afternoon but kept coming. A few hours before my shift and first job assignment were complete, my supervisor quietly gave me a note. I finished the call, and Sandy held it where I could read it. I had been selected as one of 30 people to stay on for a few more weeks. I was also allowed to leave early since call volume had decreased. With two thirds of my fellow employees leaving the job for the last time, I left my table in place for the next day.

Arriving promptly Tuesday morning, the large room filled with cubicles sounded silent. I got in my position as I had for several weeks and waited. Not much later, my phone activated and I did my routine greeting. However, I didn't know what to do next as enrollment was closed. I said the keywords, "Let me ask my supervisor," and Sandy promptly summoned him for direction. One final enrollment week was being offered June 16-20 for those that missed the first time. I just had to tell any callers to call back then.

With very few calls and sight limited to my cubicle, boredom quickly set in. Some staff read books, but I didn't have enough space on my table for the book board along with keyboard, mouse, and phone. My computer didn't have any games or outside internet access, but it did have Microsoft paint. The calls I was given could be an hour or more between and lasted a minute or less. Therefore, I started painting what I could see- my keyboard. I carefully used the square tool and added rounded corners to match the keys in front of me. After I was satisfied with one, I duplicated it according to the number of keys I had. When my supervisor would occasionally pass unseen behind me, I could hear comments on my accurate work.

My art project progressed as the week continued, but I was also thankful to be given the option to leave early most days. In the month I had been working, it was difficult to cover my regular life's needs. After my shift, I could get groceries or run errands, but I needed to be home before my caregiver's shift was over. My medical supply company also closed shortly after I got home. I had my helper take inventory of supplies one evening and then try to get home in time to place the order the next day. Finding a time for my monthly ventilator maintenance checks was also a challenge, but I got it worked out.

Since I had income, I wanted to stop the county rent assistance for my apartment. However, my case manager advised me not to since it was only a temporary job. I did report my earnings to Social Security as required so my SSI would be decreased proportionately. Criteria 508 also continued to give me occasional websites to evaluate. I was allowed three hours to evaluate a site, but I only needed 30 minutes of one evening after supper to complete the task.

I was thoroughly thrust into the working world and getting used to the strain on time and energy. Voc Rehab wanted to meet with me to discuss the progress on finding permanent employment. So, on Friday, June 6, I took time off from my morning shift for a meeting. Instead of heading west to work, Sandy and I drove to the Jessie Parker Building near the state capitol. Going to work every day had become routine and it felt odd not to be going. We went to a meeting room and joined Michal (my Voc Rehab counselor), Guy from Easter Seals, and Mom.

It had been a little over three months since I earned my Associate's degree and I had applied for several positions and had been on a number of interviews, but had not received any job offers. Since I had been working 40 hours a week the past month, I hadn't submitted any applications for further interviews.

Michal said she had been talking with Guy about employment prospects. He hadn't given my name or details but talked with a few friends who owned businesses. They said hiring someone like me had potential to significantly increase their cost of medical insurance. Due to the expense, they would never hire someone with my disability. Guy said this would likely be the scenario for any company that interviewed me. Based on this information, Voc Rehab had decided to stop helping fund my nursing or job search. It was unlikely I would ever find work, especially with the type of insurance I needed. They recommended that I no longer look for work and it would be best if I moved to a care facility.

Sandy was then handed a paper with phone numbers to area nursing homes. Michal had contacted several of them and the longest time any had for taking a new resident was four weeks. Voc Rehab would therefore keep my same coverage in place for an additional four weeks, ending on July 4, 2003. I pointed out that since Guy had been hired, I had not received one interview through him. I also reminded everyone I had taken time off from a job to be at this meeting, and I had been selected to stay on longer due to my performance.

Michal asked, "Does Adecco provide insurance?" I was not aware of any, so had to reply with no.

Mom added that very few nursing homes take someone who is vent dependent. Did this list include facilities that would take someone with my needs? Michal didn't know as she hadn't asked. She was aware that I may not agree to go to an institution, but this was what they recommended and were willing to offer.

Not long after, Sandy and I were in the van headed to West Des Moines so I could clock in for work. The day was slow, and I was given the option to go home after only a few hours on the clock. My mind wasn't thinking about my job responsibilities, so I gladly returned to my apartment.

Within a few hours, my future had again gone from looking hopeful to looking uncertain. I didn't know what would happen in the immediate future or even where I would be living. I had hoped to continue looking for work around Des Moines but didn't know if I could.

The next few weeks were already scheduled for my nursing care, but everything beyond that was unknown.

18

UNCERTAIN DIRECTION

When David was being pursued by King Saul, he wrote Psalm 11. Verse three says, "If the foundations are destroyed, what can the righteous do?" With part of my funding coming to an end, I didn't have all the resources I needed for caregivers and live on my own. I could only trust on the sure foundation of God.

I missed two years of CHAMP Camp due to being in school. When applications became available in early 2003, I gladly signed up. Our group would leave for Ohio on June 20, but I needed time to pack. I worked one more week at ADP and left on June 13. I explained that I had originally been told the assignment would end that day and had made plans that couldn't be changed. My supervisor seemed to understand but I felt bad leaving my first job two weeks early.

Sandy had heard me talk extensively about camp and agreed to be my day assistant for the week. I went back to Pella on Friday the 13th and spent the next week packing my supplies while Dad did van maintenance. Since I started school, it had been sitting in parking lots in the cold winters and hot summers. As a result, it was showing some wear but still ran well.

It felt good to be back at camp and see the people I had spent many summers with. There were new faces as well as some regulars that had moved on from camp. Every activity had one to two counselors who were in charge, called program specialists. Since I enjoyed fishing during my camper years, I was asked to be one of the specialists at the waterfront.

My role was to make sure each group knew the rules as well as keep track of fishing bait and what the campers caught. At the end of the week, awards would be given to the camper who caught the biggest fish and who caught the most. I was with the younger boys' cabin again, but I would be at Lake Crumb every morning for the four trail groups.

Orientation was thorough and my fellow counselors and I knew what to expect when our campers arrived. One of the boys in my cabin was Devin. He was almost eight years old and, like me, had received a spinal cord injury when he was three and was a vent dependent quadriplegic. Another first-time camper in my cabin, Luke, had something I wasn't familiar with, Spinal Muscular Atrophy. Luke could only make a few sounds and move his eyes, so he was unable to communicate verbally. One of the other counselors made a sign with words and pictures of the regular camp activities. She wanted to see if she could help him communicate by looking at the choice he wanted.

The campers all arrived to the extreme fanfare that had my parents questioning camp my first year but that I now helped produce. I had warned Sandy, but she still wasn't sure what to think. As night came, Karen took over my care from Sandy and I recruited Big Brian, or anyone, to help toss me from my chair to my bunk. Along with my bedside vent, there were six campers with ventilators in the same room. Even with the rhythmic tumult, it wasn't hard getting to sleep.

I woke up Monday morning and was in my wheelchair before most of the campers were up. It increased my time sitting, but I could help control the ambulatory kids that needed less specialized care while the other counselors helped with medical needs.

By Tuesday, we had the routines down and everyone knew how to help each kid. With the lights on and radio pumping out morning tunes,

I rolled by Devin's bed to see if he was doing okay. My eyes fixed on his chest, and I didn't see any movement except breathing. I stopped a passing counselor and as I jerked my head in his direction, I asked, "Did he fall asleep again?" She answered, "No, he's bopping to the music."

My gaze refocused to his head and I saw his head bobbing back and forth in time with the beat. I hadn't thought before that I look the same and, from neck down, didn't move according to my head. Another counselor came around the corner pushing Devin's power wheelchair, and I quickly moved so he could be released from the captivity of his bunk.

On dance night, most of the campers moved to the music as much as their bodies or mobility aides allowed. When the "Chicken Dance" started playing, more counselors joined the kids to form a pulsating combination of legs, wheels, and medical technology. I mainly sat on the fringes with a few other counselors getting a rest and refreshment. In previous years, I was always part of the group spinning and moving around. But as a college graduate and nearing my 22nd birthday, I was more aware of others watching me. It somehow didn't seem proper to perform in such a manner, even though most everyone else was. A couple of the other long-time counselors spoke of seeing me "cut a rug" before and I joined in on "YMCA" and a few other songs, but not most.

The week soon ended with me helping present fishing awards. Mom and Dad picked the three of us up after enjoying their own time in the area. I was soon asleep as the van traveled back to Iowa on the familiar roads from central Ohio.

Seeking Employment Continues

As the country celebrated Independence Day, I officially lost part of my funding that had allowed me to live independently for more than two years. Insurance would pay a maximum amount per day for care through the agency and a maximum per week of private hired care. It was also less expensive to hire an LPN than an RN. Mom and I looked at the numbers, and I could continue to live in my apartment if we utilized more private hours. Most of my agency nurses were also LPN's, which helped decrease expenses. It was a precarious house of cards that could easily collapse, but it would work for a short time. The arrangement would continue to use a lot of insurance funds and I still needed to return to Pella every weekend.

I decided to try to go through the summer to find work with insurance and reevaluate before fall. I again started to apply for any position that I thought I could perform, whether it was related to Information Technology or in another area. Wells Fargo had several offices around Des Moines, and I got to find several of them. On the phone, one recruiter gave me his location multiple times, emphasizing another office was across the street. If I went there, I would arrive late, and that would not be in my favor. I arrived in the correct location a few minutes early, but still didn't get a second interview.

Some interviewers acted like they didn't want to hire recent graduates with little work experience, but they still had to say an opportunity was given. After getting past the security guard, I interviewed in a downtown location while Sandy waited outside the door. The cascade of questions included wanting to know if I had ever confronted a supervisor, and how I handled the situation. I only had one job with such a hierarchy, and I didn't have any trouble that needed to be addressed. I responded that I never had a situation where a supervisor was in error and couldn't give a real-life example. The same questions were repeated from different angles, wondering how I corrected a supervisor. Instead, I switched tactics and gave examples of when I needed to confront a caregiver.

After 20 minutes, I was glad to be finished with the interview and I was frustrated, wondering why I had been asked to come. The security guard told Sandy it must be going well since it took so long, but he was incorrect. I received the familiar form letter from Wells Fargo thanking me for my time, but I wasn't selected for the job.

Soon after CHAMP Camp, I developed a bladder infection. Thankfully they were rare but I needed a round of antibiotics. After I completed the medication, my stomach decided to strongly express a dislike for the drug.

Karen took over the evening shift, and I started having diarrhea shortly after. It wasn't something I had experienced before, but I didn't want to eat or drink to add fuel to the fire.

After hours of nearly non-stop runs, Karen called Sandy for help. I was now having trouble speaking or making coherent thoughts. I knew I should drink and tried to get some water, but I choked violently and coughed when the liquid hit my stomach. My two caregivers decided it was time to go to the emergency room, and they devised a plan to transport me without having a big mess in my chair.

Normally, I talked to hospital staff on my own. Unfortunately, I barely knew what was going on around me and my vision was narrow and full of shimmering lights. Karen reported to the emergency nurse, and I was taken to a room.

Just as when my leg broke a few years earlier, another late evening call was made to my parents. Dad stayed home but Mom ventured out, driving through the nearly empty downtown city streets in Des Moines. When she arrived around midnight, I had been on fast-paced I.V. liquids for over an hour. As she walked in my room, I gave a cheerful, "Hi mom!" It looked like nothing had happened but the hospital decided to keep me overnight for observation. Several hours later, the morning nurse came to make rounds and asked a few questions to check my level of awareness.

Nurse: "What time is it?" Looking at the large clock on the wall behind her head, I answered, "9:05." She then went on with, "What day is it? Where are you? Who is the president?" I answered the next two correctly and for the president, I responded, "Dubya."

Everyone I knew around my age referred to President George W. Bush by his middle initial, W. The confused look on the young nurse's face told me she didn't understand. I changed my answer to Bush, and she left satisfied. With the nurse's station directly outside my hospital room door, I could hear her recount my confusing response. Her fellow nurses explained the answer and I was allowed to leave and return to my apartment.

My "plumbing" issues persisted for a few days, but much more controlled. I spent three days naked in bed making sure to drink plenty of water and not dirty any clothing.

Immediately after this experience, I went to an interview for a help desk position at a local fresh food distributor. My body wasn't ready to be in my chair and I immediately got light-headed when Sandy got me up. Answering questions, I sounded like I was intoxicated as I attempted to respond. I tried calling Guy at Easter Seals to see if he could explain the situation to them, but I didn't get a response.

July progressed with numerous interviews, but no job offers. I received a letter from Adecco that they were now offering medical insurance. The temp agency would pay the monthly premiums when an employee had an assignment, but the cost would be out of pocket when not working. The minimal information provided didn't look like good coverage so I didn't look at it further.

Every 60 days, Iowa required nursing agencies to recertify clients and make sure everything was correct on the person's care plan. Erin, who had been removed as my caregiver for attitude disagreements, was now my nursing supervisor. She had recently done my required update but the new paperwork didn't get to me. After some searching, Erin realized she accidentally slipped it under the door of my neighbor's apartment. She retrieved it from the occupants and correctly delivered it to me, explaining the error. I shrugged it off and was glad the papers had been found.

A few days later, Sandy felt ill during her shift and had to leave early with Erin filling the time until Karen came. She couldn't understand why I wasn't mad and upset about the paperwork mix-up she had done. The paper contained all my personal information about all my cares and procedures. I explained I understood it was a mistake and was not done intentionally. Getting angry wouldn't change anything and wasn't how a Christian should act. My reaction didn't make sense to her but it wasn't a problem again.

Three years after graduating, Pella Christian High School contacted me about needing a webmaster. I accepted the offer to manage their website and was thankful to get more web work while I waited for permanent employment.

My county DHS worker suggested I talk with Senator Tom Harkin's office. He had helped write the Americans with Disabilities Act and was well known for helping people with disabilities. Maybe the Senator could offer advice or might know resources I could utilize.

I made an appointment with his office and, a few days later, found my way to the federal building in downtown Des Moines. As I approached the metal detector, I wondered how I would get through security. A guard ushered me through another entrance with a few checks of my equipment before Sandy and I found our way to the Senator's office. We waited by the entrance, and I could hear someone listening to messages on an answering machine. One Iowan asked if there was anything that could be done to curtail New York Senator Hillary Clinton's spending as she traveled promoting a book. As I quietly laughed at the comment, the notetaker realized guests were listening and shut her door.

Another lady came and took us to a meeting room where I explained the past few years. I told her about my job search since graduation, Vocational Rehabilitation's response, and how I was still looking for work. The staffer said she would report everything to her boss but said I could try a place called Central Iowa Employment and Training Consortium (CIETC). They helped people find jobs and maybe had openings.

Round Two at Work

A few days later I was at CIETC talking with the CEO, Ramona Cunningham. I gave her my résumé and answered questions as we talked about my history. A few minutes in, she stopped me and said they had a temporary position available in their IT department. One of their staff would be out for several weeks due to surgery and I could work until she returned if I was interested. I quickly accepted the offer, but I was also required to attend the weekly job fair on Wednesday mornings.

I learned CIETC was a division of Iowa Workforce Development which offered state benefits to employees, the exact medical benefits I needed. The head of the IT department showed me their main room, but it didn't have enough space for me. I was given my own office a few doors down from theirs. It was large enough for me to easily drive around and have my own desk. My bedside table fit beside the desk and, if I parked correctly, my feet would go underneath as if I was in an office chair. Another small table was just behind me where my caregiver could sit and have a view out the window facing the parking lot.

My first job was to get five new computers ready for distribution to job coaches. I needed to install a different operating system than what they came with and then the machines would go to someone else for further work. I asked for help with the first one, but soon saw it was the same process Tom and I had done to my home computer in high school. All I had to do was put in a CD, answer a couple of setup questions, then watch progress bars as the system installed. My new supervisor left, and she soon brought four more computer towers and two monitors to my office.

After more than an hour of watching progress bars and occasionally answering questions, the first computer was ready. I told Sandy what cords to unhook, and then directed her on how to set up the next tower. I started the process again and ate my sandwich I brought from home while I waited for the automated process to continue. Looking at my desk, I contemplated the possibility of updating multiple computers at once. The second computer finished shortly after my last bite of lunch, and I had Sandy organize a type of assembly line on the floor. Finished computer towers were on one side of the room and computers that needed work were on the other side.

Setting up computer three, I had Sandy move the tower and monitor further on my desk than the first computer had been. As I started the installation, I also directed her to set up the fourth computer on my desk. They both fit, along with a monitor for each. When computer three moved on to automated tasks that didn't require my input for a while, I switched the keyboard and mouse and once again started the routine. The fourth machine was well into its automatic work before I had to finish the previous machine.

My time for the day was up before I could get the last computer started, but I managed to work 8.5 hours and finish four of the five computers. Punching out for the day, I was told no overtime was allowed so I could only get paid for eight hours of work. On my second day on the job, I finished the final computer and was a little disappointed I could only do one machine at a time.

I finished the computer setup faster than my supervisor expected, but another IT member soon trained me on my next task. Whenever a counselor met with a client, they wrote what services they were receiving. The IT department then entered the interaction into the computer. I was shown the system that was used to enter information into the database and the reports from the counselors.

For every interaction, I had to enter the client's name, social security number, and what they did. Some people received assistance with childcare, others received tuition help, and a variety of services. It was simple data entry, but I made sure to enter everything carefully and check the correct boxes.

Unlike my first job, this was in an older building in downtown Des Moines. There was only a small staff room with a microwave and a few chairs and no cafeteria. I brought a sandwich or microwaveable meal for lunch and ate it in my office looking out the window. While waiting for clients, some of the counselors and other staff would drop in and chat with me while I worked or ate.

There was a total of four people in the IT department, including me. I always wore a watch but couldn't see it on my arm under my table. I could almost tell time without looking at it though. Every hour, at nearly the exact same time, several of the staff would leave the building for a five- to ten-minute smoke break.

Dave was one of the counselors and quickly became one of my most frequent visitors. We usually talked about my job search, school history, and different topics of the day. Along with helping clients, Dave also maintained the CIETC website. He joked that I was trying to get his job but without counseling people. Dave said a lot of good job coaches had been let go over the previous years due to budget constraints, which is why an office was available for me to use. He said he could watch a client skip and run across the parking lot to enter the building but develop a severe limp by the time they got to his office on the second floor. They then needed financial help due to having too severe of a disability to work. Several times, Dave said he wanted to bring these clients down the hall to meet me but didn't know if it would help.

Wednesday mornings meant attending the weekly job fair. I sat at the edge of a room full of people that were receiving assistance from CIETC. As I looked over the crowd, I wondered what faces belonged to the paperwork I entered. Job recruiters from UPS, Mediacom, and others would talk about openings as well as benefits of working for their company. Mediacom employees would only pay $5.00 per month for benefits and receive full cable television packages and internet. Most openings were in sales, going door-to-door, but some office jobs were open.

Anyone working with UPS had to start in a warehouse sorting boxes for a few years before moving on. If someone wanted to drive a brown delivery truck, it first required five years of sorting and a perfectly clean driving record. I noticed every week that few faces changed. Several in the group wanted to help with temporary jobs at the upcoming Iowa State Fair, but I started to feel most were perpetual job seekers in order to fulfill requirements for government assistance.

One vocal person in the room seemed to know the Des Moines bus system perfectly. If an employer gave their address and it wasn't near a bus stop, she would loudly respond with, "Oops!" I thought she would be a great fit for the Metro Transit Authority but was certain it had already been suggested.

Since I was at work during the day, I left my home air conditioner turned off. The system was only an over-sized window unit that had been built into the wall of the main living area. That meant the cool air had to travel through the room, kitchen, and down the hall before getting to my bedroom. Leaving it off saved electricity but made for a warm house to return to as July turned to August.

One day, I returned home from work and had Sandy turn on the air and then get me in bed. Since the room was hot, I had Sandy take my clothing off and put a fan on me so I wouldn't overheat. Just as I started cooling off, there was a knock on my front door. Leah and her husband were in Des Moines and stopped to visit. I hadn't seen her since her last day helping me before I left for college. It was nice to visit, but I didn't think I should remain in my birthday suit. Sandy put shorts back on me while we caught up in my bedroom turned sauna. I started to think it may be better to partially leave the air running while I was gone to keep my apartment a little cooler and avoid further surprise meetings.

Back in my office, paperwork slowly came to me, and I would almost have the information entered before the counselors returned to their room. By lunchtime one Thursday, I had already completed my tasks for the day and the afternoon looked just as slow. I talked with Dave by the staff microwave about the slow morning and he suggested I leave early. His suggestion took me back to lessons I learned from Dad.

As I was growing up, I often saw Dad go into the Town Crier early in the morning and come home 12 or more hours later. If work was busy and deadlines approaching, he worked to ensure everything was completed. At slow times, he didn't stay any extra and did various assignments for Mom at home. I had the same concept about my work. To me, it wasn't right to sit in my office and get paid to mainly look out the window. It felt like I was stealing from my employer to do so. I told my supervisor I planned to leave early so that work could maybe accumulate in the afternoon, and I could get it entered the next morning. She warned that one of the others may get the paperwork instead but didn't say I had to stay. I left a few minutes later, nearly three hours early and worked on web updates at home.

The next day, I was happy to see a small stack of papers waiting for me to enter. They were quickly finished but I was given a new project to keep busy. The new computers that I had helped set up were being distributed, with one going to an executive and everything needed to be transferred from their old computer to the new. The updated computer had a CD burner, but the old one only had a slot for a 3.5" floppy disk. I would need to carefully transfer every file, just a few MB at a time.

At home, I very carefully organized my computer's documents into multiple folders. I was thankful to see this person did the same and I didn't need to keep track of random documents. After one folder was transferred to multiple floppy disks, I put them in corresponding folders on the new computer. Sandy and I got a system going of numbering disks, then putting them back in the same order to transfer. The assignment took a little over a day, but it felt good to be productive and help my team.

My fellow IT workers couldn't understand how I got so much work done more quickly than they did. As I continued to get more data entry complete, I started getting more visits from the other technology workers. The all-female department started talking about each other to me, and I soon learned all the gossip in our section. One person said the other didn't have any formal training in technology and thought it was odd for her to be in such a position. Another commented that she had wanted time off but having a female supervisor sometimes caused problems. As the visits and conundrums continued, I kept working when papers arrived and nodded in response as I partially listened.

My night nurse, Mary, continued helping me in Des Moines and Pella, and I grew to know her well over the years. I told her about the situation at CIETC and she grinned. Mary's theory was that my fellow employees thought I was a mole. They maybe thought I worked for the state, or another company, and was planted to find problems in the IT department and recommend staff adjustments.

The idea didn't sound likely to me, but this was only the second time I worked at a full-time job. I wasn't familiar with office politics and regular interactions between staff. In late August, my time at CIETC was halfway through and I still didn't have any permanent plans in place.

Adecco called after I got home one afternoon and had another job assignment for me. I declined, citing I was working another temp job elsewhere. When the Adecco representative asked where the job came from,

I remembered their rule that I couldn't work for another agency. I briefly explained my meeting with Senator Harkin and the representative seemed satisfied. She said to let her know when I was available. Sandy's daughter had also signed on with Adecco and was called, likely to do the same assignment I was asked about. It was helping a company with web work and other technology updates. However, it abruptly ended weeks earlier than expected and her daughter could barely retrieve personal items from her desk before being ushered out.

With data entry at CIETC barely keeping me occupied, I was given the additional task of evaluating the counselors' performance. My supervisor gave me a list of clients assigned to each job counselor. I went through every name to see when they were last contacted and what services they were receiving. Clients attending school didn't need much interaction but others required at least monthly visits. Most of my checks found everyone was busy, except my frequent visitor Dave.

Dave let me know my supervisor got in trouble when I went home early and was tasked to make sure I stayed busy. The additional assignment helped, but I still had ample time to get everything else finished. I was told more jobs were done by the others that I could be trained in, but they didn't want to overwhelm me with too much work. Downtime allowed me to get out of my desk and to be able to fully tilt my chair. The summer of working and interviewing had taken its toll with another large pressure sore developing on my butt.

A few weeks before my temporary assignment was complete, the person I was filling in for returned part-time. She was friendly, easy to talk with, and hardly complained about the other staff. Soon after her return, I had a visit from my counterpart citing I needed to adjust how I entered the client interactions. The way I had been trained was backwards as to what should have been done. So, instead of marking yes to an activity and no to others, I was marking them incorrectly. I pointed out it was how I had been shown, but I would correct it for my final few days.

After my day job, I worked on updates for my web clients. The principal at Pella Christian High emailed me that he heard I was working and wondered if I would continue doing web development. I confirmed my job status but that it would soon be finished, and I would have more time for prompt response on web work.

I prayed almost nightly that I could be hired somewhere and stay living on my own. I was thankful for the years I had been given but wanted them to continue. I enjoyed making my own decisions as a responsible adult and giving my parents freedom for not having to help me as much. However, I would do whatever God had planned for my future.

As August neared its conclusion, my job assignment was also complete. As I went to the lunchroom on my last day, my wheelchair stopped responding to my attempts to drive. I tried turning it on and off, but it didn't change anything and Sandy had to push me back across the hall to my desk.

Just after I finished my final employee evaluation, Dave popped in to talk. He had lamented several times how he looked forward to getting a new building some day and listed the problems with the current facility. I was late getting to my second-floor office one morning due to the elevator not working, but otherwise I felt it was adequate. I told him about my chair trouble and he volunteered to help, if needed, when my shift was over.

About an hour before I left, Dave said he needed to leave early. I had my tasks almost finished and chose to do the same so Sandy could utilize his assistance. Before leaving, Mrs. Cunningham came to my office, along with a few other staff members. The CEO said she and everybody loved my work and that I had been a great help. Unfortunately, they didn't have the budget to hire me permanently.

After our goodbyes, Sandy pushed my table to the elevator and van while Dave pushed me in my uncooperative chair. It was a challenge not to roll off the van lift, but they got it without trouble. Back at my apartment, my wheels started sporadically working again and I was able to get out of the van without help.

Returning to Pella

I completed my classes in February, but AIB didn't have a graduation ceremony until September. A few days before officially graduating, I returned to campus to get my cap, gown, and to plan logistics with President Nancy Williams. A ramp had been made for me to get on the stage, but I couldn't grab my diploma as the other students could. I showed her how to tuck the award between my lap and arm rest so it would hopefully not fall off descending the ramp. After trying a few ideas, it seemed to be the best option.

Seven months after completing my degree, I officially graduated and received recognition for it. Taking pictures with my entire graduating class, I was easy to spot as the only person using a wheelchair. It was nice being on campus again and seeing my former instructors, even for a short time. It would be my last time visiting AIB or experiencing dorm life.

With no more job prospects and pressure wounds getting worse, it seemed best to move back to Pella with my parents. I did not renew my apartment's lease beyond September and all my belongings were moved for the final time. Combining my plates, silverware, pots, and pans with my parents' utensils made for a lot of superfluous supplies. Most of it was stored in boxes in the basement to be sold later at a garage sale. Other than a TV stand, my furniture had been borrowed from my grandparents and was simply returned.

My parents and I had developed our own separate routines that had to be adjusted. Living at home, I no longer needed nursing coverage for every hour. It saved insurance funds, but meant Mom or Dad had to stay up until my night nurse came at 10:30, even though 9:00 had become their routine bed time.

I called to cancel my renter's insurance and utilities in early October, just after my lease expired. Budget billing worked well, and I received some money back. I had lived on my own for almost three years, earned my diploma, worked two temp jobs, and had countless interviews. Now back in my bedroom in Pella, I felt a sense of defeat. I ended up right back where I was after high school and only had a plaque on my wall and another pressure sore from the experience.

In November I had surgery to close the sore with another muscle flap. This time, Dr. Rouce started by taking out all the bad areas and left an even larger hole to stabilize. Another surgery would be done in a few weeks to close the area with muscle. Between procedures, I had to stay in the hospital. I was allowed to sit on a specialized bed and could operate my laptop. The hospital said not to have valuables in my room but I wanted something to do.

Since I couldn't operate a call light and my vent needed supervision, I had sitters. As I sat in bed flying planes on my flight simulator, I had someone from medical transport sitting with me. As he sat with earphones in his ears, I soon heard loud snoring from his direction. The sound prompted passing nurses to check in and see if I was still breathing correctly.

While in the hospital, I got to know everyone. As my birthday neared, there was some talk of sending me to a nursing home for further recovery. The nurses worked it out so that didn't happen, but that made my 22nd birthday my last day in the hospital. One nurse made a chocolate dessert that she called "better than sex" cake. I didn't have experience to compare, but it was very good.

I was home before December and continued bed rest as ordered. The year had started off on a high but now ended flat. I wasn't sure what to do next but knew I didn't want to sit around and play games.

The new year would start a new adventure that had already begun.

19

TANGLED WEB

King Solomon wrote numerous proverbs to show that God desires us not to waste time and to live a productive life. In Proverbs 6:6-11, we are told to look to the ant as a work example. They stay busy, working in summer and preparing food for time ahead. Without fully realizing it, God had already provided a plan for me to continue working and serve Him in all situations.

I continued checking website accessibility for Criteria 508, but they didn't have much work for me. The company frequently wanted me to purchase more books or software to improve my skills and have further testing capabilities, but at my own expense. I decided they weren't a good fit any longer and chose to part ways. The four websites I obtained while living in Des Moines still needed webmasters, and I needed something to do.

Medicaid and Social Security had strict restrictions about how much money I could earn and have in my name. Owning a business would be impossible, so Mom and I would work together. She would be the official owner and help with paperwork and I would do web development for clients. I decided to use the name Vander Molen Technology, or VMT for short. I wasn't sure what to charge but picked an hourly rate that I thought sounded reasonable.

In spring 2004, I was able to sit again and be active. Pella Christian High wanted their website redesigned and they chose to use a company called The Design Center. They would make the site's design, then I would make it functional and continue to do updates after it was complete.

I was soon sitting in the teacher's lounge at school for our initial meeting. Four years earlier I was taking tests in this same room. Now I was considered a professional helping the school. The small web committee consisted of two faculty, Cheryl, from The Design Center, and me. We discussed what was needed on the site as well as different design options. After a few weeks of working with everyone, I decided I didn't care for committees. Despite some frustrating starts, it eventually led to a complete design to be given to the school for approval. It looked like something I could make work, so I agreed to the final project. This was more complex than what I had done before, but I kept working at it, piece by piece, and eventually came out with a working site that looked like the intended design.

While this project was going on, I also started working on the site for Pella Christian Grade School. Without advertising, I was starting to gain clients and earn a little income.

Since I was working but keeping an eye for full-time positions somewhere, I started working with Vocational Rehabilitation again. John was my new counselor and based near Pella. He was an older man with many years' experience in helping people. At our first meeting in my parents' family room, I couldn't help but notice he seemed nervous and on edge as we talked. He let me know that due to my past records, Voc Rehab would only help me with items related to VMT and not seeking other employment. He also was required to report everything they did with me to the governor's office. That explained his nervousness, but I wondered how the report requirement was added. I suspected it had something to do with Senator Harkin's office but wasn't told.

I had been using my same IBM laptop for nearly four years, but it was generally best to replace computers after three years. Voc Rehab agreed to a new computer with software for web development. I heard Apple computers had better graphics than Windows and were good for my type of work. I wasn't very familiar with their options, but I knew someone who was: Tom.

With the busyness of college life and living in different states, Tom and I hadn't communicated very much in the last few years. I emailed him to break the news I was looking at switching to an Apple and needed some guidance. Less than a minute later, my phone rang with an excited Tom on the other end. He said I should have warned him to sit down first, but he was more than happy to help. After looking at a few options, we figured out a good laptop that should work well. We also looked at software like Microsoft Office and the best options for web development.

A few weeks later, I had my new machine and a variety of boxes and CDs to install software. It took time to get my documents transferred from my old computer and new programs setup, but it was fun getting familiar with a different type of computer. I would also be able to communicate with Tom more easily but none of my games would work on it. Tom showed me how to set up a section where I could also install Microsoft Windows. Then I could still have my familiar entertainment and test new websites on most types of web browsers. It was the best of both computer worlds with one simple machine.

Whenever possible, my parents liked to get away on their own and often went on dates outside of Pella. These excursions often included getting groceries and household supplies from different retailers. On one outing that included shopping in Knoxville, near Pella, Mom noticed a sign hanging on the door at Pamida. It said a man from the area, named Ken, was a vent dependent quadriplegic living in a nursing home in northeast Iowa. He enjoyed talking with people and provided his email address.

I remembered hearing about him from local small town talk. Ken was a few years older than me and had been injured when I was in my early teens. We had a mutual night nurse for a few years as well, and I thought

I could start corresponding with him. Mailing him, I found Ken was easy to talk to and, sharing the same diagnosis, we understood our mutual challenges of daily life. However, most of his family had abandoned him and he only had state funding for insurance. That meant he didn't have the resources to live independently and had been forced into a nursing home a few years earlier. I couldn't imagine living in such a situation, but I could at least be a friend through email.

Summer came with volunteering at CHAMP Camp. Sandy and Karen came again, working 12-hour shifts. I felt much more comfortable this time and was able to get into the group activities more and provide more help with the campers. The concerns from the previous year were behind me and it was a recharge of energy working with the kids and seeing my friends.

A few weeks later I was back into the regular world, working on business needs. The principal of Pella Christian Grade School had moved on to another school in Michigan, and an interim was in place until a new person could be hired. He had been told I was the school webmaster and asked to meet with me to discuss changes.

Sandy and I arrived at the building to find the front doors held open by bricks. We got to the office a few minutes before my scheduled meeting and were greeted with a locked door. It had been several years since I had been in the building, so I showed Sandy around a little and located the picture of the graduating class of 1996. I was easy to find among my classmates, but there were now eight more graduating classes after mine.

Twenty minutes passed and still nobody came for our meeting. I sat in khaki pants and casual business attire as we waited in the hot non-air-conditioned halls. I started to wonder if the principal and secretary were in another room, so the two of us took a full tour of the facility to find every outside door open, but the building was vacant. Arriving back to the front, a parent came and asked us if the secretary or anyone was around. As we hadn't found a single person, we sent him on for another time. I considered going home to reschedule but didn't feel comfortable leaving the building open with nobody inside.

Finally, an hour after our scheduled time, the principal arrived along with a few other staff members. They had left for lunch and had forgotten about our meeting. As they unlocked the office, I followed them in and was thankful for the air-conditioned space. The interim administrator was a little surprised to see someone in a wheelchair, but I introduced myself and what I had been doing the last few months for the school. He asked me to redesign the site like I did for the high school, and I headed for the van less than five minutes after getting in the office.

I started the work of rebuilding the site the next day. I wasn't told to update any information, so after completing a new site template, I started copying the text and pictures from the old design to the new. Each grade talked about regular activities for the year and highlighted some of the special topics covered.

When I got to the page for second grade, I saw the last item listed for special activities was disability awareness. It made me wonder what they did and if there was a possibility that I could help. I quickly switched over to the list of staff and the same guidance counselor I had in grade school was still there, Mrs. Handthorn. She confirmed they still did the awareness section but it only consisted of watching a 30-minute video.

Mrs. Handthorn let me borrow the DVD so I could get an idea of what topics it included. The program was done by Joni Erickson Tada, and mainly covered her disability and answered questions from a class of kids. Joni was a quadriplegic but she could breathe independently and had some arm movement. She had a Christian ministry based in California and I was somewhat familiar with her. However, I figured I could likely do better than a video and decided to volunteer to speak with the students after school started.

As I continued to rebuild the grade school's site and work for my other clients, I was contacted by The Design Center. They liked the work I did for them on Pella Christian High's website. They had been working with another company in town for web development, but that developer was ceasing web work and moving to medical technology. I had casually been talking with Cheryl, the owner of The Design Center, about helping them; she finally agreed after seeing my work.

When the school year started, I completed the redesign for the grade school. I also started working on projects for The Design Center. Just as before, they designed the site, then I built and maintained it after the development phase was complete.

Disability Awareness Presentations

Several weeks after school started, I was scheduled to speak with the second graders. I made a presentation based on the video I had watched and my life experience in dealing with the public. I wanted to include portions to have the kids do something so I would keep their attention, but also cover material to help them learn. I had never seen an instructor bring notes to class when teaching, so I also needed to memorize my routine.

The day came, and I rolled into class with Karen beside me. I came in during recess to have a brief planning session with the guidance counselor. It was only a few minutes before the bell rang and 20 kids came trotting into the room. Mr. Joel was introduced as the school webmaster, and then it was all up to me. To my surprise, the students actually paid attention and seemed to be listening. They even eagerly asked questions when I allowed them. Then came the time to show mouth writing.

I demonstrated how I write my signature but forgot they hadn't covered cursive yet. One student responded, "I can't read it, but it looks neat." After my show and tell, it was time for the class to practice what they saw. They weren't quite sure what to expect, but everyone got out a marker and paper as I directed. After the students wrote their name with their hand, they put the markers in their mouths and tried to write like they saw me. After one attempt, I added a tip to not use the middle of their mouth, but their side teeth on the same side as their dominant hand. The second attempt was a little better, but still nothing legible in the room.

When the demonstration was complete, I continued with my memorized talk. While it ran through my head and out my mouth, I hardly noticed the kids were still laughing and showing off their new writing skills. I was well onto the next point before Mrs. Handthorn redirected the students' and my attention to what was happening. After several questions, I wrapped up 40 minutes after I began. Navigating through the school, I was soon in another classroom of 20 second graders. This time, I learned from previous mistakes and had the students put their paper and marker away after writing.

The Best Man

My volunteer week at CHAMP Camp didn't go well for my skin. A pressure sore developed in the same area as the previous one, and steadily became worse. Working with my plastic surgeon, Dr. Rouce, he suggested another muscle flap surgery was needed. In September, less than a year after the previous flap surgery, I had more muscle taken from my right leg to put in my butt. I was becoming very familiar with the process of staying in bed for several weeks afterward, but it still wasn't fun.

With my air mattress, I sat up in bed to work on my laptop. It wasn't much different than my regular routine, except that I didn't get up in my chair for church or anything else. Along with helping on clients' websites, I also found a company that produced books and podcasts teaching web programming and current trends. Learning on my own was a challenge but it helped with business needs.

The new Apple computer had different messaging software and allowed easier communication with Tom. We hadn't talked much during our college years but could now text or talk by video. He was nearing the end of his four-year degree in Michigan and was looking toward the future. He had done more than just study and work in school and had spent significant time with another student.

Tom had dated a few times in high school, but he would always eventually conclude we would stay bachelors. That idea changed though, and he was now engaged. Rianna, his wife-to-be, was from the Toronto area and the wedding would be near her family.

Through our messaging, Tom asked if I would be attending the ceremony. I quickly thought of all the packing and work it took for the routine trip of going to camp for several years. Going out of the country with all my stuff would be a lot of work. It would be great to see Tom get married, but I imagined it would be like previous weddings I attended. I would see the bride and groom for a minute or so in the congratulatory line, and then not see them again. I didn't want my parents to go through the work and expense of taking me and just feel like we occupied seats.

I replied that I would like to go, but it was most likely that he would get a nice card instead. Tom responded that he would let the wedding planner know they were back to square one as the best man wouldn't be able to come. This revelation was unexpected, and I was surprised to learn of his plans. At supper the next night, I told Mom and Dad about our conversation and being asked to be Tom's best man. They were also shocked at the prospect but said they would work to make it happen. I let Tom know the good news and he again contacted the planner with an update.

My head swirled with thoughts of my position in the ceremony and what responsibilities I would have. The only thing I had heard of best men doing was putting on a bachelor's party with questionable entertainment. Planning such an event half a country away didn't seem like a possibility, but I would see what could be done.

Walking by Faith

With the start of 2005, I continued working on more websites for The Design Center as well as my own clients. It was fun working with different companies and organizations and learning what they did. However, I felt limited in what I could offer them. I continued studying material from Sitepoint, but it felt like I never had the right skills when needed.

In October 2004, actor Christopher Reeve died about ten years after receiving his spinal cord injury. In that decade, he raised great awareness about injuries like his and increased interest in research on potential cures, treatments, and knowledge in general. After his death, many people in the medical field said he had lived an average life span for someone with his injury. Mr. Reeve had the same injury level and abilities as me. The comment reminded me of quad friends I had lost and the brevity of life with major medical concerns. I was thankful for the life God had given me so far, but always wondered how many more years I would receive.

February 20, 2005, marked the 20th anniversary of my family's car accident. It was a Sunday and, as usual, my parents and I attended church in the morning and evening. Just before the evening congregational prayer time, Pastor Zeilstra asked if anyone had requests for needs or thanks. I had already told him about the anniversary, and it was part of the petition.

My church gave thanks for the years God had given me and all that I had been able to do in the previous two decades. Life had not always been easy, but my family had been brought through it with friends and our church along with us. We didn't know what God had in store for me but would continue to trust His plan.

The weeks and months passed with Kid Care continuing to cover my night hours as well as some days with Sandy. Mary continued helping at night as she had for several years. However, family problems and her own health issues often resulted in frequent nights without help.

Whenever someone couldn't fill a shift, my parents had to cover the time. Karen would come around 9:00-10:00 in the evening to do my night routine and let Dad go to bed. When she left by midnight, Mom would take over until nearly 2:00 in the morning when Dad got up.

During my school years, I went to sleep when Karen finished. Now, I stayed awake with Mom so she could stay alert more easily. Playing computer games or working on a web project until the early morning hours wasn't too hard for me, but it was starting to get harder on my parents.

Mom couldn't move me, so I stayed in one place in bed until Dad woke up. He would then turn me, and I slept until my day nurse came at 7:00. Karen helped cover some nights when she could, but it was hard to find further help.

Planning for Tom's wedding continued with the date set for October 8, 2005. It would be Canada's Thanksgiving weekend and sounded like it would be a beautiful time of year. The ceremony was going to be held in a small church in a suburb near Toronto. Tom said there were a few steps to get in, but shouldn't be an issue for a small ramp.

After college graduation, Tom moved from Michigan to Madison, Wisconsin where his fiancé had already started graduate studies. They both took the five-hour drive to Pella so I could meet Rianna and get caught up with Tom in person. I was soon sitting in bed with my best friend on one side and a woman I had never met on the other. Tom and I chatted away about the last few years while Rianna listened and added some comments. A few minutes later, Tom excused himself to get a drink and left me alone with his bride.

I wondered what to say to a woman I hardly knew anything about, but asked how school was going. She had received her B.S. degree and was working toward a Ph.D. in biochemistry. Rianna started talking about parts of a cell and proper function and my mind soon glazed over with confusion. Tom returned a few minutes later with a slight grin and I was glad to change the subject to something I understood.

Travels and Opportunities

Before leaving the country, it was time for another volunteer week at camp. Karen was no longer able to go, so I had to seek other help. Mary agreed to do nights, with Sandy on days. However, since they were both employed through Kid Care, I didn't have enough insurance money for all-day care. Mary volunteered to take partial vacation time even while working so I could attend. With two nurses along, my parents and I made the familiar trip to central Ohio.

Most years, we stopped at a hotel in Dayton overnight and completed the journey in the morning. The overnight pause never seemed to go fast enough as my excitement continued to build for another week of working with the campers and counselors who had become good friends.

Twin boys were part of the campers in my cabin. They used breathing support at night but were otherwise completely mobile under their own power. I soon became the main counselor assisting them. I made sure they brushed their teeth, changed clothes, and got to bed on time for their nightly routine.

Keeping track of the twins and overseeing the waterfront were not my only concerns. My two caregivers had never worked closely together, and both had different ideas of how to do things. One would fold a pair of shorts and put them on a shelf. The other would see them, refold, and place them on the opposite side of the same shelf. It became a battle of wills with me as referee. I was thankful their shifts didn't overlap and made a mental note not to have such an arrangement again. However, the scenario would soon be repeated, and it was too late to make changes.

Since I was a delegate for the Youth Leadership Forum in 1999, I kept in contact with the organizers. YLF was still held in Ames every July on the campus of Iowa State University. For one lunch during the week, delegates were matched with a counselor, or member of the community with a similar disability, that could be a mentor. I had helped in the mentor lunch the previous two years and the other counselors encouraged me to return as a leader.

I figured since I enjoyed helping kids at CHAMP Camp, I could do the same with YLF. I applied over the winter and was accepted to volunteer for the week with Sandy covering days and Mary nights. Now I had less down-time at this camp which decreased caregiver interaction and my caregivers' behavior was much improved. This time, YLF paid for the cost of my assistants so they could both get their regular hours without insurance restrictions.

Less than a month after returning from Ohio, I was getting settled in a dorm room at ISU. Thankfully, I didn't have any large web development projects going on and Tom agreed to help with any updates while I was gone, both to camp and YLF. Orientation for YLF was brief compared to what I was familiar with. Every counselor was a former delegate, which meant every counselor had some type of disability. I was the only quadriplegic but there was a paraplegic and others with learning challenges.

Delegates also outnumbered counselors. Instead of 2.5 counselors per camper at CHAMP Camp, the average was one adult responsible for 2-3 teenagers. Counselors were expected to be up by 7:00 for breakfast every day and end each day with a meeting at midnight.

Immediately, I knew I couldn't be up in my chair for that many hours straight and I let everyone know I wouldn't be able to attend the night meetings. They understood my restraints and we reviewed all the high school students that would be coming. Nobody had extensive medical needs, but one teen had a heart condition and we needed to make sure he limited his activities. Another young lady had trouble with schizophrenia and needed certain routines to help her get through the day.

After a Saturday night pizza party near campus for counselors, the high school juniors and seniors arrived on Sunday. There were no outbursts of a welcome committee, just a sign-up table and directions to assigned dorm rooms.

Throughout the week, different classes were held to help the teens transition to adult life. It felt familiar to when I attended six years earlier, but it had some changes. The late July week was hot with outdoor temperatures around 90° with even higher heat indexes. The buildings were well air-conditioned in the low 70's. Going from outside to indoors felt like rolling into a wall in both directions that happened multiple times a day.

As the week progressed, the teens became familiar with the route from the dorms to the classroom building we were using. They started going out on their own, even though the college required a counselor to be with them. It became difficult to keep track of everyone but nobody got lost.

Tuesday morning had a session about sex education that a few counselors could skip if they wanted. The constant temperature changes and sitting upright in my chair was getting hard on me, so I opted to miss the session. I sat outside of the building during the hour-long activity, fully tilted back. The constant warmth of the sun felt good on my face and Sandy and I could take a much-needed break.

By Wednesday, the group took the regular trip to the Iowa capital building. Before that, we were bussed to a Marine helicopter base in Boone and toured the facility. I enjoyed seeing how maintenance was done on the machines and flight plans made by the pilots. I got the best of my two interests in one location as well. As the group watched a Blackhawk helicopter start its engines and takeoff, I also watched as a Union Pacific train passed on the horizon.

After the helicopter base, we left for the capital to take a tour and listen to the lieutenant governor talk about legislation. Just as in the previous years, the guard at the entrance to the capital gave me a confused look at the metal detector. A swipe with a wand cleared the wheelchair users for a roll through the capital. I had expressed concern on where I could use the restroom with my female caregiver. One of the counselors worked at the capital and, thankfully, she arranged a place.

Getting escorted back to our group by security, a man approached us and started talking with Sandy, ignoring me. He touted some company he was with that was working to solve "disabilities like his," pointing to me. He gave her a business card after the sale's pitch and promptly disappeared. Our guide said such confrontations weren't allowed in the capital, but he let it slide.

The evening concluded with supper at the Iowa Historical Building with a wounded veteran giving a presentation. One delegate was quite vocal in her opinions on the military and another young lady tried to keep her quiet. On the hour bus ride home, the second delegate rode directly behind me sobbing the entire way back. She was sure nobody liked her and wanted to go home. Another counselor and I tried to calm her, but not successfully.

With long days, my vent started to alarm low battery during evening activities. I was up in my chair longer than at CHAMP Camp and there was not enough time to charge my batteries overnight. To keep getting air, I had to sit in the back of classrooms, along with most of the other counselors, and have my vent plugged into the wall. It allowed me to get through the day but made extra work for my nurses and restricted how active I could be.

I was glad when Friday morning came, awards were given, and the week was complete. I was concerned about the lack of organization I had seen and that some of the delegates' medical needs were beyond our capabilities. One of the administrators said it had been noted before YLF started that one delegate should be excluded, but the board thought everything would be fine. In retrospect, they agreed more care was needed in selections, but I decided not to return as a counselor.

Breathing Issues

The last few days of YLF, I needed more suctioning than usual. Going from hot to cold and back again was hard on my lungs. I hoped it would clear up when I got home, but it didn't.

On the following Tuesday, I had my regular appointment with my pulmonologist, Dr. Hicklin. I generally saw him twice a year and chatted for a few minutes about life and any concerns I had. He would listen to my lungs, and that was the extent of the appointment. I expected the regular routine this time, but also to mention the unsettled lungs and extra junk.

When we exchanged our familiar pleasantries, I talked about what I did the previous week at YLF. When Dr. Hicklin listened to my lungs and heard about my experience, he didn't like what he heard. Instead of returning home as I expected, I would be staying in the hospital.

While listening to my lungs, Dr. Hicklin heard extra secretions deep down in the lower lobes. The best course of action was to go in with a camera and suck out the extra mucus. After getting settled in my hospital room, I was asked about being sedated, as most people were, but I declined. The procedure didn't sound much different than what I always did when suctioning and thought I would be fine.

My vent was removed and pure oxygen directed down my trach. The respiratory therapist then put his special suction tube down into my lungs to clear them out. After about 30 seconds I wanted to move to try and take a breath. The oxygen was keeping my stats where they should be, but my brain was saying I needed to breathe. Without the vent on, the only way I could bring in air was to shrug my shoulders. However, I knew that much movement would cause problems for the suction equipment and possibly hurt my lungs. So, I tried to signal for them to stop as my body started flinching with the battle of wills going on in my head. One part of me wanted to breathe while the other knew to stay still. Nearly a minute after starting, the therapist stopped and let me get a few breaths from my vent. He said I did very well, but it would need to be done again sometime in the future.

Mom was also anxious for me to get out of the hospital and back home. In four days, we were planning to have a 55th wedding anniversary celebration for her parents. It had taken several months of planning to get all my cousins, aunts, and uncles together for the weekend and arrange family pictures. If I was still in the hospital, then I would be missing from the activities and family picture archives.

After a day to recoup, the deep suctioning procedure was done again on Thursday. I was better prepared and knew what to expect, but still denied sedation. The same internal battle surfaced of wanting to breathe, but I was able to suppress the urge and let the therapist finish. This time, everything cleared out better and my lungs started to return to normal. With Mom's nerves near maximum, I was released on Friday afternoon, less than a day before the big party.

As August started, summer activities decreased as we looked forward to Tom's wedding. A lot of planning remained, I was having physical problems after a busy summer, and the trip ahead would prove to be more than expected.

20

WEDDING BELL BLUES

Genesis 2:24 says men and women leave their parents to be joined together as one couple. I had been to weddings before, but never had a significant role in one. As Tom's day came near, I looked forward to the happy times ahead. Unfortunately, they wouldn't last long for me.

While volunteering at camp and YLF, my pressure sores returned. Visiting Dr. Rouce again, he did what he could to try to avoid another surgery. He recommended I do as much as possible to reduce wrinkles and constrictors. The doctor said it was best to wear pants, or shorts, with nothing else underneath. Underwear was another layer to add problems that I did not need. My parents didn't like the idea but, in an attempt to help, allowed the commando dress code.

As October approached, the sore continued to get worse and surgery was needed. I didn't want to cancel on Tom for the wedding on short notice, so Dr. Rouce agreed to do another muscle flap procedure in late October.

I gave The Design Center and my other web clients notice that I would not be available to do updates for a week and would not have my usual backup. I told them I would be out of the country and unavailable.

Sandy agreed to help me overnight for the trip and the four of us were soon packed and headed east. I had never traveled during the fall before as Mom was usually busy helping at my family's grain elevator. Harvest was the busiest time of year at Pella Feed Service, with the year's crops being harvested and brought in. Leaving on October 4, four days before the ceremony, we saw several farmers in the fields bringing in the summer's growth.

We stopped overnight in Michigan before continuing to Toronto. The fall leaves were starting to turn and were beautiful. I enjoyed being in a state I had never visited and seeing new sights. The next day, before crossing the border, we made sure there wasn't any food in the van and my medications were in their correct bottles for easy inspection. At the border crossing, the security guard took our photo IDs and asked us what our plans were. We answered his questions and were soon on our way again. None of my medical supplies needed screening and nothing in the van was investigated.

Looking out the van windows, the scenery didn't look much different than the previous day's travel. However, the road signs gave a clue to the different location. Speed limits were much higher, at least 100 or more, and distances to upcoming towns were posted with further distances. However, the numbers were no longer in miles, and we could only guess the speed limit and just kept up with other vehicles.

Toronto roads had five or more lanes going in one direction with cars and trucks everywhere. It made me thankful to live in small-town Iowa and not have to deal with such conditions daily, but it was also part of experiencing new areas.

After a second day of driving, we arrived at our hotel for the next few nights. Mom got two adjoining rooms so Sandy and I could be in one during the night and my parents in the other. In the morning, Dad could bring me over to their room if needed so Sandy could sleep.

When the van was relieved of luggage, our small group went to find supper. Not long after sitting down at a nearby restaurant, Pastor Zeilstra and his wife greeted us. They had departed our church that summer and we hadn't seen them since August. It was odd being so far from home and being greeted with familiar faces. They had come a day earlier than needed so we would have someone around we knew. The groom's parents assumed Tom was in the area but hadn't heard from him.

Changing from the day to the night routine took Sandy some adjusting, but we started our second night together well. We both liked the room temperature warm but couldn't decipher the thermostat's numbers in Celsius. We guessed 22° and left it at that.

When morning came, I only had one task to do the entire day, to get fitted for my tuxedo. Dad found the shop, and Mom brought in a pair of dress pants that fit me well. It would be easier to compare the two pairs of pants than try to get me out of my chair, lay down somewhere, and then change clothes. I had given my measurements several weeks earlier, but my pants from home were different in length than the proposed suit pants.

Next, Dad attempted to get the tuxedo's coat on me while I was sitting in my chair. He tugged and pulled on the fabric as much as he dared without ripping it, but my right arm could not go through the sleeve. The shop owner took the adjustments, but rehearsal was the next day with the wedding on Saturday. She wasn't sure if everything could have enough adjustments in time for the ceremony but would try.

After the fitting failure, my parents and I had a free day to do whatever we wanted. Mom had researched tourist activities in Toronto and had a list of possibilities and some attractions she would like to see.

Visiting a different country and new area, Dad and I had different plans, watching trains. He drove around looking for rails and found a vehicle manufacturing plant. One area had large parking lots full of new cars and trucks and some were being loaded onto train cars. It was fun to watch the loading process, but the three of us moved on and found a place to sit by some busy looking tracks. It wasn't long before Dad was dozing in the driver's seat while Mom tried to keep entertained and not think about the places we could be visiting instead.

By late afternoon, the three of us returned to the hotel to do my stretching exercises and personal cares. Sandy had been able to sleep fairly well and joined us for supper. The tourist day in Canada concluded with driving through a large park overlooking Lake Ontario. Sandy first noticed squirrels running around, but they were black instead of the brown variety from home. The sun set as we sat in the parking lot of a GO Transit commuter rail station. It was the end of the passenger line, and we watched trains stop, unload, and head out in the opposite direction. Dad and I enjoyed the day of Canadian rails, but Mom wasn't so sure.

Tom's Wedding Rehearsal and Ceremony

Friday meant rehearsal followed by the bachelor's party in the evening. The small church was a short drive out of the city and through the rolling countryside. It looked like it might be pretty, but the skies were overcast with a gentle soaking rain. Upon entering the church, I was greeted with several imposing stairs. Tom had given various numbers of steps the previous few months, but said they weren't too steep. With the large obstacle in front of me, I wondered if his eyeglasses needed a major adjustment.

Dad unloaded the wood boards that had travelled with us from Iowa and set them on the stairs. The temporary ramp had been thoroughly cleaned so to be suitable for such an event. Tom made an appearance to check on ramp progress and confirmed he had arrived. I attempted to ascend the steep incline and made it up with Dad and Tom pushing behind me. My assistive devices took up most of the staircase, so we decided I would come up before the rest of the wedding party and the boards would be put somewhere else. After the ceremony, I could go to the back of the sanctuary, carefully back behind the last bench, and wait to leave after everyone else had gone.

Tom had two other guys standing with him, neither of whom I had met before. At one point during the service, the wedding party needed to leave the front steps and sit on the front benches. There wasn't room for me to turn around and not hit someone, so I had to back up without turning to look. I warned the other groomsmen to be careful and to watch their lower extremities, as I couldn't see behind me when reversing.

Running through the proceedings, everything seemed in order. It was my responsibility to hold the bride's ring until ready. Tom didn't want to dig in my pocket for it, so he decided to put it on my finger for easy retrieval. I wasn't sure this was a wise choice, but I let him decide. To help calm the groom's nerves, I tried to distract him with other thoughts, such as a new Apple computer coming down the aisle. He wasn't certain it was a good comparison or that his bride should hear such a suggestion.

After rehearsal, the wedding party headed to supper and then a bachelor and bachelorette party of sorts. It was a simple meal and a good time to get caught up with everyone and hear stories about how Tom and Rianna met. After eating, Tom arranged to have a party at his soon-to-be-in-law's house. We would be in the basement, but Tom said there was a gentle slope to the backyard and just a small bump by the walk-through door. It would be a simple task to get me in and out of the house.

I trusted Tom's evaluation and Dad arranged to follow someone to find the party. The sun had set, but the rain continued at a harder pace as we drove through the dark Canadian roads. The van was low on gas and we managed to stop at a gas station along the way. The price seemed very low until Dad remembered it was in liters instead of gallons. Estimating the familiar cost, it was fairly high priced. Dad got as little as he thought we needed and continued through the moonless trip.

Arriving at Rianna's parents' home, I couldn't see much in the dark except a wet lawn. Tom directed Dad and me to the side of the house, through the grass, and down a fairly steep hill. My wheels didn't have much grip going down and I mainly had a controlled slide.

Driving my chair a little further through the yard, I got to a small cement patio outside a sliding glass door. The small bump Tom said would be easy to get over was easily a foot high. Dad attempted to get some of the grass and mud off my wheels before entering the house but could only do so much. Dad then helped pop my front wheels over the step into the house and he and Tom picked up the back of my chair to get it in.

Sandy stayed with me at the house while my parents toured the area for a couple of hours. It took work to get in, but I was sitting in the basement of a home in another country surrounded by people I didn't know. Tom and the guys took over the basement with Rianna and the girls upstairs. The homeowners provided punch and other drinks, but I only took water after hearing the punch was spiked.

Tom convinced me to play poker, without money, with a few of his friends from college. I had only played the game once before and hardly knew what a good or bad hand was. It wasn't long before I lost all my chips, but everyone was friendly and fun to get to know. A few hours after I arrived, it was time to depart through the same route I entered.

Getting down the steep embankment was easy, but then I had to get up the rain-soaked hill. Dad warned me not to spin my tires and just go at a slow pace. While holding an umbrella, he helped push while I tried to slowly drive. Rianna's father also came to help get me up and out of his yard. Just at the steepest part, my forward movement stopped. I gave my chair a little more power, and my wheels spun in the mud. With more pushing and spinning, I made it to the top just as Tom came to check on our progress. I left a few deep ruts in his future father-in-law's yard, but he said it was only progress toward a proposed landscaping project.

Once back in the hotel, Sandy and I quickly went through my night routine so I could try to sleep. Saturday morning came with the wedding only a few hours away. Sandy's shift finished at 7:00 a.m., but it was too early to get in my wheelchair for the day. Dad picked me up from my bed, carried me through their hotel room, and laid me in his bed. I breathed on my own for a minute, with Mom holding the ambu bag while Dad moved the bed vent to join me.

The Dutch are known for cleanliness and keeping everything neat and organized. At special events, it was extra important to have everything polished to perfection. Dad followed our ancestry and now applied it to my chair. The previous night's adventure left my wheels caked in mud and it needed to be clean before appearing at the ceremony.

Mom gave me a report of his progress as I laid in bed waiting for Dad to get me ready for the day. He took the phone books from our two rooms and propped them under my rear wheels. With the makeshift chair lift,

Dad cleaned the grooves of the tire tread with the hotel toothbrush. He didn't want dirt all over the floor, so he carefully picked it up and dumped it in the trash can. The project had started long before I woke up, and it took well over an hour after I was transferred to meticulously clean every surface so it would be presentable again.

Before the wedding, pictures were scheduled for the bride, groom, and wedding party. As the time drew near, Dad turned his focus from my wheels to getting me ready to go. When my limbs had been stretched and hair washed, we began the arduous task of getting my tuxedo on. Pants and undershirt weren't too hard, but the tuxedo coat was a challenge. Dad got my left arm in and the coat around my back, but the difficulty was with the final arm. After a lot of pulling the coat and bending my arm, it reluctantly slipped on. Dad carefully tossed me in my chair and figured out how to place the tie around the vent tubes.

Friday's rain clouds cleared out for a sunny, but cool, early fall day. We found where the bride and groom were taking pictures and got me out of the van. Tom saw us and called for me to join him down a small hill through the grass. I thought briefly about the mud but concluded the morning sun had probably dried it out some. I started to head from the dry rock path toward the field and heard Mom yell, "No!" I quickly stopped and looked for a different path that didn't require off-road traveling.

The photographer had everyone get arranged in various configurations for pictures in the park. I was thankful my altered suit fit, and I looked like the other groomsmen, although sitting.

After the wedding party had sore mouths from smiling, we headed to church for the ceremony. As soon as we arrived, there were yet more pictures to take. When that round was complete, I went up the steps into the church so my ramps could be put away. The pastor then approached me with a document and said I needed to sign the marriage certificate as the best man. Dad had wandered away for a minute, so I explained to the pastor how I sign. He was a little reluctant to stick his own pen in my mouth, but it was our only choice. The quality of my signature depended heavily on how steady the paper was held. This man's seminary school evidently didn't practice such a task as I attempted to sign a moving document. I ended up getting something resembling my name, but not my best.

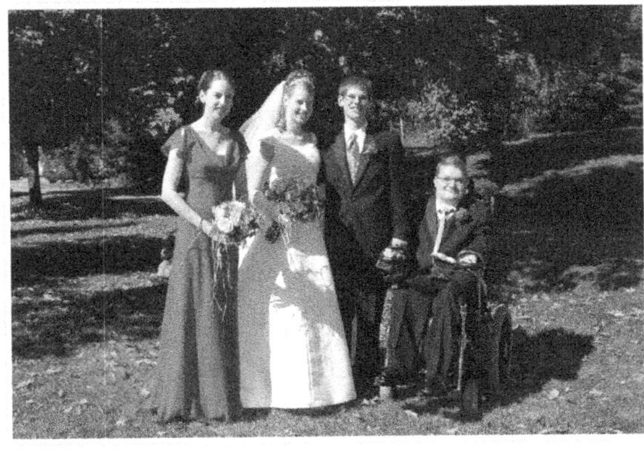

I navigated to the front of the sanctuary for final preparations as guests started to arrive in the small facility. As we discussed, Tom put Rianna's ring on my hand for easy retrieval. As he slid the ring on a finger of my left hand, I made sure to answer, "I don't." We were great friends, but not getting married. The photographer made sure to get pictures of the process as well.

Now that my job for the day had started, I went to my parking space behind the last bench. The rest of the wedding party waited in the basement until it was time to enter. I smiled and nodded as guests walked by with curious looks, but eventually the ceremony began. I drove up the aisle beside the maid of honor and took my position beside Tom.

With a bird's eye view, I watched my best friend take his vows and take his wife's ring off my finger. I expected my arm to shake and jump with a muscle spasm in response to the touch, but it didn't happen. Everything went well and we were soon retreating down the aisle, after the new couple briefly had their first kiss.

As the church slowly emptied, I sat in my spot patiently waiting for ramps so I could depart. As I waited, the pastor came to me for another signature now that the vows were complete. His practice from the first round helped, but not by much. Dad got the boards in place again after the crowd departed and he and another groomsman helped me back down the steep decline. I was thankful to be done with stairs and steep descents. My parents and I then picked up Sandy from the hotel and went to the reception hall.

We arrived before the bride and groom, so I found my spot at the head table. On every table was a centerpiece consisting of a part of a cell; protein, nucleus, and several names neither my parents nor I could read. Each name came with a short description of its function. It was a unique arrangement that could only be done by someone working on a doctorate.

After everyone arrived and was seated, the bridesmaids and other groomsmen started telling stories and gave prepared speeches. I didn't know a speech was part of my job description and had apparently missed it at other weddings. I thought of something while my turn approached. I reiterated being at my grandparents' 55th anniversary that year and looked forward to celebrating this couple's anniversary. It was short but seemed to pass the test.

My parents and I stayed long enough to see the start of dancing after the meal. One of the bridesmaids asked me out to the dance floor, and I agreed. However, my only dance experience was at camp, and I had no idea what to do with someone that wasn't familiar with wheelchairs. Wearing long pants, I couldn't see the end of my footrests to see how close I was getting to her legs. I carefully guided the front of my chair from side to side somewhat to the music and attempted to keep my focus on her face instead of lower dress. After a couple of songs, we stopped dancing, and I was glad to head back to the hotel.

It was a long day, and one I won't forget. Through all the activities, I didn't get much opportunity to tilt my chair. As Sandy got my suit off, it was apparent my pressure sores had not done well. Blood and other drainage had oozed out of the bandages and onto my rented clothes. Thankfully, with the shirt tucked in, the tuxedo pants stayed clean, but the bottom of the shirt didn't fare as well.

On Sunday morning, my parents wanted to leave early. However, I learned on Saturday that it was also my job to see that everyone returned their tuxedos. Thankfully, Tom's parents were willing to wait until the rental location opened so we could get going. Sandy attempted to sleep in the van as the four of us headed back toward Iowa.

Returning Home

Just before crossing the border into our home country, we stopped to see Niagara Falls. Sitting outside near the railing, it was neat to see the water gushing over the edge. As the fall air blew across my face, all I could concentrate on was the cold. I tried to enjoy seeing one of the wonders of the world, but soon had to return inside the visitors' center. I only stayed outside a few minutes viewing the attraction that some people travel across the world to see.

Crossing the border at Buffalo, New York was the same process as getting into Canada. The agent questioned Mom's place of birth as he looked at Sandy's passport. A quick explanation of the hidden passenger in the back satisfied him and we were cleared to enter the United States.

The route home was different than when we had gone to Toronto. Our first hotel was in Altoona, Pennsylvania. On Monday morning, my parents and I let Sandy sleep for a few hours at the hotel, and we headed to a nearby landmark known as Horseshoe Curve. The mountain grades required railroad engineers to add numerous bends to the rails and at one section included a 180° curve. It became a popular destination for railfans and included a museum, park, and type of elevator called a *funicular* that brought visitors up to the rails.

Mom and Dad had visited the park a few times while I was at CHAMP Camp and were familiar with it. I was looking forward to seeing it as much as they wanted to bring me. Sitting in the parking lot, I couldn't see the tracks above us through the van's roof, but I could hear train wheels screeching around the corner. After paying the entrance fee, I drove onto the lift and took a sideways trip to the top.

Having rails halfway surround me was fun, as well as watching a train negotiate the curve, but the weather was the same as the day before at the falls. The cold, damp, fall air whipped on my face as I sat in the elevated park. I wanted to stay and watch trains, but my coat wasn't warm enough and we soon went back to ground level. We entered the small museum and gift shop at the bottom and the warmth inside the building was a welcome relief. Dad drove back to downtown Altoona and found a place to sit by the tracks to give Sandy more time to sleep.

As we sat, Dad kept opening his window as he thought the air felt good. His opinion of ideal temperature was also great for snowmen, but I had different preferences. Sitting in the middle of the van behind the front seats, the cold breeze seemed to go directly on my face. I started shaking my head to keep moving and to stay warm. The shaking rocked the entire van, so Mom would frequently remind him to keep the window closed.

By lunch, Sandy was ready to go, and we continued driving west. Our next stop was in Dayton, Ohio, at the same hotel we had used when traveling to camp a few months earlier. I liked being in a familiar area and closer to home. It had only been a week, but it was filled with once in a lifetime memories. At least, I reminded Tom, it would only happen once.

Another Muscle Flap Surgery

In November, on the day after my birthday, I had muscle flap surgery again to close the pressure sore on my right butt cheek. This was the third surgery in three years in the same area. Dr. Rouce said he left some muscle on my leg to use again for the next time. I didn't think it was funny but was glad to know some remained. I was getting tired of constantly dealing with pressure sores and surgeries that didn't seem to work. This time, the doctor also took a bone sample and tests came back with an infection. He put me on an I.V. antibiotic that needed to continue while at home.

Christmas was approaching and I would still be on bed rest and not allowed in my chair. Mom and Grandma Labermen arranged for the entire family to come to our house for our regular celebration, all 40 of them. It was a tight squeeze to get everybody in, and the house was filled.

Beside my bed was an I.V. pole connected to a line in my arm. At one point, Dad quietly had everyone leave my room while he changed canisters. Other than that, I had frequent visitors coming through my bedroom.

For the kids to open presents, they were required to be where I could see them. Watching my cousins' children and younger cousin's faces light up when opening gifts made me feel part of the celebration.

With the close of 2005, it had been a full year. Events that were difficult to participate in were made possible by God's grace and my parents working to make them happen.

As another year started, I endeavored to make changes that weren't always the best decision.

21

ROUND TWO

In Matthew 6:34, Jesus said, "Therefore do not worry about tomorrow, for tomorrow will worry about its own things. Sufficient for the day *is* its own trouble." When difficult times come, this can be hard to remember. I knew the verse but did not take it to heart and I allowed worry to cloud my decision making.

Most people look forward to a new year and starting with a fresh look on life. As 2006 began, trouble with caregivers continued to increase. The previous few months, Kid Care had an increasingly difficult time covering my night shifts. Nurses didn't want to make the drive from Des Moines to Pella, and several were unwilling to work with someone that was ventilator dependent.

Mary continued as my primary night nurse and trained anyone new that the agency sent. During the 8.5-hour shift, she would start to show my regular night routine as I also talked through my needs and assured them that I was able to explain all my procedures. It became frequent for a nurse to train one or two nights, but then not come for their first shift alone. Others would leave halfway through training, citing they were uncomfortable working with a vent.

With every person, I tried to emphasize that I would gladly answer any questions and that my parents were just on the other side of the house, if needed. Mary also told potential caregivers that I was able to breathe on my own for short periods if conditions were correct. Despite these assurances, few stayed on for very long.

Rhoda had helped me during junior high and high school, and she came back to help some nights. She also had a sister, Audrey, who lived in Pella and was a retired schoolteacher. Audrey agreed to help some nights and cover shifts as needed. Neither of these women had formal training in healthcare but were able to learn and completely take care of my needs. Since they didn't have nursing licenses, they couldn't work for the nursing agency, but my parents could hire them privately. My parents paid my providers out of their pocket, but the amount given would be reimbursed from insurance. The necessary paperwork kept Mom busy, but it allowed my shifts to be covered. It was also less expensive than nursing agency rates and extended the time I had before reaching my lifetime cap with insurance.

During the day, I continued working in web development and increased my number of clients. The Design Center and I built more sites for churches and small businesses. Between their clients and mine, I was responsible for maintaining over 30 sites. Some only required updates a few times a year, but others had weekly changes.

Tom helped me with regular updates, or constructing new sites, when I started getting behind with work. He became an unofficial second employee of VMT and was a big help. We made sure to have regular employee meetings that consisted of playing computer games over the internet while maybe discussing work needs.

Early in the year, the application for camp arrived and I gladly filled it out. Sandy agreed to help me during the night and Karen would help during the day. With the paperwork complete, I looked forward to another year of helping the campers. About a month after everything was signed, Kid Care started asking questions about how camp was run and how insurance handled the funding.

My insurance policy allowed for a case manager who knew my situation well. I spoke with her often when correcting a payment error with supplies or nursing. She knew about my volunteer trips, but since I was using an Iowa based nursing agency, and doing all my regular cares, it wasn't a concern. They paid the same just as if I was home and didn't need to adjust anything.

That answer partially satisfied the agency, but they also wondered if camp was under the direction of a doctor and what licensing was required. Dr. Chuck was the head physician and helped the campers first, but also assisted the counselors if a medical need arose. Since it was a volunteer week and not at a medical facility, the nurses, respiratory therapists, and other specialties didn't need to get Ohio licenses if they were from a different state.

Kid Care didn't care about how the other counselors worked, but said Sandy had to get an Ohio nursing license. Without it, they wouldn't let her help me at camp. I needed to be independent in my care to volunteer as a counselor and couldn't do that without Sandy's help. Thankfully, she was willing to do the work required and started studying for an Ohio nurse's license.

Pursuing Higher Education

I studied web development trends and technologies on my own time but was still unable to build everything my clients needed. I also continued volunteering with the Rock Island Technical Society, doing some site updates. My main contact was still fellow railfan Dick Tinder. He taught computer courses at Simpson College in Indianola, and I thought it would be a good way to increase my knowledge and get my Bachelor's degree.

By April, I had completed the enrollment information, given my AIB course information, and had gone to an orientation class for adult students. Indianola was about an hour drive from Pella through winding country roads. Orientation was three meetings at Simpson's three campus locations.

The instructor leading the class was friendly and I easily understood everything he covered. As the orientation continued, I learned Mr. Little was in charge of campus accessibility and helping students with disabilities. AIB hadn't had such a person and I looked forward to having an easier time getting help. As he took us on a tour of the main campus, he was careful to point out ramp locations, accessible bathrooms, and the one area on campus that didn't have wheelchair access.

Tuition was part of the three-section course, and the part I wasn't sure how to manage. Going part-time, I knew the cost would be less than traditional students, but I did not want to rely on my parents' assistance again. The last orientation evening was in West Des Moines where Simpson's evening classes were held. Dad came as my assistant as I didn't have anyone else available.

It was a very warm night for April, but I was thankful Dad was willing to take me. The final activity of orientation was writing thoughts about the class and future schooling on a small piece of paper. Trying to whisper to Dad what to write didn't sound easy or like something I wanted to do. Instead, Mr. Little allowed me to go home and email him my response.

Whenever the temperature rose, the van would have trouble running at low speeds or when idling. Using premium gasoline usually solved the issue, but this night's heat was unexpected. As Dad and I got in the van to drive the 50 miles home, it reluctantly chugged to a start. We encountered a few problems when going to Des Moines, but the problems appeared to be worse. Driving through the streets of West Des Moines, the motor chugged a few times, but it got us to the interstate. At highway speeds, it worked better, but we didn't dare try to go all the way home with the motor threatening to quit and leave us stranded. After a few dozen miles, Dad pulled off to another suburb east of Des Moines. Every stop light and stop sign could mean the engine would stop and not be able to start. Dad slowly coaxed the van into each intersection, trying not to fully stop, while we thought of all the gas stations in the area and guessed which ones would have premium fuel.

After driving past a few stops, our quest for high-end fuel was not found. The two of us debated on routes home that had the least requirements of stopping. Now late in the evening, the dark Iowa countryside seemed to close in as I thought of other people with wheelchair equipped vans who could pick us up if we got stranded. We approached highway 163, our road home, from a two-lane road that only had stop signs at the intersection. We prayed there wouldn't be any opposing traffic that would require us to stop, and we could keep moving.

Half a mile away, we could see the four-lane road ahead and car lights. Dad slowed on a slight uphill grade and it looked like we had a break in traffic. He decreased speed as little as possible to turn and, coaxing the van, headed toward Pella. I dozed a little for the next 30 miles as the motor was running better at highway speed. As our destination approached, we saw emergency lights approaching in the rear-view mirrors.

Dad reluctantly slowed to let an ambulance pass and heard the engine sputter. He thought this chance encounter might doom our trip and leave us in the middle of open fields. Thankfully, the engine revived and got us to our exit. Back on city streets, the stop and start scenario began again. A few blocks into town, we approached a red light and the engine died as we slowed down. Dad was able to coast into a parking spot on the side of the street as he decided what to do next.

Our ailing van had nearly gotten us the 50 miles home, but now it refused to start. The parking spot we were in was directly across the street from the BP gas station with premium fuel. The motor started long enough to get us across the road, but not to a fuel pump. My watch beeped at 10:00, indicating that my night nurse would be coming in 30 minutes. From this point, my chair could get me home using nearly two miles of sidewalk through town.

My cousin Brian, also Dad's coworker, returned home from bowling to his house, which was directly in front of where we were parked. Reluctantly, Dad asked him and his roommates for help to push the van. With all the men adding muscle, they got the 3.5-ton vehicle to the gas pump. The station was closed, but the card operated pump topped off our tank with the premium fuel we needed. With the additional liquid in the tank, the motor started up with no trouble. Dad thanked me for leaving class early and we got home just as the night nurse pulled into the driveway.

The next day I contacted my Vocational Rehabilitation counselor to see if I could get any financial assistance to return to school. John said that, based on the decision of 2003, it was unlikely for me to find work, so he would not approve any help for school.

Mom and I talked about the situation, and felt I was being discriminated against due to my disability. We also thought that if any other quadriplegics tried to get help for employment, my situation could be used against them to also deny them funding. I found Amy's contact information in my address archives. She had helped me in high school to prepare for college and I hoped she could offer advice again. Amy directed me to an advocacy group that helped people with disabilities get funding for different needs.

I didn't get the information until late in the workday, but I called the phone number I was given to continue making progress toward school. A woman answered the phone and gave her name, but I missed what she said. I attempted to succinctly explain my situation but didn't really know how to start and tried to make sense. The voice on the other end of the phone replied, "You don't know who you're talking to, do you?"

With a hesitant tone, I slowly replied, "no." She said it was Waneta, one of the counselors I had worked with at YLF. The name and face came to mind, and I was relieved to have someone familiar who knew me. Waneta said she was heading out and had hesitated to take my call but would get in touch with me soon.

Champ Camp, Car Troubles, and Goodbyes

Camp came in June and all of Sandy's licensing was complete. Kid Care covered her expenses, but she could not be on the clock helping me except in Iowa or Ohio. Therefore, we could not stop overnight in Indiana or Illinois on the way home and would need to drive 600 miles in one shot.

Driving to Ohio was very routine with Dad rarely needing to look at a map. The summer solstice was a few days away, but the temp quickly rose and felt like it was much later in the season. After several hours on the road, we neared our regular stop for lunch before getting to the busy Indianapolis area. The Hen House, a restaurant with a tall red barn shaped sign, signaled our exit. Dad slowed as we reached the off-ramp and departed the interstate. The van suddenly chugged and died before reaching the stop light at the end of the exit. Sandy and I had experienced our own van problems and were familiar with the scenario. However, it was a first for Mom and Karen and they weren't sure what was happening. A Shell gas station was nearby, and Dad was able to partly drive and coast to a fuel pump.

He got everyone out of the van to walk to the neighboring Arby's that we visited annually. I started down the sidewalk, only to see that it ended before our destination. I didn't want to try to go down a four-lane road in the wrong direction, so I slowly bumped through the grass until encountering a 6" curb. An employee from the restaurant saw our plight and quickly came out to help me negotiate the bump.

Dad topped off the van with fuel and came around to join us. After lunch, we continued east to our destination of Dayton, Ohio. As always, traffic in Indianapolis was busy and moving well over the posted speed limit of 55 mph. The chaos of cars was familiar, but we liked it when it was behind us.

Almost past the city, Dad took the exit to Interstate 70 that would take us directly to Dayton. Just a mile after entering the highway, traffic was completely stationary. Dad quickly negotiated the van through traffic from the left lane to the shoulder three lanes over. As soon as he stopped with the rest of the vehicles, the engine died. Cars and trucks slowly shuffled forward around us as the van convulsed with small amounts of movement.

From previous trips, we knew this section of interstate was busy the entire 150 miles to Ohio. It was unlikely we would make it there, especially not before Sandy was due to be on the clock. An on-ramp was just ahead of us with vehicles reluctantly entering a freeway that resembled a parking lot. We eventually drove past the ramp, and Dad concluded the best course of action would be to reverse up the on-ramp, using the shoulder.

The rear windows of the van were covered with luggage and were useless for seeing anything. Dad used the rearview mirrors with Sandy attempting to look behind us as we slowly progressed backwards. After 15 minutes of stopping, restarting the van, and inching our way up the narrow shoulder, we made it to the top of the ramp. We were now greeted with another four-lane road, traffic lights facing the opposite direction, and trying to back onto the road with limited visibility.

Dad knew he would only get one chance to get the engine going again, so we sat and monitored the lights and traffic to time their frequency. Finally, Sandy said it looked clear for us to move, and Dad got the van running and quickly reversed while traffic was stopped. A turning school bus nearly sideswiped us as Dad quickly halted. He somewhat calmly commented on the situation before trying again, this time successfully entering the road and driving in the right direction again.

The gas tank was nearly full already, but Dad got us into a fuel station and topped it off. Looking at the atlas, he and Mom saw a secondary road that nearly paralleled the interstate. It was approaching 4:00 in the afternoon and the day's heat would start decreasing soon. Highway 40 would be slower driving but might actually get us there.

Travelling on the new route, the van did fairly well. Going through small towns in eastern Indiana felt like an entirely new trip. It was more scenic and less stressful than our regular interstate route. As the sun set low on the horizon, temps cooled, and the van started running better. We made it to Ohio before Sandy was scheduled to take over, with time to spare.

When morning arrived, the five of us made the short trip to Recreation Unlimited near Ashley, Ohio. When Mom and Dad dropped Karen, Sandy, and me off for our week, they would have their vacation, which would also include fixing the van before returning home.

Like me, several campers had graduated and were too old to return as kids, but they still wanted to attend and experience the week. Two other alumni campers had also been volunteering as counselors, but now there were too many of us to effectively run the camp and care for the campers. To remedy this, an alumni week was held at the same time as camp. Some could serve as counselors, but we were mainly considered adult campers for the week.

CHAMP Camp normally used two of the three bunk cabins at Recreation Unlimited. This year, alumni campers and our support teams lived at the third cabin and didn't have much interaction with the kids. I chose to continue volunteering as a counselor during the week and helped with fishing at the waterfront. It was fun seeing some of my old friends from my years as a camper, but some were missing as they had passed away. One alumni camper, Greg, introduced me to Camrin, his girlfriend. Greg was three years younger than me, but we had spent much time parked close to each other under ceiling fans in the non-air-conditioned cabins. Another alumni camper came for the week but hadn't gone through the application process. His surprise appearance prompted some in-house fundraising for his caregivers' room and board. Some of the alumni participated in the activities while others discussed forming a governing body to start an alumni camp. My full interest was in working with the kids, so I didn't spend much time with the alumni activities.

At the end of the week, four campers graduated and were surrounded by those of us who had been before. They were told about future possibilities of outings by graduates and maybe a weekend camp. It sounded positive, but I was doubtful anything would happen.

Administrators from CHAMP Camp told us they would no longer allow counselor applications from alumni campers. A camp dedicated just for us would be the only way we could experience the summers we loved. After seven years as a camper and five years volunteering as a counselor, I couldn't imagine no longer having camp. It had become my only regular trip outside Iowa and was an important part of my life. The thought of not returning and having to say goodbye to a place and people so familiar felt like losing a piece of my heart.

By Friday, it was time for families to arrive and everyone to return to regular life. My parents enjoyed their week on their own, but one day was spent with the van in a garage. The fuel pump had been replaced as it was likely the cause of the engine's problems. Before camp, Dad had looked at having it done in Pella, but didn't like the estimated charge. He was very pleased that the cost in Ohio was half the price of previous quotes. The long drive home went without any problems, except occasional snoring from the three of us who had been at camp.

Mounting Stress and Worries

Back home in Iowa, I returned to solving other problems. I talked with Cheryl from The Design Center, and she was willing to be a witness to my work ethic and how school would help. Her only concern was that I continued working with her on web development and not look for other employment. I scheduled a meeting with Waneta and John at my house to see if an easy resolution could be made, but the meeting wouldn't be until early October.

Power wheelchairs were designed to last around five years, at least according to insurance. Mine was now nearing ten-years-old, twice the amount of time it should have lasted. Dad did very well at keeping it working, but he was beginning to have trouble finding parts. In 1996 Mom said the next chair would be my responsibility. I knew it might take a while to find a solution, so decided to start the process.

In late August, one week before classes started at Simpson, I had an evaluation of what chair I needed. Since I hadn't stood in several years and already had broken a bone, I wanted to try a standing wheelchair. They weren't very common, but a few companies did make them. The occupational therapist wasn't sure it would work for me but added it to my list of requirements. It also needed to be the same length as my current chair, including the vent tray.

I declared my major as computer science, taking two classes at a time, one with a technology emphasis. I would commute to Indianola three days a week for two hours of class. Mom thought it sounded fine, but only as long as the weather was good. If it was snowing heavily or had the possibility of ice, then I would stay home.

With my monthly social security income and wages from VMT, I could just barely cover tuition. I would have to pay in segments during the four-month semesters. Adding the cost of fuel for the van would make the venture more difficult, and if my work income decreased, I wouldn't be able to pay. If I couldn't get help, then my goal of getting my next degree would not happen.

Considering my course credits from AIB and taking two classes at a time, I would graduate in 4.5 years. At the current rate of use, I would also reach my lifetime cap for insurance at about the same time. The scenario sounded very familiar to what I had gone through for my first degree and was not something I wanted to repeat.

To an outsider looking in, my life seemed to be going well, but I was struggling to cope with the world around me.

To an outsider looking in, my life would have seemed to be going well. Unfortunately, I was struggling to cope with the world around me. I frequented an online forum called Care Line. The site was for people with all levels of spinal cord injuries. Members ranged from newly injured individuals, people with many years of experience, family members, and caregivers. It was helpful talking with others that knew what daily life was like, and where I could say what was on my mind. I could also help families who recently received an injury and didn't know where to begin.

Ken and I also continued to communicate through email and occasionally on instant messenger. He typed much slower than me and I felt bad replying more quickly. I wondered if I somehow was showing I had more abilities than Ken and I didn't want to hurt his feelings.

Living in a nursing home for six years, he had experienced poor care. Ken had nearly died a couple of times due to being denied suctioning and almost drowning in his own fluids. He also had been in bed for over eight months. The nursing home said they didn't have enough staff to get Ken in his chair. However, since he had been abandoned by his family, Ken thought the nursing home just ignored him since nobody helped monitor his care.

School started at the end of August with my thoughts going in multiple directions. Even just starting, I liked what I saw of Simpson. I brought a few of my bedside tables to use in my classrooms and met with Mr. Little. He already knew I would need to do tests in another room so I could tell my assistant what to write. In class, note takers were also common and this had been arranged before I asked. It was a welcome start to have disability resources in place.

At home, everything wasn't going as smoothly. Mary frequently called to say she could not cover her night shift due to health or family problems. Kid Care couldn't find other nurses to cover the time, and they often went open. My daytime help, Rhoda and Audrey, could do scheduled night shifts, but not with short notice. Karen had a daughter-in-law, Sara, who worked as a Certified Medical Assistant overnight at a local nursing home. After a short interview, Karen and I trained her to do my cares. Unfortunately, Sara could only help on occasion when her primary job allowed.

With little sleep and extra stress, the combination was having an effect on my parents and me. Mom would get ill from not having her regular sleep schedule and needed additional rest and several days to recover. The routine continued where Mom and I stayed awake until nearly 2:00 a.m. when Dad took over. With my bedroom lights on and staying active, it helped Mom stay awake. However, not getting turned to my side as much as usual allowed junk to build up in my lungs that I then had a harder time getting cleared. Little sleep also made for an irritable family. Starting school again was something I looked forward to, but Dad said it was a waste of time and money.

When my day nurse left at 5:00, my parents and I ate supper in my room. The rest of the evening they left me to myself unless I needed something. Even though they were just down the hall, we all enjoyed having our personal time away from nurses and having some peace. Alone in my room, on my computer, I could work on websites, homework, or anything else.

By September, the increasing nursing problems had taken a toll and turned my thinking to the future. I knew the status with little care could not continue for my parents or me. Thinking of Ken and his living conditions in a nursing home, I didn't want that for my future. I reasoned that the best course of action, if everything continued its present course, was to discontinue my vent and trach and end my life. I was thankful for everything my parents had done for so many years, but I wanted them to be free of having to help me.

I reasoned that the best course of action, if everything continued its present course, was to discontinue my vent and trach and end my life.

The online forum I had been frequenting to help others with spinal cord injuries became my source of help. I posted what my living situation had turned into and wanted to look for resources to prepare for whatever was to come. Writing online was the one way I could live a private life, on a public forum, without my family and caregivers watching and knowing what I was doing. The exercise helped to calm my thoughts and consider my options.

My two courses at school were a basic computer introductory class and persuasive writing. I found both subjects to be relatively simple and didn't require much work. It felt like I was living one life that I showed those around me, and another life I mostly kept hidden from everyone I saw in person.

I confided in my nurses Sandy and Mary to tell them what I was planning, and also Tom. With working full-time and a year into marriage, Tom was busy. However, he still helped me with some web work and was always available to listen.

Several members from the online forum offered support and understood what I was going through. Some gave suggestions to contact the media or church to try to find more caregivers. Others offered resources for people looking to make living wills or end of life decisions. One member, Brenda, had access to state resources that could help people affected by spinal cord injuries. Through email, I told her my history and how I was looking to end breathing support. She found a lawyer in Iowa City who did living wills and was willing to help, so I called him to see how to proceed.

Part of my goals through Kid Care was to get exercise by practicing my frog breathing or breathing on my own. I didn't have energy to do anything other than breathe, so I didn't do it very often. However, Sandy and I experimented with a plug that completely sealed off my trach, called a decannulation valve. With the vent off and the stopper in place, no air could go through my trach. It allowed me to pull air in through my nose and mouth by using my neck muscles.

Being free of tubes and vent noise was very relaxing. If Sandy left to use the restroom while I was breathing, I would stop to see if I could go long enough to pass out. I could get up to a full minute without taking in air, but my instinct to breathe became too strong after that and I would gulp in a few breaths.

> *In my mind, I kept telling myself that ending my life was not according to God's will.*

In my mind, I kept telling myself that ending my life was not according to God's will. However, further contemplation always lead me to conclude it was the best option. I had already lived twice as long as the statistics gave me, and this would just prevent future problems. I talked with the lawyer from Iowa City on the phone and agreed to work with a student from the University of Iowa. We set a date to meet at my house and go from there.

I told Mom that Kid Care was requiring clients to have living wills. Since I was already on a vent, we had to be careful with wording and that's why a lawyer was involved. When one lie comes, more are required to cover them up.

As I worked on being freed from this earth, the October 5 meeting came with John and Waneta. When the two sat down at my dining room table they acted like old friends that knew each other well. Waneta started by asking what could be done to help me with school. John said that Voc Rehab would agree to assist with the cost of technology related classes. The stipulation was they had to potentially help my work with VMT. Anything outside of that, or toward looking for other employment, would not be approved. It wasn't what I expected to hear, and I was preparing to have a legal hearing. This solution would help me with school, but anyone else in a situation like mine might get the same treatment I had experienced, of being told to just go to a nursing home. I agreed to the terms so I would get assistance for the semester I already had started. It felt like a win and a defeat at the same time.

With multiple projects happening at once, I still managed to do adequate work in my classes. It took some adjusting to get back into a school routine, but I seemed to fit in. In English, the students were assigned to write papers on various topics. For every assignment, first drafts were given to another student to review. They would give suggestions for changes, and then the completed project was submitted for grading, along with suggested critiques. One time during the semester, every student would read their paper to the class. Everyone then gave written feedback before the final product was submitted. My full class review would come in late November, just before my 25th birthday.

Before my writing review, I had my first meeting with the lawyers from Iowa City. My official representative was Karla, a law student nearing the end of her courses. Her instructor, who I had spoken with on the phone, came along and did most of the talking. I explained again what life had become and what I expected the future to be like. I would complete a living will, but wanted to look at what it would take to get my trach removed and stop receiving breathing support. I explained that I didn't want to hurt my family and wanted to keep everything quiet. Mr. Sanders said that we could work on the removal when the directives were complete, but the media would likely want extensive coverage. I didn't want to be a public spectacle and decided to add a clause to that effect to my directives.

We went through who I wanted to have as my contact person. It needed to be someone I trusted, preferably around my age, and not a close relative. From Mr. Sanders experience, close family sometimes doesn't honor someone's wishes, especially in difficult circumstances. I didn't have many people that fit the requirements but suggested Ken as a possibility. However, he was quickly dismissed since he couldn't come and be present for me in an emergency. Tom was my primary choice, but I added a couple of cousins just in case he wasn't available.

Every section of the advanced directives had different medical procedures and I had to declare what I did or did not want done for each item. It took nearly an hour but the three of us got through it. A clause was added about nursing homes. If I had to live in a facility as a permanent residence, the clause indicated what treatments I would continue or stop.

When every section was complete, papers would be sent to my contacts for signatures and the directives written in legal terms. When that was finished, the lawyers would return for signatures and provide me with the paperwork I needed to have available. What I was originally seeking to do was not going to happen as I planned. However, it was the best solution and I felt better about whatever may come.

In school, the due date for my paper's full class review was quickly approaching. Stem cell research was a popular topic in the news as a potential cure for spinal cord injuries and other ailments. I wrote on the benefits of using adult stem cells for treatment and research instead of embryonic cells. For research, I thought it would be good to interview Rianna, Tom's wife. She didn't have any experience with stem cells, but I got her thoughts on the issue and whether it was morally wrong to use embryonic cells for testing. If nothing else, I thought interviewing someone who had a biochemistry major sounded good in my citations.

When it was time to read my first draft, Sandy arranged all three pages of my report on the table in front of me. I could turn the pages with my stick if they were stapled together, but this would be easier and faster. Just as I was ready to start reading, Mr. Smith directed the class to read my report to themselves. He didn't have me read it out loud like all my other classmates. I was baffled as to why he changed the routine for me, but I didn't question anything. I quietly read my own writing while everyone else did the same.

A week later, it was time for another exam in Mr. Smith's class. As usual, I went out of the room so I could tell Sandy what to write for answers. This time, Mr. Smith followed us and handed the test to Sandy. He said, "You read it to him, so he knows what to tell you to write." After the test, Sandy and I talked about these instances, and we guessed that he thought I was illiterate. It would explain why I didn't get the opportunity to read my paper in class, but I wondered how he thought I did my schoolwork. I didn't ask him about it, though, as the situation never came up again.

In early November, between classes and legal work, I tested a possible new chair at Advanced Rehab Technologies in Des Moines. It was a regular wheelchair with four wheels and a long support beam from front to back. I had seen similar models at camp. However, it was too long to fit in the church elevator. I came back in early December to try again after adjustments were made. Unfortunately, it still didn't fit the space requirements even after extensive modifications. I didn't like making them start over again, but the chair technicians would look at other manufacturers and get back to me.

Two days later, Mr. Sanders and Karla returned with my completed living will directives. They didn't allow Sandy in the room as we went over everything one last time. It all looked correct to me, and Sandy was allowed back to the room to help me sign. Official copies would be sent to my regular hospitals and documentation to my designated representatives. If I ever needed to change contact persons, then the entire process would need to be started again.

It had been a busy year with new experiences, but I was reminded of my past years when I watched the local evening news. When I lived in my apartment in Des Moines, the last place I worked was at CIETC. It was no longer part of Iowa Workforce Development and had been purchased by a local college. Investigations found that my former boss, Ramona Cunningham, had not been honest with her pay or with a few of the board members. She had improperly spent over $1 million and was now in custody and facing federal prison time.

I remembered the last thing she said to me three years earlier, that I would have been hired if funds were available. Investigations didn't say when the spending spree started, but I was sure the misappropriated funds could have covered my salary as well as a few more counselors. If I had been hired, it was possible that I would have lost my insurance through the state and would have had to go to a care facility like Ken.

As December continued, a family at church had twins that came earlier than expected. The Van Hoerkels also had a young daughter, Rae, and needed help with childcare. James, one of the twins, went home after a short time in the hospital, but his sister Elaine needed to stay longer. If James was to be allowed in the NICU, he couldn't be in childcare with other kids. Mom and a few other families volunteered to watch them instead.

It had been several years since I had cousins that age around me. It was fun having an infant and 2.5-year-old around the house. Mom fit in well as an adoptive grandmother and remembered how to walk while holding a baby. I imagined what it would be like if I had married and had kids. My parents and I loved children, and I knew they would be good grandparents. Now that I was back in school and around more people, I wondered if I would find someone to date.

My first semester back at college finished on December 11. With all the activities outside of school, my grades weren't as high as I had hoped. As 2007 approached, I prayed it would be a better year and not as difficult.

Unfortunately, major challenges were ahead that would change everything I relied on.

22

ON THE HUNT

Paul was chosen by God to be His messenger to the Gentiles. After his conversion to Christianity, Paul served God through many trials. In 2 Corinthians 12, Paul prays that a torment may be taken from him. God's answer was "my grace is sufficient for you." It can sometimes take adversity to remember that God is in control. I was given the opportunity to learn this well.

Classes resumed at Simpson in January 2007 with one programming course in Java and a history class. Driving back roads to Indianola three days a week in the winter wasn't always fun, but weather remained favorable most of the time. The regular schedule meant Sandy went with me on Mondays and Wednesdays and Karen accompanied me on Fridays.

The hour-long commute gave me plenty of time to talk with my caregivers. I had known them both for years and could easily discuss any topic. I was thankful I had great care and could be independent without relying solely on my parents.

Kid Care continued to provide my nursing services even though I had aged out of their system seven years earlier. Sandy was the only day person they provided and Mary the only help at night. With Karen and Sandy, 5-6 days per week, 8-9 hours a day were covered. Nights were a different story.

As a single mother, Mary liked having overtime, and covered the 9.5-hour night shift five days a week. The remaining two nights were filled by Rhoda or my parents. Winter weather added to the problems as Mary couldn't always make the 20-mile drive to get to work. It wasn't an ideal routine but time was mostly covered.

Late in January, I went to wake up my Apple laptop and nothing happened. I tried a few different options, but nothing worked. Tom was more familiar with Apple computers, so I found his phone number and gave him a call. Using the phone to contact him was an oddity so he knew something had to be wrong.

Tom walked me through a few more options to get it to turn on but nothing worked. Turning to Apple support it was determined my hard drive had crashed. I lost everything I had on the computer, work files, nursing billing records, schoolwork, and personal documents. It took a few weeks to regenerate my information, but some was lost forever. I learned to store all important files so they were always backed up, preferably somewhere online or on a separate hard drive.

CHAMP Camp again adjusted their policy of not allowing alumni campers to apply as counselors, now a maximum of two would be accepted, based on first come first serve. As soon as applications were open, I filled mine out and hoped I was quick enough to be one of the two chosen.

The Van Hoerkel family from church continued to be regular visitors. The twins, James and Elaine, were now home, but Elaine continued to have health problems. Some of her challenges included needing help from a suction machine. Since I had a suction machine at my dorm in Des Moines and at home in Pella, I had an extra one I wasn't using. On Saturday, April 7, while Sandy was covering my daytime hours, Mom and Dad took my extra suction to the Van Hoerkel house but they weren't home. My parents put the machine on their enclosed porch and left for a day of watching trains and spending time together. About an hour later, I got a call from Dan, my church's new pastor. Elaine had been taken to the hospital in Des Moines that morning but had passed away on the trip. Dad was their elder, or church contact person, and needed to know. My parents had just recently purchased a cell phone for emergencies, and I called it to let them know the update. They were shocked by the news and returned home.

Easter Sunday was the next morning, and at church the Van Hoerkel family sat on their usual bench directly in front of us. Rae promptly scooted under the bench to sit with my parents while four-month-old James squirmed in his mother's arms to join his older sister. Since not many people had the opportunity to meet Elaine, her mom asked me to put together a presentation of pictures for the funeral. This wasn't how I expected to use my knowledge of PowerPoint, but I was glad to be able to help the family any way I could.

Just a few weeks later, the spring semester finished at school. I had completed my first year at Simpson with a total of four classes. After summer vacation, I looked forward to taking more courses in August.

Continuing to work toward a new wheelchair, Advanced Rehab Technologies had another system I could try, a Permobil. The two companies each sent a representative to my house with a chair to try. I had seen this brand of wheelchair at camp, but it was rare. The system was completely backwards from my current chair with large drive wheels in the front and small turning wheels in the back. The demonstration model looked okay, but I wasn't sure about getting used to steering from the back instead of the front. I saw on their website that they did have a standing option. I asked the Permobil salesman if it would be possible to test that model. I explained that it would be good for my bones, and it would have a shorter overall length when upright. He answered that people who used ventilators weren't paired with standing chairs. It was uncertain how long vent tubes would need to be and I would not be able to test one. However, they left the demonstration model so I could try it for a few days.

As I attempted to drive it, the turning felt awkward, and it seemed like it barely had enough strength to move. Dad looked at it carefully and said the chair's main weight was on the smaller wheels instead of the large ones and he didn't like the chair's manufacturing. With my vent tray on the back, it was also two inches too long for the church elevator.

Back in Des Moines, the chair technician with Advanced Rehab said they could possibly shorten the vent tray, but cutting into it would mean the chair was mine. I decided this would not be a good option and needed to look further. The technicians and company were great, but they didn't have experience with a chair brand that would cover my needs. Advanced Rehab said they would not be able to help me and not to contact them further.

About the time I returned to school, I started going to Pella Hospital for physical therapy. I did a stretching routine multiple times a day but couldn't remember the last time I saw a physical therapist for an update. It was likely I was doing the same routine since coming home from the hospital over 20 years earlier and thought adjustments were probably needed. Insurance only allowed a limited number of physical therapy sessions per year, and I had to be careful how many I scheduled.

After getting transferred to an elevated mat, I carefully watched how my feet, legs, arms, and hands were moved. If my lower half was given a deep stretch, I could somewhat feel the muscles. It was a great sensation to feel my feet and not just see them. After a 30-minute session, my limbs and entire body felt very relaxed, and I had fewer muscle spasms.

Two people were needed to lift me between the exercise table and my wheelchair. The physical therapist normally picked up my legs and lower half while Sandy got my armpits and upper half. On May 7, after a regular session, I was halfway between the table and my chair when the therapist lost my lower half. In the blink of an eye, Sandy caught me and managed to get me safely in my chair. Dropping me could have resulted in broken bones or other injuries, but thankfully everyone seemed to be okay.

Later in the day, a few minutes before the end of her shift, Sandy sat me up in bed when my afternoon care routine was complete. The pant leg on my shorts bunched up on my leg as I went upright. Sandy pulled on the material to straighten it out and recoiled from pain in her arm.

Kid Care called the next day to inform me Sandy had hurt her arm and would not be back for three weeks. Karen and Rhoda could help cover some of Sandy's hours, but my parents would need to take off work and cover the extra time. I was thankful it was early May and hoped everything straightened out in time for camp.

Three weeks passed with a mix of people filling in the time Sandy had been scheduled. We were looking forward to days getting easier again when the nurse scheduler called. Sandy would be gone another week and my case manager from Kid Care would be calling soon.

June 1 came with no word from anyone at the nursing agency, so I called the scheduler to get an update. Sandy had signed paperwork saying she would be my caregiver at camp. Her Ohio license had also been renewed, but Sandy needed to return soon to help pack and get me ready to go on my volunteer week. After expressing my concerns, the voice on the other end of the phone spoke up. She wasn't supposed to tell me, but none of the supervisors would call. The scheduler told me Sandy had requested not to come back for concern of injuring her arm further. Kid Care was responsible for covering 8.5 hours every night and 8-9 hours five days a week. With Sandy gone, only five nights were filled, and the remainder would be left to my parents.

Thankfully, I was selected by CHAMP Camp to be one of their two alumni counselors, but with two weeks to go until camp, it looked like it would no longer be possible. I had just finished reading the book of Job and how he was tested by God through tragedy. In the end, he received more blessings than he had at the beginning of his life. The thoughts I had a few months earlier of removing my vent and being done with life quickly came back to mind. However, I reminded myself to trust in God's plan in whatever may come.

Rhoda's sister, Audrey, stopped over to say hi and see how my family and I were doing. She hadn't worked with me for several months due to other responsibilities, but we remained friends and kept in communication. Audrey wasn't fully aware of everything that had happened, but was disappointed to hear about Sandy leaving and the uncertainty about camp.

After further discussion, she volunteered to help take care of me during the night. Karen was covering my day hours and she offered to bunk near me and assist with some of my night cares and continue to help during the day.

Mom gave Audrey a tearful hug as I quickly and gratefully accepted her offer to help. Audrey would miss a national teachers' meeting she had planned on attending, but knew how important my volunteer week at camp was. Karen also heard about a nurse, Miranda, who had left an organization in Pella due to burnout. She was possibly willing to get back into nursing and could help cover my open days.

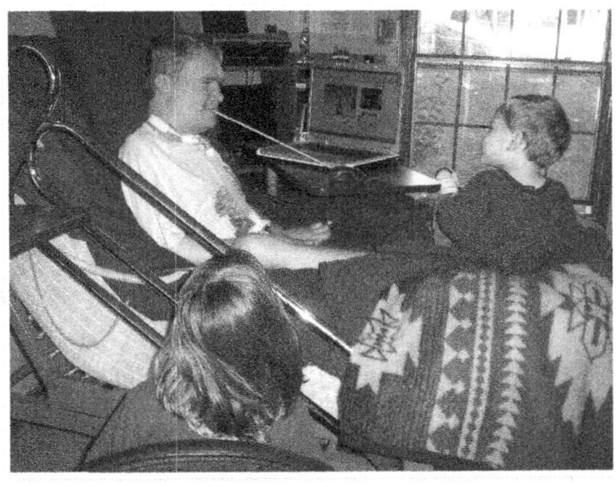

With everything going on, it was a nice break to have friends come for visits. Rae and James Van Hoerkel came over, along with their mom, Ruth. Karen had me up in my chair so I could help entertain Rae while Mom and Ruth chatted. Her third birthday was coming up in a few weeks and we liked having the kids around the house. At first, the active toddler wasn't sure why I couldn't play with her on the floor, but she quickly adapted to activities on a table I could reach. After frequent visits, she soon got used to my equipment and that it was just part of me.

As the family prepared to leave, I noticed Rae bend down in-front of me, stand up, and give me a confused look. I paid closer attention to her actions and saw her stoop down, tickle my feet, and look for a reaction that didn't come. Ruth attempted an explanation to the confused child, but I watched her repeat the process again and gave the laugh she had anticipated.

With camp quickly approaching, Mom, Karen, and I started the extensive packing process. With five people and their luggage in the van, it made for tight quarters. I needed to be sure to have all my supplies for the week, but extra air space needed to be removed from the bags to make room.

Just three days before leaving for Ohio, Mom and I arranged an interview with Miranda, the potential assistant. She was very boisterous and talked a lot, but was friendly. As I sat up in bed with my legs stretched in front of me, Miranda would grab a foot and shake my leg for extra emphasis on something she said. I waited for the resulting muscle spasm but my legs didn't react. After the second foot shake, Mom warned her that such activity could cause problems and it was quickly stopped. Miranda had some experience in working with trachs, suctioning, and my other cares, but not with spinal cord injuries.

Mom and I thought everything went well, so we agreed to start training after I returned from camp. Miranda was an RN but we thought it was best to hire the nurse privately instead of through Kid Care. Then the hourly cost would be less for insurance and she could start working sooner.

CHAMP Camp and Parents Day

A few days later, after packing the van, we made our way east to Ohio with Karen and Audrey as my assistants. This would be my sixth year as a counselor and fourth in charge of fishing. The week was planned to have a pirate theme for the dance and camp decorations. Getting in the spirit, Audrey packed an inflatable full-size pirate as her date for the dance. The widowed retired teacher told her adult children she was seeing a man named Piraté. They were happy for their mother, until pictures after camp told the full story.

My bunk was in the back of the boy's cabin, a short distance from the campers' beds. Dad helped Karen unpack and set up my bedside vent, humidifier, and various supplies, in places where Audrey could find them in the dark. Karen declined to sleep in a separate, quiet, air-conditioned cabin, and took a bed directly beside me in order to help at night, if needed.

After a weekend of counselor training, campers arrived Monday to the usual loud chants and cheers. I wondered if Audrey could sleep through the noise, but also was glad she could experience camp. On Tuesday afternoon, my trail group went into the woods for stream study. Some campers traded their wheelchairs for bean bags by the water and others walked around carefully searching for crawdads. Every year, it was a competition to see which group could catch and release the most crustaceans.

Cory was a new camper, and he normally used a walker. As some campers scoured the water, another counselor held his hands and helped him walk down a metal ramp to a platform a few inches above the stream. I was parked in this same location watching for escaping crawdads that I could direct campers to find. I moved over to try to give more space, but quickly became Cory's standing aide. He gladly held onto my arm and played with my watch while I chatted with the hardly verbal boy. I made sure not to move my chair and gladly helped Cory stand in place. After about 20 minutes, he reluctantly received help to his walker for the journey back to the cabin.

That night, Cory became ill and had to spend extra time in the cabin away from commotion while he rested. This wasn't the first time such a scenario had occurred with the campers. I somewhat jokingly told my fellow counselors that if a boy started using me for support, it could be a sign of upcoming sickness. I wasn't sure if the kids felt like I was a comfort or if my help made them ill, but I didn't want to test my theory.

On Wednesday morning, everyone had an early wake-up time to get to a unique activity. Camp arranged an accessible hot air balloon that could give everyone a ride. As the sun rose, I watched campers carefully back their wheelchair into the large basket. Along with a couple of counselors, they soared up 60-70 feet until the aircraft was straining at its tethers.

Once all the campers had gotten a lift, counselors were given the opportunity to take a ride. I asked to go, and Karen and I were soon on our way up. The burner felt hot a few feet above my head, but at least it was only short bursts. As we reached our maximum allowed height, the basket lightly rocked at the end of the ropes. It was a quiet rest floating above the ground with everyone below looking small. After several seconds motionless, we were soon descending and back on solid ground. As we landed, multiple counselors leaped onto the basket to keep it from bouncing. I never expected to be able to ride in a hot air balloon and was thankful for the chance and excited to see the campers experience it.

Not long after breakfast, everyone was off to different activities. It was also visitors' day with some counselors' families and camp donors coming for a few hours. Mom and Dad had been dropping me off and picking me up from camp for 13 summers, but never got to see what happened during the week. Mom's parents made the drive to Ohio to celebrate grandma's 77th birthday and join my folks for a few days touring Amish country. But on this day, the four of them visited CHAMP Camp.

For me, each day started out on the fishing docks on Lake Crumb. After collecting my parents and grandparents from the front gate, Karen and I ushered them through the campgrounds to the water. When the campers arrived, I gave the same safety instructions and order of events I had memorized years ago, but it was fun showing my family how I helped.

Mom, Grandpa, and Grandma chose to take the pontoon boat tour of the small lake. Dad remained with Karen and me, tracking how many fish the campers caught and trying to stay clear of freshly baited hooks flying through the air. The boat tour concluded before my time at the waterfront ended, so one of the camp leaders took my family on a golf cart tour to other activities.

We met up at the boys' cabin an hour later to recap their visit. My parents were glad to finally see camp in its entirety and not just when everyone was leaving. Grandma told me she had a hard time not crying seeing so many children with vents and medical needs, and she was thankful that such a place existed and for everything the campers were able to do.

During the down time between morning activities and lunch, some campers received medical treatments while others hung out in the cabin's common area. A game of UNO was starting, and another player was needed. I said my goodbyes to my family, thanked them for coming, and joined the game.

On Friday, my parents returned to pick us up to return to Iowa. Although physically exhausting, Audrey said she greatly enjoyed the week and wanted to look at next year's schedule to see if she could go again.

The Freedom of Breathing

After another Saturday night with no nurse, Miranda came to train with Karen on Monday morning after camp. I was impressed with how well she learned my cares and was willing to drive my full-size van. My schedule put her on two days a week, and it looked like days would be fully covered, but nights continued to be short with Kid Care only providing Mary. Rhoda helped as well, but it still left frequent openings. Sara, Karen's daughter-in-law, was able to do more hours, she was also fully trained, and by July she was a regular on the night schedule.

VMT was slow with few updates for existing clients or large projects for new sites. Tom talked with a couple at his church in Madison, Wisconsin about helping me with web development. I already did their church's website, and the man was interested in a website for his seed company. Soon, Tom and I had a very large site to build and carefully keep track of information to get it on the right pages. I never knew how many varieties of tomatoes, sweet corn, and other garden vegetables existed. After a few months' work for both Tom and me, the site owner was happy with the work, and it went live to the public.

When classes at Simpson started at the end of August, everything was going well. Introduction to Database was a fun class with basic programming. It was a course I could see might apply to VMT for future sites. My second course, Literature and the Human Condition, didn't seem to have any real-world application, but all I needed to do was read classic literature.

Having most of my nursing shifts covered again made for a great summer. Mom and Dad could do their own activities during the day, and I could get out when I wanted and have time away from my computer. The only times my parents watched me were Monday-Thursday evenings, all day on weekends, and when someone was sick.

With the change in caregivers, I had to adjust who I utilized for certain cares. Every other week, I changed my entire trach. Sandy had been the primary person for this, and we had gotten into a familiar routine. While sitting up in my bed or wheelchair, she would position a mirror in-front of me so I could see my neck. In one swift move, Sandy would disconnect my vent, take out the trach, lay it on a table, and insert a clean one. In the few seconds without the breathing aide, I would look around the hole in my neck for any red or sore areas. Everything usually looked good, but other times I spotted areas to monitor.

A month before Sandy left, the swift change was interrupted when she realized the clean trach was missing lubricant, but the old one was already out. As she promptly grabbed the K-Y Jelly and applied it, I shrugged my shoulders in an attempt to breathe. I received a good gulp of air through the hole and mouthed, "I can breathe, you don't need to hurry." Sandy replied, "I thought you would be able to." After about a minute sans-trach, the clean hardware was easily inserted.

Now with Sandy gone, I chose Mary as my trach change nurse. Doing it at night meant for later bedtimes, but I didn't mind. It became our regular routine to be slow in reinserting my clean trach, giving me more time to inspect for problems. After talking with my ENT, he allowed me to leave it out for up to ten minutes at a time.

I had to change the trach alternating weeks, but I was allowed to do it as often as I wanted. I started having it out a few times a week and quickly worked up to my maximum allowed time without it. Another talk with my doctor got my order changed to an unlimited amount of time without the trach, as long as the new one went in easily. As a result, my night routine changed in that when Mary came, she would get me undressed for the night, cathed, then sit me up in bed for my Bible reading. After getting positioned, I had the vent turned off, the trach plugged, and trach ties taken off my neck. I figured out how to do my self-breathing, so I didn't pop out the trach until I was ready. Looking ahead in the night's reading, guessing how long it would take, I took a larger breath and blew out the trach about halfway through reading.

For 22 years, I had constantly heard the ventilator running beside me and having air shoved in my lungs. I also had full feeling of my throat with an ever-present feeling of the trach, sometimes with painful rubbing. Now, for a few minutes, I could be free of it all. Sitting in bed with no vent sounds, trach ties, or trach was very calming. I could quietly read the Bible in peace and get into a rhythm of shrugging my shoulders to pull in air. If it was a short passage, I brushed my teeth before replacing the trach. Sucking on a straw to rinse my teeth felt funny on my throat, but it worked.

By July, I worked up to 15 minutes of leaving the hardware out. The formerly round hole in my neck would become more oval and partially close. Putting my head down toward my chest and slightly lowering my chin would make my neck look completely solid. It felt good to be without breathing assistance, but I reluctantly let Mary put in a clean trach every time. I sometimes had to move my head around to get the trach to go in, but it usually slipped back in without trouble.

More Chair Choices

I heard about a wheelchair provider in eastern Iowa, The Upright Chair. They only had one model available, but it had the option to stand. Mike, a company representative who used the chair, came with his wife the day after school started. Rolling into the living room, he demonstrated the chair's function by pushing a handle and standing up. He explained the three different options: manual, semi-electric, or fully electric. I would need a fully electric option where I drove and operated the standing feature by joystick instead of by hand. However, standing was the only position the seat could do; it could not tilt or recline.

After taking my measurements, I was offered to test the demonstration model. It wouldn't fit me very well, but I wanted to at least give it a try and see how it felt. Dad transferred me from my wheelchair and sat me in the demo. It was made for someone larger than me and did not have a place for my vent, so Dad put the vent on the floor beside me. To have enough tube length, he added a section from my bed vent.

My knees didn't reach the support frame that kept them in place, but some towels filled the gap. More padding supported my arms, and I was somewhat comfortable. Mike's wife said they didn't recommend standing barefoot but I wasn't concerned about it. My main hesitation was whether my legs could handle my weight.

With a few slow turns of a lever, I was soon standing. It had been over ten years since I stood, but my body seemed to do well. They asked if I felt light-headed or experienced any other issues, but I felt fine. Mike said the chair couldn't move while standing but he added that it was very stable. He thought they could meet my length requirements with a vent tray on the back but couldn't guarantee it.

As I stood chatting, I liked the feeling of being upright. I could talk to everyone at eye level instead of looking up their nose and feel more like part of the group. Dad noticed my right foot was partially turned out to the side and started to head toward me to straighten it. I told him not to touch it and I kept repeating "no" as he approached, but he straightened the foot anyway. As I knew would happen, a muscle spasm started shaking my entire body when the foot was touched. With my full weight on my legs, I envisioned the next sound being a bone breaking. As my body vibrated uncontrollably, I quickly had Mrs. Mike put me back down. I was sitting again within a few seconds, but I didn't want to attempt going up again. Even with the moments

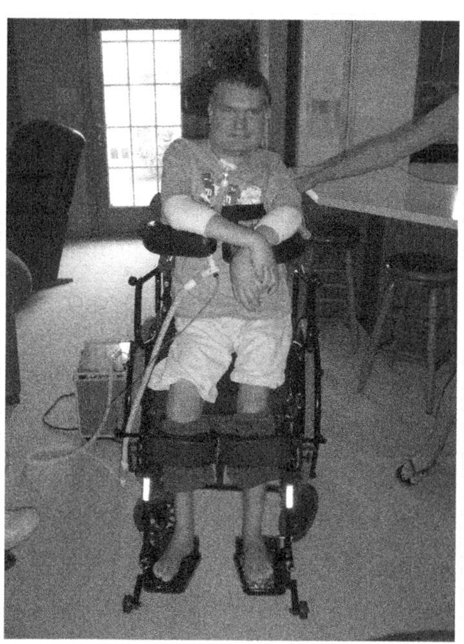

of terror, I thought the demonstration went well and I was returned to my regular seat.

After the chair salesman left, my parents and I discussed our thoughts. I loved the standing ability but didn't like it being the only option. I was used to tilting when getting positioned and while riding in the van. We also didn't know about length and whether it would fit in the church elevator. I wondered if standing partially would decrease the length but I wasn't sure if that disabled driving. Dad thought the chair design looked basic and questioned its durability. With these thoughts in mind, we decided to continue looking for another option.

More Changes

With all my nursing covered, Mom and Dad managed to go on an extended vacation. They took a ten-day trip to Oregon, traveling by Amtrak, and leaving me in charge of the house. Along with going to school, I needed to plan my meals and be responsible for getting the mail and trash. It felt like I was back living on my own in Des Moines. I loved it.

They returned on September 1, and we had all enjoyed the time to ourselves. Dad got the mail when he unpacked the car and found a letter from Kid Care. I read it, and the contents instantly changed everyone's mood. The nursing agency had decided to stop serving my county and would be ending services in two weeks. The next day, Rhoda called to let me know she was quitting. Her music business was increasing, and she no longer had time to help with nights.

I had recently heard in the news about a man in his early 50's who had received a C4 spinal cord injury and was on a vent. Eight weeks after his injury, he decided to stop receiving breathing support and died shortly after. I really wondered if that wasn't the best option for me as well, but I knew God was in control no matter what happened.

Losing the nursing agency and Rhoda would mean little to no coverage for night hours. My parents couldn't stay up every night and function the next day at work. Therefore, unless another agency could be found, I would need to go to a nursing home.

Life can change quickly, going from good times to bad in a short time span. I wasn't sure where to start looking, but I needed to find a solution in less than two weeks. Like so many times before, I didn't know what my future would hold.

23

CHANGING OF THE GUARD

> Matthew 6:8 says that God knows our needs before we even ask. Remembering this can be a hard thing to do, but forgetting this promise in difficult times leads to increased anxiety and confused thinking.

With thoughts of my life drastically changing, I couldn't sleep. It was Sara's regular Saturday night shift, and she wondered why I was restless. I directed her to read the letter sitting by my keyboard. She then understood my frustration and offered to help in any way she could. Having my trach out and breathing on my own had become my best calming mechanism, but I knew Sara was not experienced enough for this. Instead, I asked her to turn the vent off for one minute.

She reluctantly agreed to the odd request, with my oxygen sensor attached. With the breathing machine off, I could only hear complete silence and concentrate on my thoughts. The sound was peaceful and a welcome change from getting a breath every few seconds. After one minute, as I asked, Sara flipped the switch and air was shoved into my lungs. The brief respite helped, but only a little.

Mary was willing to go with me to another agency, but she also talked about how much she could make going to a career outside of home care. I searched online for nursing agencies around Pella. The list wasn't extensive, but I only needed one to say yes.

Calling one provider, I briefly explained my situation and care needs. Unfortunately, it turned out they didn't serve my area. I continued to contact more agencies, but I only received more refusals. Most companies only did short visits to check on people, not full multi-hour shifts. If they did shift work, it wasn't offered in my area, or they didn't do nights.

The deadline given by Kid Care for losing coverage was September 14. By September 11, I still hadn't found a company that would take me. I contacted Kid Care and they were willing to extend the deadline, but I needed to continue looking for a replacement.

I finally found a company, Iowa Health Home Care, based in Des Moines that was willing to cover my hours. After class, I met with two nursing supervisors in the back of Simpson's library. The study room didn't have a door we could close, but I tried to stay quiet so not everyone in the library could hear. Attempting to remember all my cares, medications, and history off the top of my head was a challenge, but I covered all the main points.

On September 20, I had a doctor's appointment in Des Moines. A nurse from the agency agreed to meet me before the appointment so we could cover final information. Her main concern was about my insurance and funding resources, but everything seemed in place. The new agency officially started on September 22, a little more than a week after my initial deadline. I prayed this agency would work well, especially without having another choice.

After the nurse from Iowa Health departed, I had a regular checkup with my urologist. It had been 11 years since I switched to a cathing routine instead of being incontinent. I had a few infections over that period, but it was going well. As part of the routine, I had also been taking oxybutynin four times a day. Dr. Rosenburg wanted me to try switching to another medication, Detrol LA. He said it was basically the same pill, but I only needed it once a day. If I had trouble with leaking, then I could switch to twice a day. I didn't want to change anything since it was working, but taking fewer pills per day would be nice.

One week after adjusting the medications, I started getting headaches. Especially in late evening, the slightest amount of stiffness or muscle spasm would start my head pounding. The headaches quickly increased to unbearable pain shooting through my brain.

Mary could barely get my night cathing done, and everything else in my routine was a very slow, arduous process. Any type of touch or movement would make the pain skyrocket to where it felt like my head would explode. She could barely get any of my cares done and I could not sleep. By morning, the pain would finally decrease, and I could once again tolerate getting touched and moved. In the afternoon and evening, I felt perfectly fine.

Iowa Home Health sent a new night nurse to train, but I couldn't do my regular routine due to pain, and Mary sent her home after only a few hours at my house. As the days progressed, the headaches got to the point where I was unable to do any web development work or go to school.

Neither my doctor nor pharmacist thought the change in meds would cause headaches. However, after a full week of extreme pain, the urologist agreed to let me switch back to my regular oxybutynin. The change wasn't immediate, but my head mercifully returned to normal a few days later. I was very thankful the headaches subsided, and I did not want to adjust medications again.

My Attempt at Online Dating

Returning to school after a few days away, I heard other students talk about dating and some were looking forward to marriage. Two years earlier, I had received a paper about my high school classmates and what they were doing five years after graduation. Many of them were married, with some already having kids. I had hoped to be married, or at least dating, by this point in life.

At night, Mary and I had many discussions as she did my bedtime routine. She was certain that if she worked days with me going to school, I would be dating someone. As Mary said this, I remembered she had three ex-husbands and four children. I was fairly sure I didn't want to take her up on dating advice.

I decided to try online dating, which was starting to get popular. I filled out a profile on Yahoo! dating but didn't want to pay for extra features. It was simple to sign up, so I also tried Match.com, and one called eHarmony. The last one had a very extensive sign-up process and was more in-depth in finding out my interests and a potential partner. I knew I was looking for a Christian within a few years of my age and someone who wanted kids. Beyond those requirements, I wasn't sure.

Within a short time, all three services had several matches for me. Some sounded like women I might be interested in, but I had to pay to get the contact information. eHarmony offered a special of three months for $60, so I paid it.

As part of my match qualifications, I specified the lady needed to be within 150 miles of Pella. I didn't think anyone, including me, would be willing to travel any further than that to meet in person. Despite this stipulation, I was matched with people from New York, Montana, and states further away. Most of the matches that came through did sound like someone I would be interested in meeting.

I found it somewhat odd that most of the people I was matched with had occupations in the health field. Some were nurses, others were pharmacists, and a few were in school to be doctors. I had lived with medical professionals around me almost all day, every day. According to eHarmony, that was the type of person I was most compatible with.

I made the first step and contacted a few of the matches. However, unless they had also paid for a full membership, they couldn't respond or see my interests. This resulted in very little correspondence with anyone. One match that had very high compatibility ratings lived in Pella. I carefully read the woman's information and decided to initiate a contact.

After several days I received the same response as the others, nothing. The profile said she was a teacher, which prompted me to look through the websites of local schools. I quickly found her listed in the faculty at a grade school. The site said she worked with junior high students as a resource and extra-curricular teacher and provided her school email address.

As days passed, I debated if I should contact the match through her school email. Would she think I was a stalker? What would I say in the message? "Hi, I'm Joel, you don't know me, but I saw your dating profile and wanted to find you." Nothing sounded good in my head.

Finally, I decided to wait and see if she would respond to further contact through eHarmony. After several more weeks, I didn't receive a response and didn't feel right using her work email. I decided it would be best to concentrate on work and school and someone would come along if it was God's will.

Moving into a New Year

As Christmas approached, I again had the same thoughts as a year before. I wanted to stop using my ventilator and trach and be free from life on this earth. Two to three nights a week I had my trach out for 20 minutes or more. It felt good and relaxing, but I also kept hoping the clean one wouldn't be able to be inserted.

Our family friends came for New Year's Eve but left before the clock hit midnight. Back in my bed, I watched as the minutes ticked by, getting closer to the start of another year. As had become tradition, I had Mary take off my neck ties and I then blew my trach out of my neck a few minutes before the hour. Unable to speak without the device, I mouthed the words "Happy New Year." A few minutes later, a clean trach was again in place.

I could honestly say that, when 2007 ended, I was not using a vent or a trach and was breathing on my own. I also started 2008 in the same condition and got a picture with my computer's camera to prove it. It was only for a few minutes for both years, but it was true.

Classes resumed at Simpson on January 7 with the same routine of every Monday, Wednesday, and Friday. In between school and web work,

I also had to keep up with medical appointments. Since breaking my leg, I had been taking a medication called Fosamax to help strengthen my bones. A bone density test showed improvement, but I still had severe osteoporosis. I wanted to stop taking the extra drug, but my doctor said I needed to stay on it for a few more years.

Sara had switched from nights to days and she, Miranda, and Karen covered day hours and drove me to Indianola for school. At home, I spent time studying and working on websites for clients. As each day and week passed, they seemed to blend together, one after another.

February 20 came, marking 23 years since becoming a quadriplegic. Reading online, I learned about new therapies and treatments that were developed to help recent injuries. Some had good success in restoring movement and decreasing injury severity. I wondered what life would be like if this information had been available when I was injured.

A few weeks later, my parents and I were at Pella Christian High School watching my cousin's drill team routine. As parents filed in and found seats on the bleachers, Dad pointed toward a man who was entering and said, "There's Gordon." It took me a few seconds to realize who he meant. You would think a man who helped save your life would stick in your mind, but I didn't recognize him. I had heard that some people ridiculed him for helping me the day of our accident. They said I was now stuck as a quadriplegic, on a vent, and that it would have been better if I died.

Some days I wondered if they were right, but God had also allowed me to do quite a lot. April 15 came with news stations reporting where you could file your tax returns at the last minute. I didn't earn enough in 2007 to have to file taxes. The lack of work made me feel like I wasn't good enough for businesses to hire as an inexpensive web developer.

One of the graduate campers died on March 31 at 20 years old. I hadn't spoken to Brian or seen him at camp since 2006. He was a fellow vent dependent quadriplegic, had helped in the ROTC, but had died from brain cancer.

Every night, I always read the Bible as part of my bedtime routine. At the time of Brian's passing, I was reading Ecclesiastes. Solomon said everything was meaningless, a chasing after the wind. I wondered what our time on earth was worth? Every day, week, and month seemed to pass without any useful progress toward any goal.

No company wanted to hire me when I lived in Des Moines. Now, churches, schools, and businesses in Pella were using other web developers to do the same thing I did, but for more money. After four years as an active client, Pella Christian High School said they would no longer be using VMT at the end of the school year. The school was changing to a competitor and doing their own updates.

Statistics said I should have died years ago as a teenager. A body wasn't meant to be motionless for so long. I reasoned that my insurance lifetime cap would be reached in about two years and I would then have no choice other than a nursing home. It was unlikely I would live very long in such a place and could be free of this world.

I was thankful God had used Gordon to save my life so many years before and the opportunities He had given me. As Solomon concluded, our purpose for our short time on earth was to serve God. I looked forward to being done with life but had been given time to do His will.

School finished at the end of April, allowing for an easier schedule for a few months. I had continued visiting with second graders at Pella Christian every year since 2004. This spring, I added Oskaloosa Christian, and hoped they would invite me for an annual visit as well. Spending 30-40 minutes with each class was fun and I looked forward to it. Teaching the kids about living with a disability helped them experience a new perspective and I loved hearing their questions.

My friend Ken's birthday came at the end of May. He and I had corresponded by email for a couple of years, but never met in person. Miranda didn't mind taking me on the two-hour trip to Waterloo, so we planned to go on May 28. I had never visited someone in a nursing home before, and especially not a younger person.

It took some searching to find the facility, but we eventually located it outside of town and then found Ken's room. Miranda and I arrived around lunch, and an aide was helping Ken eat. As he sat in bed, I noticed he couldn't move his head very much and I tried to sit as directly in front of him as I could. Ken was easy to talk with, and I looked around the room as he told us his life's story.

I could get in fairly easily, but the space was tight. The only outside view was one window in the far back corner with a curtain partially draped over it. However, it was impossible for Ken to see it, or anything other than his computer, a wall, and the door into the hall.

Ken talked about his history of growing up in the small town of Tracy, near Pella. As a teenager, he got into a single car accident that broke his spinal cord at nearly the same place as mine. Since he was under 18, medical decisions were up to his family. Most of his relatives, except his mom, said to let him die. Ken lived with his parents for a few years, but experienced physical abuse and other problems from them. He then went to school at the University of Iowa, in Iowa City, and nearly finished his degree. But before he could graduate, Ken's medical insurance ran out and he had to completely rely on state funding. The only way Iowa would pay for the necessary services was if he lived in a nursing home. Ken tried to go through the courts to live independently but was forced into the facility in October of 2000.

Since then, Ken's family had abandoned him except for a few distant cousins. Days were spent with no visitors and doing what he could on his computer. I knew he had barely ever been out of bed and as far as I could tell, also didn't get dressed.

After an hour of talking, I offered to pray with Ken, and then Miranda and I started toward home. From our email conversations, I knew a lot of Ken's history already. It was good to hear and see him in person and much easier to communicate. Seeing his living conditions made me more appreciative for the blessings God had given me and I tried to be sure to keep in regular contact with Ken.

Back to Summer Camp

June came and we prepared to go to camp. Miranda agreed to cover my night hours while Sara would help during the day. A little over a week before my volunteer time, the Van Hoerkel family came for one of their regular visits. Soon after they arrived, a game of Chutes and Ladders was on my table with me on one side and Rae on the other. Preventing the board from toppling to the floor was a challenge, but I managed to keep it in place with my stick. Sara kept herself busy in another room while the moms chatted.

Since I was playing with his sister, James toddled over to see if he could help. The 17-month-old stood beside me looking up and wanting attention. When Rae took her turn, I pointed my mouth stick down toward my side. James reached up to grab it, but his fingers couldn't quite reach. The two moms sat chatting a few feet away and seemed oblivious to my plight to entertain two children with one mouth stick.

No matter what I thought, the kids seemed satisfied with my efforts. I wondered if I had been blessed with children, would daily life be similar to this? James soon lost interest in the stick and went to explore other areas of the room. Rae and I continued our game, but she also got bored before the conclusion of our match.

Despite my attempts, she had never wanted to ride on my lap before. That changed on this day, and she finally took interest. With Sara's help, I gladly allowed her to perch on my legs. Mom was very uncertain if it was a wise idea to have Rae on my lap. With a month to go until her fourth birthday, she was getting bigger and heavier. Mom envisioned broken legs from the added weight, but I was certain everything was fine.

For the next half-hour, the active girl ascended and descended my legs several times as I navigated around the house. She quickly figured out how to get up and down on her own and insisted on taking a random blanket on our excursions around the house. Unable to see the bottom of the cloth, my concern was getting it caught in my wheels and getting stuck or pulling my passenger off.

My lap eventually became boring, and my leg bones survived the experience. When it came time to leave, the kids did not want to go home. Apparently, this visit was a test to see if the youngsters would like being around. It was assumed they would get bored in a few minutes, but that was obviously not the case. My attempt to entertain young children had won them over more than expected.

During my afternoon medical cares, I did my regular skin check as Sara moved a mirror over my naked body. Concentrating on my legs and hips, everything looked fine, and I was glad that acting as a stroller went well. However, the next day a tiny open spot appeared on my upper right leg where my passenger had been sitting. I couldn't see it with mirrors, but I was assured it didn't look serious and would likely be gone soon. With camp a few days away, I wasn't as certain, but hoped it would heal.

A week later, June 14, the van was again packed full and headed east to Ashley, Ohio. Both of my caregivers had heard about camp and seen pictures, but this would be their first experience. The route that was very familiar to my parents and me was a new adventure for them.

After one night in the hotel, I was back at Recreation Unlimited and free from parental monitoring. Graduate camper Ryan was a fellow counselor with me in the younger boys' cabin. Derrick also returned as a counselor after graduating the previous year. He had been one of the boys I watched my first year as counselor. Seeing him in the new role as a responsible adult made me start to realize how long I had been with CHAMP camp.

The days before campers arrived, orientation included team building, getting to know all my fellow counselors, and extensive coverage of the boys in our cabin. Each one had somewhat different care needs and diagnoses, but also some similarities. One of the new campers would be a six-year-old named Dylan. His paperwork said he only used breathing support when sleeping and was completely mobile during the day. However, Dylan was unable to hear and only spoke through sign language or writing on a small white board. Sara looked forward to refreshing her sign language skills, but I wondered how I could best work with him. I usually helped with the kids who were ambulatory, but I had to communicate by voice.

Monday morning, the campers arrived to the great fanfare that was part of camp tradition. Sara and I volunteered to get two kids through the check-in process and help ensure all medications, equipment, and changes in care needs were documented. Miranda's sleeping accommodation was close to the entrance, a new building complete with air conditioning. I hoped the greeting party wasn't too noisy and wouldn't wake her up after working overnight.

By Tuesday morning, all the campers and counselors were ready for the first full day of activities. My day started, as it had for several years, in charge of fishing at the waterfront. Sara was okay with helping bait hooks and taking fish off lines, so we prepared for a great morning. Dylan was one of the campers in our first group and he was happy to experience his first-time fishing.

As the campers got ready, I had Sara set up a bamboo pole for the boy's first fishing attempt. She wanted to give him a regular rod and reel, but I explained this would be best to start. Dylan quickly signed something to Sara, but she didn't understand him. Two more slower attempts didn't help, so he reluctantly wrote down his question. A few simple words explained his desire, "Want catch blowfish."

I hid a grin but said through Sara that we unfortunately wouldn't catch any blowfish in the pond. She then explained how to toss in the line and wait for a fish to bite. The inquisitive boy shrugged his shoulders to say okay, walked to the edge of the dock, and threw the line and pole in the water. As Sara used another pole to fish the bamboo rod out of the pond, she understood why I had given directions to use a rod that would float. More specific instructions were given and only fish were retrieved from the water for the remainder of the activity.

The theme for the year was the 1970s and counselors had come equipped with hippy costumes. For talent night, counselors were responsible for making up a cabin skit. We borrowed dresses and makeup from female counselors and dressed our boys up as girls. After he was decked out with a feather boa and makeup, one camper drove his wheelchair to me. Michael assured me he was never doing this again, but it was hard not to laugh at the nine-year-old's comment. We were first up for the night and the entire camp laughed as our cabin went on stage. The campers and the counselors sang, "Girls just want to have fun," to the delight of the audience. Once off stage, as wigs were removed and dresses taken off to reveal the kid's regular apparel, it once again looked like I was in a boys' cabin.

The week quickly wrapped up but Miranda had a lot of back pain from the low bunks. I decided that if these two came to help me another year, it would be best to switch their roles and have Miranda do days, when I was in my chair, and Sara do nights.

Heading home, the three of us slept as the van progressed toward our hotel in Illinois. While Miranda got me undressed and started my night routine, I asked Sara to check on the sore that appeared just before camp. She said it was a little worse, but not bad and didn't appear to be doing anything. I was thankful to hear it wasn't drastically bigger, but it hadn't gone away either.

Back Home and Back to School

Back at home, I enjoyed the warmth of the season and continued working on websites. However, the work was decreasing with some days having very little or nothing to update.

By July, the sore on my leg had increased in size despite trying to stay off it. I returned to Dr. Rouce after a few years away to see what he recommended. I had gotten to know the doctor and his nurse Sheila quite well after spending so much time with them. She was surprised to see Sara with me, and I explained the change in nursing coverage since my last visit. When the doctor came, he had already been informed of my recent history and looked at the new area.

The physician prescribed an antibiotic cream and dressing change twice a day. Since it was small, he would try to glue and stitch it closed in a few weeks. I reminded him I often react badly to adhesive, but he was confident it would work. I trusted the doctor's expertise and waited to get surgery scheduled.

School was approaching again, but I didn't receive any information on tuition expense. Gas prices were getting close to $4.00 per gallon and I wasn't sure I could afford the cost of college and commuting three days a week. I contacted Simpson, only to find out they didn't have my FAFSA and income information. It had been filed back in March, but for some reason didn't get to the school's business office. I quickly filed again but thought it might be best to take time off and give my body a rest. This would start my third year back at school and take me closer to finishing my bachelor's degree.

Talking with my Voc Rehab counselor, he said they could help with my fuel expense instead of tuition for select courses. Looking at the numbers, I would get more money with this program than with tuition help. I agreed to the switch and, if my paperwork went through, I could start class on August 27.

Before I started anything, I needed to have the opening near my groin closed. The procedure was scheduled for August 15 at a small surgery center in West Des Moines. A few days before my scheduled time, the facility called to get my information. It was a new building, and they hadn't worked with someone on a ventilator. The anesthesiologist wanted my nurse to come into surgery with me so she could monitor my breathing. It didn't sound like I was heading into a safe situation. My wound was healing very well with the prescribed treatment, and I wasn't certain the procedure was even necessary. However, with returning to school and being up in my chair more, the area could get worse. I thought it would be best to have it closed, so I kept the appointment.

Two days later, Sara came at her usual time of 7:00 and got me ready to go to Des Moines. After a quick morning routine, Mom got in the van and the three of us headed west.

I should have cancelled the appointment and let the area continue healing on its own. It would be another trip to the city that ended with different consequences than planned.

24

DOWN AND OUT

In Hebrews 12:10-11, God says that he disciplines us for our good. It doesn't seem pleasant at the time but produces righteousness. It took another cycle of trials before I took this to heart.

I had originally been told to be at the surgical center by 11 a.m. for my appointment. However, the scheduler changed it to 7 a.m. the day before. I explained I couldn't get there that early with my caregiver's schedule but would come as soon as possible. My party of three arrived at the facility to find a large, crowded, waiting area. As soon as she saw me, a receptionist behind a desk called me over. I guess they had been told to look for a guy in a wheelchair that morning. My paperwork went through quickly and we were taken to a private waiting room.

Sara and another nurse picked me up to transfer me from my chair to a bed and quickly got me prepped for the procedure. The anesthesiologist, Dr. Kadmere, introduced himself with a thick Indian accent. Since I could speak well, he said Sara didn't need to come back with me and he would just use a mild medication to reduce muscle spasms. Since the doctor wasn't doing major surgery, I thought the plan would work.

I was transported to the operating room where my I.V. was connected to a bag of saline. I watched the anesthesiologist insert another liquid just before Dr. Rouce started. I felt the familiar numbness and tunnel hearing I had experienced from other surgeries just before falling asleep. This time though, the feeling stopped, and I stayed awake. After a few minutes, it completely wore off and I felt normal again. However, the surgeon was continuing to work and my legs were jumping and kicking nearly non-stop.

Dr. Kadmere seemed oblivious to my flying legs, so I asked for more of the sedative. He promptly administered more and my lower limbs relaxed as the numbness returned to my head. I hoped the first prompting would be the only one, but the same scenario happened several more times. I reminded Dr. Kadmere that he needed to give me enough to keep my legs from jumping.

Finally, Dr. Rouce finished his work in gluing and stitching the area shut. My bed was rolled through the halls back to the first room, where Sara and Mom waited. Since I barely had any sedation, I was released much faster than usual and was allowed to sit in my chair as normal.

Two weeks later, classes started at Simpson with my paperwork all complete. This semester, I was taking Statistics and Principles of Accounting. I thought my accounting courses from AIB would allow me to skip the introductory class, but it was still required. On the first day, the accounting instructor asked if anyone was an accounting major. None of my classmates, which included several football players, raised their hand. Therefore, he would make it a very basic course.

I was thankful for one easy class, as Statistics looked to be more of a struggle. Sara said she enjoyed math and could help me, but she only came to school with me on Fridays. The first few weeks were basic math that was very simple, but the course quickly became difficult to understand and to get the calculations correct. By October, I started needing assistance to keep my grades up. I was getting through the material, but everyday life was distracting me from my studies.

My concerns about closing the pressure wound with adhesive came true. The once tiny spot was now very large, but not deep. I continued to see the doctor, but his treatment was no longer working. Some of my nurses said I should get a second opinion, but asking other doctors confirmed that Dr. Rouce was the most qualified person in central Iowa. To get some exercise, I had been practicing breathing on my own and doing head lifts while lying flat to increase my neck muscles. I stopped both of these practices and increased my protein intake, but nothing made a difference.

In addition, web development was very slow with only a little over six hours of work halfway through the month. My thoughts returned to wondering why I was still attempting to go to school or why had God allowed me to live so much longer than other quads.

As fall progressed, it was decided that I needed to have surgery again and be on complete bed rest afterward. Before my flat time started and being stuck at home, I went to a concert in Des Moines featuring the Trans-Siberian Orchestra. The wheelchair seating had my parents and me by ourselves with lights sometimes pointed directly at us. It was fun hearing the band live, but Dad didn't care for the bright lights and very loud music.

My final test for Simpson was on December 8. Accounting was familiar and simple for me, and I passed with a high grade. For Statistics, I was thankful to pass the class and hoped my next courses in January would be easier.

Two days later, I was again in surgery for the same pressure area. Before going in, I prayed that something would go wrong and I wouldn't survive the procedure, but I wasn't even fully sedated. It was hoped that having the area closed again, and staying out of my chair for a few weeks, would allow me to return to school in January. I didn't mind missing the cold December weather and I was allowed to briefly join my family's Christmas celebrations. Pastor Dan from church visited shortly after the surgery, but I didn't let anyone know about my wishes to be done with this world, except Tom.

Sitting or lying in bed was my regular location anyway and I could easily control my computer for work and entertainment. Even though he lived in Wisconsin, Tom and I could play our online games together and talk, at least when his wife let him. However, he had family Christmas gatherings in Canada and Michigan which meant I was back to being on my own, with nurses and parents.

My legs had a major increase in muscle spasms and were constantly kicking and flying around. Two of my nurses said there was another skin opening where it looked like some stitches came lose.

Dad's Accident

On Christmas Day, I didn't attend church, but went to Sully to spend a few hours with Mom's side of the family. We usually had lunch once a month at the Laverman's house, but only with family in the area. It was fun seeing my cousins and their kids who lived further away and getting to hear what they had been doing. On Christmas night, though, I was told my skin didn't do well with me sitting in my chair.

Dad's family was having their Christmas party the next evening. December 26 was a Friday, with Sara working her regular 10-hour shift. Despite the holiday, Dad had a few things to finish at work while Mom did insurance paperwork in the basement. The phone rang around 10 a.m. and Mom answered it in her office. Shortly after, she used the house intercom system and asked Sara to go to Mom's bathroom and plug in her curling iron, explaining she would be upstairs soon.

With nurses in and out all day every day, my parents didn't get much privacy. Their bedroom and bathroom were the only place my caregivers didn't go which made Mom's request very strange. Sara went to run the errand and Mom soon appeared through the basement door. The phone call was from Dad's boss at the Town Crier. Dad was finishing his work and cleaning his printing press before heading home. Somehow, the machine he had worked on for over thirty years had Dad's arm trapped between two large rollers. Emergency services were on the way and Mom needed to meet him at the ER in Pella.

After a quick visit to the restroom, Mom left with Sara and me at home. We didn't know what was happening or what injuries Dad had received. We could only sit and wait. I sent an email to my church's prayer coordinator and waited for news from Mom. The coordinator was used to receiving requests about me, but not about Dad. Mom called a few hours later to let us know Dad had finally been extracted from the machine and was in the emergency room. Everything appeared to be okay, but he was receiving I.V. fluids before coming home.

A few hours before Sara was scheduled to leave, Mom returned with Dad trailing behind. Recounting the story, he said he was using a rag to clean ink off the rollers of the printing press, just as he had done for decades. This time, the rag got caught between two rollers and as he reached to get it, his arm got pulled in. Over the years, Dad had completely torn the machine apart while doing maintenance. Since it was older equipment, he knew it didn't have modern safety features to stop it in case something odd happened. For some reason though, it did stop before pulling Dad's arm through the mechanisms. Dad said the EMS crew tried different methods to free him but couldn't extract his arm. When he started losing feeling in his hand, Dad told the first responders where they could make cuts in the metal drum to get him lose.

As the day's events unfolded, I didn't feel anxious, sad, or anything. I wondered whether my lack of emotion was related to my thoughts about wanting to be done with life or something else.

With Dad's hand and my pressure sore, we decided to stay home from the second Christmas party. I was thankful everything turned out well because it could have had a major impact on our lives.

Spring Classes Postponed

I ordered my books for school early so I would be ready to start on January 3. With the new development on the skin opening, I went to see Dr. Rouce for his recommendation. He again stitched shut the area that reopened, and assigned an additional two weeks in bed with limited time in my chair afterward. This meant I had to cancel spring semester at Simpson and wait until the next school year to return.

Tom was still gone on his Christmas family trips and I hadn't received any contact from my church since the initial procedure early in the month. The latest development confirmed in my mind that I was only on a spiral of increasing problems until the end eventually came. I contacted Iowa Legal Aid to see what I could do to stop my breathing support and be done with this life. The attorney who returned my call didn't understand my situation and gave me the number for a suicide hotline. In talking with Mary, she agreed to contact a lawyer who could maybe help.

During New Year's Eve, I again had my trach out as 2008 left and 2009 started. There was a small skin growth around the stoma for the trach that had been growing. I hoped if I had the trach out long enough, it would prevent it from going in. However, it didn't cause a problem, and the hardware went back in easily so I could be attached to the vent again.

With my parents in the family room and me sitting in bed on my computer, I could use my chin to reach the vent tube where it connected to my trach. The connection was held on with two rubber bands. Since second grade, I had continued using the speaking valve to talk more clearly. It also provided enough resistance that the ventilator's alarm didn't always go off when the tube disconnected at my trach. Moisture from the vent's humidifier would also build up in the circuits causing further resistance. From experience, I knew if I could pop the tube off my trach, the low-pressure alarm was unlikely to go off. Mom or Dad regularly called back to me, "Joel, are you okay?" I would answer "yes," and all was well. However, they sometimes went 15-20 minutes without checking in. I thought I could wait until they asked, pop the tube off, then wait to pass out. This way, nobody would have to help me remove the vent and everyone would be free of me.

I pushed and rubbed with my chin on the tube's trach adapter, but it wouldn't come lose. After my chin was hurting too much to touch the tube, I stopped trying. I wondered if there was anything else I could do that would help improve my outlook on the future.

By the end of January, the pressure wound didn't look any better. The doctor wanted to try something called a wound vac to help promote circulation. A plastic seal would go over the area and then connect to a machine that provided constant suction. I had heard of the device helping other people and was willing to try.

For nurses from the agency to run the wound vacuum system, we had to use someone who was trained on it. However, they had trouble finding anyone willing to come to Pella multiple times a week. Finally, a nurse who lived in town agreed to come three days a week to change the dressing.

Getting a secure seal on my upper leg, near the groin, was difficult. If everything was working correctly, then my attachment shouldn't make any noise. With any slight leg movement, the vacuum would turn on or would alarm that there was a leak somewhere. After a few weeks, the wound vac nurse had her own medical difficulties and was no longer available. Since I had already started on the system and needed to continue, a nursing supervisor reluctantly agreed to make the one-hour drive and change the dressings. This was only a short-term plan and one of my regular nurses would need to be trained.

Mary continued to miss many nights due to various issues but seemed to be the best one to instruct. She was already fixing it at night when it didn't work, and it should be easy to get certified. Dr. Rouce also ordered an additional medication to help decrease my muscle spasms.

With all the time in bed, and little work to do, I had plenty of time to research and read. I found a study that showed some people with high-level spinal cord injuries had taken a B12 vitamin and a medication called Theophylline. Some participants were able to regain control of breathing while others had severe reactions that weren't listed. It sounded like something to try, but I needed a doctor's approval and a drug prescription. I printed out the research information and mailed it to my pulmonologist. A month of talking by phone passed before he agreed to let me try it to see if anything happened.

I started the new medication on February 19, the day before the 24th anniversary of my family's car accident. Theophylline was a steroid that was regularly used for people with asthma. Shortly after my first dose, I could feel my heart rate increase and simultaneously felt tired.

The same day, I was asked to be part of a phone conference about something called a Diaphragmatic Pacemaker System. It had recently received FDA approval for people with high-level spinal cord injuries who used ventilators. I didn't know much about it, except that it could help get me off the vent. Synapse Biomedical was the producer of the system and they were conducting several conferences. On my call was a representative from Synapse, a few other quadriplegics, and Lazlo, a man who was using the system.

It was explained that four wires were implanted into the patient's diaphragm, two on each side, and they came out to a port on the side of the chest. The port then plugged into an external control box. When everything was connected, the wires received a small electrical charge, making the diaphragm contract and the patient take a breath. The salesman said, as part of natural breathing through their system, it helped patients decrease instances of pneumonia. This was achieved by taking deeper breaths and using more of the chest than a regular vent. It also allowed for the sense of smell to be used again and improve tasting abilities. Some patients got off the vent completely while others still used it at night.

Whenever Lazlo spoke, I noticed he had long breaks in his speech. It reminded me of how I talked before I started using the speaking valve and how several kids talked at camp. I was also concerned about swallowing and if I would have to time it between breaths. Lazlo said it wasn't something he thought about and he didn't have any trouble with it.

I remembered my parents said when I was injured, they had been told about something called a phrenic nerve stimulator. This device sounded similar, but my parents were told it would severely damage my nerves after a few years and I would always need a ventilator, even if a cure was found for spinal cord injuries. Apparently, my reservation was well known as the respiratory therapist salesman said that was the first thing he asked. This pacemaker worked differently in that stimulation was applied directly to the muscle instead of the nerve. The phrenic nerve did need to be intact for the system to function, but it didn't carry the same risks.

About an hour after the call started, everything had been explained and current questions were answered. I recorded the company's information and said I would think about it. I liked using natural remedies and treatments as much as possible, which was why I did exercises multiple times a day instead of just taking more medication. I liked the idea of breathing without the vent, but having wires implanted in me didn't sound very appealing.

Through online discussions I had become friends with Bill, another vent-dependent quadriplegic. He was from Florida and we were doing a Bible reading plan together. I enjoyed helping him to understand Scripture better and answer his questions.

Bill took part in a different phone interview with Synapse, but it sounded like he had the same primary participants. He also noted the long pauses in Lazlo's speech and was concerned about the system affecting speech quality. I liked being able to talk continually and only pause when I wanted, not when my breath forced me. If someone didn't see me, they couldn't tell I had a disability, let alone used a vent. I had only interacted with several of my clients by phone and email and didn't see a reason to disclose my physical challenges.

With these new developments, I contacted the lawyer I had been given through Iowa Legal Aid to let them know I would not be needing his services. I told him I would be looking into the pacemaker system and see if anything developed with the medication trials. He said his office didn't currently have the staff to help me anyway. If I needed anything later, I could contact them again.

Tom was happy with my change of mind and having new goals to pursue. I had also been talking online with a few individuals with spinal cord injuries and their families. They were also glad that I made a change of thought.

The pressure sore had improved enough that Dr. Rouce finally allowed me to start getting in my chair again. On March 1, I was able to attend church for the first time since early December. Sitting in my designated bench, I felt like I stuck out like a sore thumb. James and Rae were excited to have all three of my family back and promptly abandoned their parents' bench for ours. Unfortunately, it felt like nobody realized I had been missing. The pastor mentioned two other members who had been away and were able to return the same day, but there was no mention of me. Going to the basement for cookies and juice after the worship service, only a few people mentioned my return.

I also received an email from The Design Center noting several areas I needed to improve in my work. With everything going on, I thought I had been doing well with web development. At least they were willing to help me improve, but I wasn't sure how much more I could do. I also hadn't looked at a new wheelchair in several months and Mom let me know she was disappointed in my lack of progress.

At night, I started having my trach out again for extended periods. I hadn't for several months, but with the roller coaster of events, it felt good to just be free of any hardware. Once again, it felt like I was living two different lives in one body. One part wanted to be done with life and do whatever was needed to get there, as long as it didn't hurt my family. The other part, the part everyone knew, was ready to continue with life and deal with anything that I was given.

A Change of Heart

During one of my parents' vacations, Rhoda had taken me to a conference in Pella about the Christian response to stem cells and cloning. It had been given by an organization called Answers in Genesis and I thought it was interesting. I started following the ministry online and loved learning about biblical creation. The ministry was offering online courses, so I decided I would take a few since I was waiting on school and frequently in bed with little to do.

The twelve-week course started in early March and went through late May. Going through Christian school, I believed God created everything, but I hadn't given it much critical thought. As the course progressed, it covered the basics of creation apologetics. It was a fascinating study of the Bible that got me thinking more carefully about why I believed in God and was a Christian.

I realized, more than ever, that I was going through the motions of Christian life and had head knowledge but hadn't really let it affect my heart. Thinking more, I better understood how God created a once perfect world, but it was now cursed as a result of sin. Consequently, problems such as spinal cord injuries and every other difficulty in life were due to original sin.

> *I realized, more than ever, that I was going through the motions of Christian life and had head knowledge but hadn't really let it affect my heart.*

With a new sense of understanding the Bible, my desire of wanting to leave the world on my own terms were gone. I knew struggles would still come, but I felt more prepared to deal with them. Since I had hidden my thoughts from most people, only a few knew the change in mind I was experiencing.

Warmer weather started to return in April, but my pressure sore was not improving. At the end of the month, I had another muscle flap surgery to close the area and spent a week in the hospital for recovery. As with every hospital stay, I had sitters in my room. They mainly just monitored me and didn't do anything other than helping me eat or assisting to move me. However, it gave me someone to talk with who didn't already know my bad jokes.

Sitters were varied in medical experience, but all of them were mainly just looking to get more hours. Talking with one sitter who had immigrated from Russia provided interesting stories as well as an opportunity to tell about being a Christian. Most acted pretty much the same, but one sitter seemed different than the others. About an hour into her shift, she helped me with lunch and asked where I lived, my history, and my parents.

These were normal questions, but she seemed to know the answers before asking. After some hesitation, she told me her name and history.

This sitter's late husband had been a respiratory therapist and ran a ventilator company. I was his first client who lived at home, and she had come with him a few times when checking my vents. Their son, who was close to my age, had also tagged along. I didn't remember any of it but was thankful to get to hear old stories I had forgotten. When my parents came to visit, they remembered more and enjoyed catching up. With new faces, hospital stays felt somewhat like a vacation.

It wasn't long before I was home again for six weeks of bed rest. I had to miss Pella's Tulip Time and wondered what summer would be like. Dr. Rouce increased my anti-spasm meds but my legs kept constantly jumping. Two weeks after surgery, everything the doctor had done broke open. To my surprise, Dr. Rouce said to enjoy the summer and we would try something again in a few months.

A Change of Plans

I still wanted to help at camp, but knew I had to keep off my butt much more than usual. In an attempt to have more opportunity to tilt, I volunteered to help in camp administration during the week. I would do my normal duties of monitoring fishing for morning activities, but afternoons would be spent updating the camp website and writing the daily newsletter. I didn't think these jobs would take the entire three-hour period and would allow me more time for pressure relief.

Packing one of my bedside tables in the van added to the already cramped space but Dad got everything in; at least we hoped. After arrival in Ohio, I was directed to the camp office and found a place for my table and laptop.

During orientation I felt out of place in familiar surroundings. I would be bunking in the boys' cabin but would miss most of the activities with them. I would see my assigned trail group one morning when they had waterfront activities. The only other time I would be with the boys from my cabin was during evening events with the entire camp.

My new assignments started just after the campers arrived on Sunday. The camp website needed updating with arrival pictures, and newsletters had to be ready for the kids' bunks by morning. The campers were greeted with whatever I could come up with along with pictures from previous years.

Camp was always the one week of the year I didn't touch a computer or use my mouth stick. It didn't seem right spending half of each day working with my regular tools and not helping with the kids. As the days progressed, I kept receiving pictures of the campers' activities so I could write articles for the newsletter and post them online. Instead of having more opportunity to tilt, the opposite happened.

I needed the entire afternoon to get everything finished and couldn't take any time to reposition. On Wednesday evening, the full camp activity was something new, exploring the ground's prairie grass. However, my vent's battery wasn't charged correctly the night before and didn't last the entire day. I couldn't go out to the prairie and, instead, was stuck in the office, on the computer, with my vent plugged into the wall. One of the counselors came back later and found five ticks on him. He said it was probably a good thing I missed it, and it was an activity that wouldn't be repeated.

During lunch the next day, I made sure to sit with Dave Carter, one of the camp founders. With his respiratory therapy experience, I wondered what he thought about the diaphragm pacemaker system. I didn't remember her, but Dave said there had been a camper a few years earlier with a similar system. He wasn't very familiar with them but gave the same good and bad points I had in mind.

The entire week had been very warm, with the only air conditioning in the office where I spent my afternoons. In the cabin after morning activities, I parked under a ceiling fan to feel the breeze and was regularly joined by Ryan, a fellow alumni camper. I had many conversations with campers and counselors over the years and I enjoyed getting caught up with a friend.

Thursday afternoon was the final activity slot for the week before closing ceremonies. A company in Indianapolis donated two soap-box derby cars for the campers to ride. The original plan was to have a staging area on the tennis courts with fun activities while campers waited for their turn in a car. However, it was too hot to sit in the sun and events were moved under an open shelter. A paved trail made a large circle around the middle of Recreation Unlimited. This became a racetrack for campers to use in their cars. Some kids could easily sit in the car's seat, but others needed a lot of support with pillows and towels to sit comfortably.

While one car was getting set up with a rider, the other would be pushed around the loop. One or two counselors pushed the vehicle as fast as they could run to get the best time. After making a loop, the pushers would return dripping with sweat and a camper, happy after feeling the speed of the run. The medical director, Dr. Chuck, frequently pushed the loop, but struggled with the heat as well.

Even sitting in the shade, some of the kids went back to the cabin early to lie down and cool off. I was also having a hard time with the heat and parked directly in front of a fan and kept having water dumped on my head. I managed to stay for most of the allotted time, until a camper needed the fan. I gladly let them use it, and Miranda and I headed for another fan in the cabin to try to cool down further in the non-air-conditioned building.

As the sun started to set, the high temperatures decreased for closing ceremonies. I presented trophies to the camper who caught the most fish and the one who caught the largest. It had been a week I wouldn't want to repeat, as I missed a lot of time with the campers. If I went again, I would need to be back to my regular role.

Miranda did better with day shift, but coming with me to camp was not a good fit for her. I was running out of caregivers to utilize at camp, but someone else would need to come as my assistant if I wanted to return.

Since I couldn't reposition in my chair very much at camp, the pressure sore got worse. Dr. Rouce didn't want to do another surgery until my legs had fewer spasms. I would continue seeing him to monitor progress, but we would not schedule any procedures until fall. That meant I couldn't return to Simpson for at least another semester, but I could do more online classes with Answers in Genesis.

I also decided to stop taking Theophylline. Taking it along with a B12 vitamin was meant to stimulate nerve communication and possible growth. However, I was now on the maximum dose of two other meds to suppress my nerves from reacting and causing spasms. It didn't make sense to be doing two opposites and the experiment didn't seem to be making any changes.

Cherokee Chairs

A week after camp, a salesman from Cherokee Chairs, based in Arizona, came to show their product. Looking online, I liked their standing chair and hoped it would finally be the right one for me. As the chair was demonstrated, I liked the look of it. It was able to stand like I wanted, but could also move while standing. That made the length issue much easier to overcome. If it was too long when sitting, then I could put it into standing mode to make my length shorter for the church elevator or anywhere else. Unfortunately, I wasn't allowed to sit in the demonstration model to test it.

As my parents and I looked it over, we talked about the need to have a vent tray put on the back with a place for an extra battery like my current system. The chair controls would normally sit on my chest, but I would need to have them on a swing away arm to not have anything laying on my vent circuit or coat in the winter. As we covered the specifications, the salesman took notes and said it was possible to do everything necessary to fit my needs. I also liked that, for the first time, I could choose what color to have my chair.

Continuing to evaluate, everything I saw looked and sounded like it would work. I wanted to go ahead with the system, but Dad wasn't sure. Since the company didn't have a retailer in Iowa, repair work would be slow and require long waits for technicians. I noted that Dad did most of my chair maintenance and I rarely used local assistance. It had already been three years since I started looking for a chair and this was the last standing option I could find.

Dad wasn't sold on it, but I didn't think it would hurt to give it a try. I decided to go with the Cherokee chair for my next transportation, even though it would require more evaluations from physical therapists, my doctor, and insurance. I was excited to finally make progress toward a new chair.

Two weeks after camp, it was a regular Wednesday evening. After supper, if Tom had free time, we played our usual game of Starcraft. As the night progressed, we chatted through an online message program while playing and I got caught up on what was happening at his home in Madison, Wisconsin. Around 7:30, my chest started feeling tight and I thought I needed to be suctioned.

Our game was almost finished, so I did my breathing technique of letting the vent give me a few breaths and exhaling quickly, attempting to move any junk in my lungs. After a couple of cycles, I didn't notice any improvement with my breathing. It had been a few weeks since Tom and I had talked, but I reluctantly ended our time early and had Mom lay me flat in bed and suction to see if it would help. After she had sucked out both lungs, with hardly anything coming up, my chest was feeling increasingly stiff. For the next few hours, the chest discomfort continued along with difficulty getting air. My regular chest percussion treatment didn't help nor did further breathing tricks. I was beginning to wonder if I should go to the hospital, but by 11:00 everything cleared up and I could easily breathe again with the ventilator.

I attempted to get an appointment with my pulmonologist, Dr. Hicklin, but he didn't have an opening for several weeks so I was given an appointment a few days later with a nurse practitioner. At the doctor's office, everything seemed fine with my lungs, but she was concerned with other problems I was having. For the previous several weeks, I would be sitting in bed on my computer with sweat pouring off my face and a heart rate over 100. As a precaution, the practitioner had me make an appointment with a cardiologist.

It didn't take long to get into the heart doctor, but he seemed annoyed that I was there. All I had to report was a high heart rate and no other systems. After a short visit, the doctor ordered blood tests and gave me a prescription to decrease my heart rate. I hoped something would help, soaking my shirt with sweat every night was getting old and I was losing a lot of weight.

As July turned into August, I wasn't improving. When I tilted back in my chair, I couldn't sit up again without passing out. I had to make multiple gradual steps to sitting. The sweating also continued and I was very quick to get angry at people around me.

The next few months would bring a new diagnosis and start a path toward major changes in what was my family's regular life.

25

HYPER QUAD BLOCKAGE

It can be easy to trust doctors and those in authority for our best interest. However, they are human and don't always get everything right. Proverbs 3:5 says, "Trust in the Lord with all your heart and lean not on your own understanding." This is where we need to place our faith at all times.

Grandpa and Grandma Labermen came for a visit, as they often did, and I told Grandpa about my new medicine and the trouble I was having. He said it sounded familiar to when he had his heart attack and had to take blood pressure medication. I tried to get used to it but taking a few minutes just to sit up was not tolerable. Therefore, I called the cardiologist to see if I could change the prescription.

Talking with his nurse, she said I could stop taking the medicine, but I needed to reduce the dosage gradually. She noticed that I had not been called about my test results from my initial visit, which showed I had a hyper thyroid, which would contribute to the symptoms I experienced. She said I would need to see my primary doctor about it and get his guidance on how to proceed. I made an appointment with him a week later and another blood test confirmed the initial results, meaning I needed to see another specialist in Des Moines.

In high school, I had bad acne all over my upper chest, face, and back. It continued through college and was still a problem. While at AIB, I saw a dermatologist, Dr. Abrahamson, to help improve my skin. He was knowledgeable, didn't mind my extra challenges, and I enjoyed him. By August 2009, it had been six years since I graduated, but I continued seeing Dr. Abrahamson in West Des Moines for treatment. While he examined my acne, Miranda started discussing my pressure sore and all the trouble with it. The dermatologist was intrigued and wanted to examine it.

With the sore near my groin, I had to get out of my chair. Miranda took one half my body while the doctor took the other half and, with much difficulty, they got me onto the examination table. Looking at the area and hearing the history of muscle flap surgeries, combined with regular pressure relief, he gave a different diagnosis. The dermatologist said I likely had an autoimmune disease called Pyoderma Gangrenosum, or PG.

He was reluctant to get involved since another doctor was treating me, however, he pointed out that each doctor has their own area of expertise. Plastic surgeons, like Dr. Rouce, are familiar with surgical solutions. Dr. Abrahamson, as a dermatologist, had seen odd skin conditions before, and in my situation, surgery wouldn't help. I decided to stop what seemed like endless muscle flaps and investigate whether a new treatment would help.

Meanwhile, I also waited to see a thyroid specialist. I finally got an appointment in early September with Dr. Khoo. Before we met, he called to discuss possible treatment options. There were different medications that could treat the issue or surgery to remove my thyroid. I had researched online and knew the thyroid was near my trach. The doctor couldn't tell I used a vent and I guessed he hadn't noticed that detail on my chart. I agreed to look at treatment options and talk in person.

When the appointment came, I was ushered into a very small room at Mercy Hospital in Des Moines. Looking at the hallways and rooms, they seemed tight and not cleaned very well. I had never used this hospital before and quickly preferred my familiar facility of Methodist.

The doctor joined my caregiver and me, and he was suddenly more interested in my complete medical history. I needed another blood test to confirm the hyper thyroid and would also need to have a nuclear test to determine the severity of the problem. Until the tests were finished, I continued sweating profusely every evening, even with fans pointing directly at my face.

In the midst of everything going on, my parents arranged enough caregivers so they could take a vacation. From September 16 to 26, I would have the house to myself and be responsible for taking care of it, as well as meals. I looked forward to it but had an extra challenge. The day before they left, the washing machine quit working. Dad would normally fix it but needed more than a few hours. Therefore, I would have to use the laundromat while they were away.

I relished the freedom and responsibility of running the house and it nearly felt like when I lived in Des Moines. My muscle spasms remained strong, they were worse if I wore shoes, but Mom and Dad wouldn't let me skip footwear in public. They said it didn't look right. Running errands to the grocery store and laundromat, I could stay barefoot while they were away. Nobody said anything to me about it and I enjoyed having easier outings with a calmer body.

Tom also had extra vacation time from work, so he came from Madison for a four-day weekend. We regularly met online to chat and play games but being together allowed for more catching up.

On one laundry run, Tom helped Sara get the baskets of clothes and towels from the van into the washers. During the forty-minute wash cycle, we left her inside and went thirty feet out the laundromat door to the neighboring drive-up coffee shop. We both ordered a drink and Tom sat on the bumper of the van while we talked and had our warm drinks. Rianna had about one year of school remaining to finish her doctorate. After that, they would be leaving Wisconsin to possibly move to Europe, New Zealand, or another state. Wherever they went, it would be further away and likely put an end to regular in-person visits. They weren't planning on kids for a few years though, so we could still have online meetings.

Our beverages were finished in time for the end of the wash cycle. The two of us joined Sara and moved the laundry back home. Tom and I had a few late-night discussions before he returned to Wisconsin, and I finished the week on my own. My parents returned on Saturday the 26th and life returned to the regular routine.

On Monday, I had my scheduled thyroid test. Arriving at the hospital early in the morning, Miranda and I were brought to an x-ray room with machines I hadn't seen before. A technician explained the procedure and a pill I needed to take. It was radioactive and would determine how much of a certain chemical was absorbed by my thyroid. The medicine was stored in what looked like a miniature nuclear containment vessel. I had seen pictures and videos of containers that transported spent uranium fuel rods, and this looked almost identical. However, I would be swallowing the contents rather than putting on a hazardous material suit for protection.

Scans were taken of my leg to check for iodine levels before I took the radioactive pill. After swallowing the medicine, I had to return in eight hours, and then again in 24 hours for more scans. It wasn't worth driving back to Pella for a few hours just to return to Des Moines, so Miranda and I stayed in the area, watching trains, planes, and just killing time. We returned to the hospital for my second test, and everything looked okay. Before heading home, the technician said I shouldn't go to an airport, as my radioactive diet would set off alarms. I replied, "That won't be a problem," but Miranda might also set alarms off since she had been near me all day. I questioned more what I had done to myself but it was too late to turn back.

Tests again confirmed that I had hyperthyroidism, likely due to Grave's Disease. Dr. Khoo started me on a new medicine to help slow the thyroid and hopefully return it to normal function. I hoped it would finally relieve my fast heart rate, nightly sweating, and the mood swings my family noticed.

I had also developed another pressure sore, this time on my left butt cheek. I was sweating so much at night that it caused me to lose a lot of weight. I had seen the red area when I checked my skin and tried staying off of it more. Despite my efforts, it still broke open. Thyroid and skin problems weren't my only challenges.

By September 2009, it had been 14 years since I started cathing three times a day, every day, for bladder management. It had worked pretty well, but Dad and my caregivers were having a difficult time inserting the catheter into my bladder. One of my helpers had accidentally used a catheter that had a sharp tip, resulting in getting blood. There were several times I had severe autonomic dysreflexia because my bladder needed to be emptied, but the tube wouldn't go in. It always went in eventually, but something needed to be done.

My urologist scheduled a procedure to clean out scar tissue from my urethra to help solve the problem. It would be a minor procedure with no hospital stay. Getting prepared in the surgery waiting room, the nurses weighed my wheelchair with me in it, then again after I was out. The math showed I weighed 102 pounds, or 17 pounds less than I had at the muscle flap surgery in April. I knew the sweating and rapid pulse was causing weight loss, but I hadn't realized how much.

The procedure went well, but I had to use a Foley catheter for a week afterward. It was a type of catheter that stayed in place and connected to a drainage bag on my leg or the side of my bed. I had seen several kids at camp use this system and my doctor frequently suggested that I use a similar system full-time. I detested having a bag of urine hanging on me and couldn't make myself look at my lower body. I was thankful when I could get rid of it again and to have no problems with my regular routine.

Keeping track of all my medical and work needs, I also continued to research the diaphragm pacemaker system with my friend Bill. I still had some reservations, but was ready for a change and I liked the possibility of getting away from the regular ventilator. On October 25, I contacted Synapse Biomedical to say I wanted to pursue their system. That night, I told my parents I decided to work on getting the pacemaker system. They were much less than enthused about my decision and loudly expressed their opinion. Mom especially didn't understand why I would want to bother with it, saying I was already dealing with two pressure sores, a new chair, and everything was working fine with my breathing. Her reaction was what I expected, but I knew it was a goal I wanted to work toward.

My thoughts earlier in the year of wanting to be done with life were partly due to not seeing any improvement for the future. This would be a change toward easier care and less dependence on the vent. At least that is what I hoped.

As November arrived, I hadn't heard from Cherokee Chairs since June. I contacted them to check on chair progress, only to learn the salesman no longer worked for them. They needed all new documentation, but I soon received a paper detailing everything I had requested. It had reasoning for the chair type, that I was dealing with multiple pressure sores, head rest, joystick, and all my details. I had to get signatures from an occupational therapist and my general physician, and then the process would begin.

I investigated financial aid in order to return to Simpson in January. The classes I needed would only meet twice a week, but they were evenings in West Des Moines. Miranda encouraged me to sign up, but I wasn't sure about sitting in my chair that much and driving in winter weather in the evening.

Instead, a few days into 2010, I applied to take online classes through a university in Arizona. I had spent several months studying online through Answers in Genesis and enjoyed it. Online education was new, with only a few schools offering this method of study, but it seemed to be the best option for my situation.

The start of another year also meant time to apply as a camp counselor. Miranda hadn't done well on the day or night shift, but I needed someone to help me during the day if Sara stayed on nights. I asked Dad about it, and he wanted to give it a try. After many summers of just dropping me off, he wanted to join me for the week and maybe help work on other wheelchairs.

My case manager from insurance called to ask about approving Cherokee Chairs. Since they were based in Arizona, it would be out-of-network and normally not approved. They also had concern about maintenance since no local help would be available. I explained that I had been looking for three years and this was the only chair I found that met my needs. I also said it was rare to get anyone to do work on my current chair, but thankfully, Dad could do a lot. I was assured the situation would be reviewed and she would get back to me. A week later, I received a call from insurance that the chair had been approved. Since it was out of network, Cherokee Chairs couldn't be paid directly. The funds would be written to the policy holder, Dad, who would then pay the chair company. My parents weren't thrilled with the situation but were willing to make it work.

Miranda and Sara continued filling daytime hours with Mary and a few other nurses filling the nights. Karen still helped as needed, but her regular time was Friday evenings. Dad could often get off work early on Friday and, with Karen helping, he and Mom could have their weekly date nights. I enjoyed a few more hours on my own and was happy that my parents could have time together.

At church, a few people had organized a young adult group for people in their twenties and thirties. Being 28, I qualified, and knew most of the group fairly well. It was fun to be with adults around my own age, but I was the only person who was single and, as usual, the only one who used a wheelchair. They usually got together on Friday nights twice a month, one for Bible study and the other for a fun night. I wanted to be part of the group, but Karen no longer drove the van, which meant everyone either had to come to my house or my parents had to stay nearby to drive us. Before inviting guests over, Mom and Dad felt they had to have the house completely cleaned and organized, so rather than deep clean twice a month, they opted to take Karen and me to church and have a short date night. It worked, but I didn't like taking away part of their time together.

I started with the online school in April. It was nice staying home for class, but I had to make sure to take a technology related course in order for Voc Rehab to help cover the cost. I looked at another school in Colorado, but their main interest seemed to be making sure I secured a student loan before expanding my knowledge.

My first course was a general orientation about returning to college and the importance of working in groups. At the end of every class, a group project was required. It counted toward 25% of the final grade and, therefore, needed to be done well. Three to four random students were assigned to work together on the assignment.

Pain, Evaluations and Surgery

As I worked with Synapse to get approved for the diaphragm pacemaker, they put me in contact with Northwestern Hospital in Chicago. For the system to work, my phrenic nerve needed to be intact. The doctor I talked with said insurance would be quicker to approve the system if they knew my nerve was intact.

Finding somewhere in Iowa to get tested was a challenge, but a neurologist at the University of Iowa said he could do it. On April 12, Miranda and I took the 90-minute trip east to see what the test involved. Dr. Shivapour greeted me with a thick Indian accent and listened to my history and what I needed. He wasn't sure how to test the phrenic nerve but wondered if my injury level had been evaluated. It hadn't been, that I could remember, and I was soon laying naked, covered with a sheet, on the exam table. Miranda and a few students had helped transfer me and I had told them about my web development work. After waiting, the doctor returned with his students, who had looked up VMT's website.

Dr. Shivapour took a device with metal spikes on a wheel, uncovered one side of my body, and rolled the device on the side of my foot. I commented he should start higher, but I watched as he went up my leg and over my hip. I put my head down so I couldn't see, and I yelped when he got to the top inch of my chest, just as I expected. The doctor asked about feeling my head and neck and concluded that my sensation level was around C4. That was a full 1.5 levels below my C2/3 injury but sounded correct.

Once I was dressed and back in my chair, the doctor explained he didn't know how to test my diaphragm without surgery. Electrodes could be used to check reaction but had the potential to puncture holes in the muscle. The doctor concluded with his thick accent, "Then you'd really be screwed!" He hadn't heard of such a device as a diaphragm pacemaker but said to contact him if it worked out. So, other than officially learning my sensation level, it was a wasted trip. Progress toward getting the new breathing system would need to come from other sources. Thankfully my pulmonologist, Dr. Hicklin, was interested in the system and would gladly give any referrals or documentation I needed.

I wasn't the only one in my family dealing with medical situations. After several years of severe pain in her knees, Mom finally agreed to have one knee replaced in early May. Her procedure was performed at a new hospital in West Des Moines that I had not yet visited. When the surgery was complete, Dad stayed with her in the hospital as much as possible, coming home in the evening to watch me after the day person left. Three days after surgery, Mom returned home with a strict schedule for exercise at home and with physical therapists in Pella.

Cherokee Chair Delivers

A few weeks later, my new chair from Cherokee was delivered. When the 53' semi-truck slowly drove past, Sara and I went out to the driveway as the driver carefully turned the large truck around on residential streets. Facing uphill, he soon had a large crate precariously placed on the trailer's lift gate.

I was anticipating that it would slide off as I recorded the event with my new GoPro head mounted camera. However, there weren't any problems, and the crate was easily maneuvered into a corner of the garage. My instructions were not to open it; the large package sat there, taunting us with its contents.

Finally, on June 16, a technician came from Cherokee Chairs. Sam was one of the founders of the company and had come from Arizona to set up the chair. I expected him to have a ramp to unload the mobility device; instead, he carefully brought each wheel down the gap from the shipping crate and skid to the garage floor. It looked like the display model I had seen a year earlier, all black and not the dark blue I specified. Dad came home from work shortly after the chair was unloaded, just as the set-up work began. We noticed there wasn't a place for my ventilator or the car battery it used for power. However, a crudely welded metal box the size of the vent was included.

As instructed, Dad picked me up from my Action Arrow chair I had used for 14 years and sat me in the new ride. It fit me well, but the vent had to sit beside me. Sam opened more boxes from the crate and produced some odd-looking contraption. He put it over my head to lay on my chest, pulling the tube for my vent uncomfortably to my side. The device was my chin control and was designed to sit on my chest. I explained that this would not work as having my vent tube go through the metal support frame pulled on my trach. Wearing a t-shirt, I could reach the controls, but with thicker clothes and a winter coat, it wouldn't work. The company owner tried to say his design was a better solution, but eventually conceded and said they would work on a swing-away control as I ordered.

Next, Sam attempted to attach a custom-made box for my vent. He had been given all the measurements of my breathing aide, but the container was the wrong size. It also included an area for a small external battery but not the car battery I normally used, and it had no way of connecting to my vent's plugin. Sam worked on constructing a wire so the vent could use the proposed battery. He asked to use Dad's soldering iron, and set up a makeshift shop on top of the freezer in the garage. He put a few wires together to fit the vent holder and the small power source, but the vent wouldn't connect to the battery.

After about an hour of tinkering, Sam left with a long list of items that needed to be addressed. Since the chair wasn't working for me and wasn't anywhere close to the specifications originally given, I didn't sign the paperwork stating that I received it. As soon as Sam was out the door, Dad became extremely irate. With a highly elevated voice, he questioned how I could have decided on such a chair and what was I thinking by going with Cherokee. He picked up the newly soldered wire to emphasize the work quality and the connections disintegrated in his hand.

Dad soon stormed off to work and Miranda and I went back into the house. I was frustrated that, after more than three years of looking for a new chair, the solution I hoped for was nowhere close. After several hours at work, Dad calmed down about the chair problems, hoping they would be resolved soon.

CHAMP Camp's 20th Anniversary

Two days later, we headed east to Ohio for a week of camp. This time, instead of the van filled with five people and luggage, there were only three of us. Sara tried to rest in the back to prepare for night duties and Dad made the familiar full-day drive east. Our small group stopped overnight at a hotel in Dayton, Ohio and arrived at Recreation Unlimited near Ashley on Saturday morning.

Mom's new knee wasn't responding as expected, but she and Dad continued doing the required stretching exercises. While we were gone, her friend Patti stayed in my room and would help until we returned a week later.

I was excited for Dad to help me at camp. I wanted him to get to know the counselors and campers I had grown close to and to experience how we helped the kids. He also was looking forward to seeing other types of power chairs and possibly helping with maintenance issues.

Saturday was the regular start to orientation, but 2010 was CHAMP camp's 20th anniversary. Special activities had been planned for the week and it looked like an exciting few days. One of the founders, Dave Carter, gave a talk about camp history and why it was started. He then spoke about the success so far, as partly evidenced by Dad coming with me. My fellow counselor and former camper, Ryan, also relied on his dad for the week and he was also included in the orientation.

One new feature at Recreation Unlimited was near the pool: a zero-depth splash pad. It allowed wheelchairs to roll up to water features and experience a small version of a water park. It was anticipated to be popular with the campers, but counselors needed to protect ventilators from water or use different approaches to let the kids have fun.

Campers arrived on Sunday afternoon to the week's theme of Hollywood. Dad seemed to get into the routine quickly and started getting to know the boys in our cabin. As I had done for several years, Monday morning started with helping a trail group at the waterfront. It was going to be a hot week and I wondered if the campers would catch many fish. Dad did well with checking fishing poles, baiting hooks, and measuring the catches.

Decorations for the Hollywood theme were all over the cabins and the grounds. Along the paths between buildings, five-point stars had been cut out and secured in the ground. Every star had a current or former camper's name on it. I found my star as well as some of the other alumni campers I remembered from previous summers. Some also included "in memory of" for kids who passed away in the camp's 20-year history.

Throughout the week, I hadn't been hungry during mealtime and could hardly eat. Wednesday morning, there was a special activity of a hot-air balloon ride. To beat the morning winds, everyone had to get up early. The boys in my cabin weren't happy with the short night, but everyone got to the balloon on time.

After all the campers had gone, counselors were able to get a lift. Dad hadn't ever been in a hot air balloon, so he, Sara, and I loaded into the basket. It was smaller than what had come a few years earlier and my chair had to be partially disassembled for me to fit. Removing my footrests worked but left my feet dangling. In the process of tilting my chair and getting in the basket, one foot got caught on the battery for my vent. Dad and Dr. Chuck saw what I couldn't and directed me how to adjust my seat to avoid breaking an ankle, which came loose, but was possibly sprained.

The tethered balloon ride went well, and we were quickly above the 50' climbing tower, but Dad thought the burner near his head felt warm. It wasn't long before we were grounded again and back to our position at Lake Crumb.

Even though it was well before lunch, it was a hot day. My trail group's afternoon activity was arts and crafts, which was my least favorite activity of camp, but at least it was indoors. As the campers worked on various projects, I parked directly underneath the ceiling fan in the non-air-conditioned building. Every window was wide open, but there was little breeze. A call went through the radios that one boy from my cabin, in a different trail group, was having overheating trouble and had to return to the cabin early.

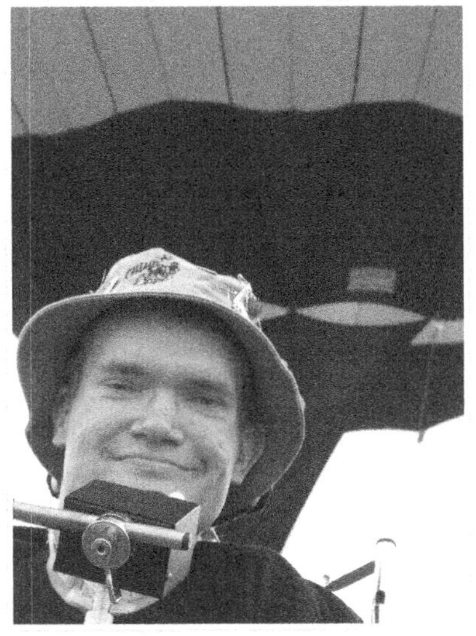

I didn't leave my position from under the fan for the entire activity and was glad when the time came to return to our bunks. There were a couple of hours before supper, so Dad laid me in my bunk and wiped my face, arms, and legs with a cool washcloth. The boy who had returned early was resting a few beds down from mine. Dad gave him the same cooling treatment since the counselor who was nearest to him had briefly dozed off in the heat.

When all the campers returned from their afternoon activities, we heard one group had been at the pool, but one boy enjoyed the new splash pad a little too much and his power chair wasn't working. Dad was intrigued and hoped he could help look at it after the day's activities concluded.

As supper neared, I was cooling off but my stomach still felt bad. For the second time, I got a gas relief strip from another counselor hoping it would help. Supper was grilled and served out by the lake. It was fun to look over the water, but space was cramped with multiple large wheelchairs, adults, and tables in one small area. The food looked good, but I only wanted a small hamburger and some fruit. Attempting to eat was a difficult task. As I swallowed half a grape, I could feel it immediately try to come back up, along with everything I had forced into me. I quickly had Dad give me a drink and I shoved it back down but didn't dare eat any more. After supper, Sara and I headed back to the cabin, but I lost track of Dad.

Wednesday's evening activity was talent night. Some individual campers had prepared skits and some cabins were performing as a group. Everyone stopped by their bunks briefly to get any supplies they needed for their shows, but I felt horrible. I found my cabin's leader and confirmed there wasn't a full cabin skit I needed to help with. I told him I was going to skip the activity, lay down and rest so I could be ready for Thursday. My bunk neighbor, Ryan, and his dad, Jeff, were ready to head out with the cabin. I asked them to send my dad back when they saw him at the activity.

An Ambulance Ride to the Hospital

He came a few minutes later, along with Dave Carter. Dad had been getting a full tour of Recreation Unlimited with Dr. Chuck when he got the message that I needed help. Dad plopped me in my bunk and took my chair to be charged while Sara took off my clothes. My belly looked like I had swallowed an entire watermelon without chewing. Looking down, I could barely see my feet over the bulge.

Talking to Dave, I said, "It's getting hard to breathe, even with this thing," as I jerked my head to my bedside ventilator, which was giving me air. Soon the head camp nurse came as Sara was trying to cath me to see if that was the problem. Taking my vitals showed a low oxygen level and numbers nowhere close to normal.

Dave retrieved one of the spare oxygen tanks and managed to get it connected to my vent with spare tubing the camp had on hand. Dr. Chuck joined the team of medical professionals around my bed. He asked how my thyroid had been and whether I had been backed up. Sara tried doing my bowel routine, but with no success. They thought it would be best for me to get checked out at the hospital and see what was going on. Dad disappeared for a few minutes and returned wearing a fresh change of clothes and cleaned up hair. He was ready to get me up and drive us to the closest hospital, but the medical directors said no. An ambulance was coming for more direct transport to the large hospital in Columbus. Dad and I weren't sure about the plan but agreed to it.

A few minutes later, paramedics arrived at my bunk with a stretcher. Dave told them what the medical team had been able to assess at our facility in the woods. I described what my experience had been the previous few hours and noted that I was normally not so rotund.

Two of the EMTs, Dad, and everyone around, helped transfer my ventilator, oxygen, and me from the bunk to the portable bed. Once everything was secure, I was carefully rolled through the boy's cabin to the opposite end where the ambulance was parked. I was familiar with the ceiling of the cabin after many years of camping, but never had been through it like this.

Sara rode with me in the ambulance as we slowly left Recreation Unlimited. A few buildings away, my fellow counselors worked to keep the campers' attention on the stage for the talent show so they didn't catch a glimpse of me leaving in a way I didn't expect. As we made the hour-long drive from Ashley to Columbus, Dad followed in the van. He called Mom on his rarely used cell phone to let her know what was happening. He forgot that a wedding shower was being held that evening, and his call on my status wasn't exactly the news the partiers expected.

Riding flat in the back of the emergency vehicle was rough, but the cool air-conditioning felt good after five days in record heat. Sara and I were kept informed of our trip's progress and we eventually arrived in Columbus at The Ohio State University's hospital.

Rolling through the emergency room's hallway, I noticed blasts of cold air hit my face from strange looking pipes. I was told the air conditioning wasn't working in the halls, and they only had cooling vents. The medics briefly stopped with my head directly in front of one vent so I could feel the cold air on my face. It was a brief rest before I was in an exam room that, thankfully, had working air.

The rough ride actually helped my stomach, and it wasn't as uncomfortable as when I left camp. However, now the taste of the oxygen was making me feel worse and I was still overheating. One of the EMTs checked on Sara and me to see how I was feeling and discreetly decreased the oxygen I was receiving. A small fan was also found that fit on the bed directly beside my cheek. It felt wonderful. The fan looked like it had been in a closet for a few years without being cleaned. If I kept my eyes closed, I could ignore the clumps of dust hanging from it.

An intern soon came to get my history and my reason for coming to the ER. He poked on my expansive abdomen, which increased my discomfort. After he left, an x-ray technician came with two large bottles. The doctor wanted to do a contrast x-ray to see how my system was working. First, I needed to drink both one-liter bottles, then wait for an hour before the test could be done. I explained I wasn't even able to eat a grape a few hours earlier, and there was no way I could drink so much fluid. The technician said I could take as much time as needed, but that was the doctor's order. I started to attempt to drink one bottle and follow orders. Sara kept encouraging me, but I only had about a third of one bottle down after an hour.

Another doctor came to check on my progress, and I told him how hard it was to drink anything. He allowed Sara to hide one bottle in the empty trash can, but said I needed to keep trying and to say I only had one bottle if someone asked. During this time, Sara and I had yet to see Dad. We asked the nurses a few times, but he wasn't found. He had taken my portable suction in the van which contained my wallet and insurance cards. Finally, after about 90 minutes, he arrived in my room, very irritated. Dad had been in the main waiting room waiting to get back to us. The receptionist said he could once I was fully checked in. Dad tried to explain he had my insurance information, but the correct people didn't get the message.

While coming to my room, Dad observed that the equipment in the halls was dirty and wasn't near the standards we were familiar with. Another intern came to apologize for the confusion and check on my drinking progress. Sara showed him the one bottle I had was getting close to halfway complete. The doctor in training looked confused and inquired about the second bottle. Sara and I answered that it was just the one. Simultaneously, Dad found the second bottle in the trash before we had time to tell him about the previous arrangement. This new intern wasn't happy with the deception and touted that I had to finish both bottles before they could proceed. Dad agreed with my earlier remarks that I couldn't drink that much fluid and he very clearly let his thoughts be known.

I explained to Dad that getting irritated with the medical staff wouldn't help me or them. However, I was thankful he was sticking up for me.

At midnight, the staff changed shifts and yet another doctor came to introduce himself. This was not an intern. He was an experienced physician who had seen more patients. My belly looked like I was ready to give birth and, as the doctor examined me, he asked about the scar near my belly button. I had already explained it to previous visitors and was now having difficulty speaking due to the pressure in my abdomen. One glance toward Sara, and she repeated what I said before.

Twenty-five years earlier, my colon had been punctured in the accident when I received my spinal cord injury. This required surgery to repair, and the scar was the continued reminder of the procedure. The actual doctor understood and thought the requirement to drink the contrast and wait for x-ray was crazy. He wanted immediate exploratory surgery and warned that I may end up with a colostomy bag depending on what he found. I agreed surgery was needed and was thankful to finally be doing something. However, I explained part of my advanced directives was no colostomy bag due to the multiple problems that I had seen other people have. From his reaction, I knew the doctor didn't fully agree with my reasoning but would honor my wishes.

Close to 1:00 a.m., a nurse came to prepare me for surgery and transport me to the operating room. The anesthesiologist said he would likely need to change my trach to a cuffed version during surgery for better airway control. I asked multiple times for him not to change it since a previous surgery had gone very badly with such a switch. However, he was unwilling to compromise, and I was soon being pushed down the hall toward an operating room, away from the only two people I knew.

En route, my one transport person said he forgot some paperwork. He parked my bed beside a wall and disappeared. My vent was perched between my legs, running on internal battery. I knew any muscle spasm would kick my breathing aid and possibly send it crashing to the floor. My ears strained to pick up any sound between breaths, however, I couldn't hear anyone talking, no footsteps, no doors, nothing. Straining to lift my head, all I could see was a long, empty corridor that appeared devoid of life, except me laying helpless on a gurney. In the deafening silence, my mind began to think. The final day of camp would be starting soon, but I obviously wasn't going to be returning. By morning, would my Hollywood star need to be adjusted to say "in memory of" instead of just my name? I prayed and thanked God for taking me this far and for giving me care through everyone. I asked if it was His will to give the surgeons skilled hands and allow me full recovery. If not, I asked for comfort for my family and to know God's will in all circumstances.

After what seemed like an eternity, my transporter returned with some papers and he continued guiding my mobile bed to our destination. Lying flat, I watched ceiling tiles and lights pass overhead with each one looking the same.

Just outside the operating room, someone else talked with me about the procedure. With difficulty speaking, I pleaded with them not to change my trach. I was told it would only be done after I was anesthetized, so I would be comfortable. I again explained it wasn't just for comfort, but safety from experience. My request fell on deaf ears, and I was soon on the final table for surgery and felt the familiar beginning stages of sedation.

The next thing I knew, I was in a different room than before. My head was groggy, but I was quickly aware of my surroundings. My eyes explored what I could find and I saw the familiar monitors of an intensive care unit, but in an unfamiliar hospital. A nurse sat in the corner working on a computer. A clock above her head was getting close to 8:00. She soon realized I was awake and came closer to check on me. As I quickly woke up, I realized I had a tube coming out my nose that I could feel going down my throat. However, I had my regular trach and was attached to my own ventilator. The nurse said surgery went well and Dad and Sara had gone to get our stuff from camp.

I was informed that the tube I had went down into my stomach and was attached to a suction machine. Everything was being pulled out to prevent anything going into my intestines to allow them to heal. I responded that whenever I was in the hospital in Des Moines, I always had someone with me. Unfortunately, no sitters were available and Wendy, my nurse, needed to work with her other patient next door. She said the hospital did have a sip and puff call system that she could set up for me. I hadn't seen such a device for a call light except in Denver and was thankful staff had prepared it for me.

Dad returned before she left. He and Sara had gone back to Recreation Unlimited and picked up my wheelchair as well as our clothes, my bed vent with humidifier, and everything else. They also found a nearby hotel so Sara could have a place to sleep. After he set up my humidifier, Dad updated me on what the doctor told him. Scar tissue from my original colon surgery had built up over the quarter century and caused the bowel to fold over and kink. I would likely be in the hospital a few days with the NG tube in my stomach until everything started working again.

That evening, Tom called Dad's cell phone to get an update on my condition. It was awkward talking with a tube in my nose and throat, but I told him everything that had happened the previous few days. He had been updating sites for my web clients while I was at camp, and I was glad to hear that it was going well. However, church had called and wondered how to do prayer updates. I had been put in charge of the prayer chain and they weren't sure how to send a request about me. I thought I had a backup person, but I explained the process to Tom.

Late in the day, it was time to let Dad get some sleep. He left to get Sara, bring her to the hospital, then go back to the hotel for the night. I was thankful they were able to stay with me because, if anything bumped the tube in my nose, it would hurt a lot and it frequently felt like it was pulling out. Sara gently helped hold it steady as hospital staff repositioned me in bed. I wasn't allowed to eat anything, except two ice chips per hour.

I did get a brief treat of water when I needed to take oral meds, but a small sip didn't go far. Sara helped through the night by washing my face and giving me my allotted ice amount. I sometimes waited until late in the hour to take my chips. A few minutes later, when another hour came, I had two more. It was a welcome relief to my dry mouth, but the wait for more seemed like an eternity.

My room was very small. Dad or Sara could sit in a chair but had to stand up whenever someone came to check on me. All I could see was the television, clock, and the hallway. Across the ICU, I could see another patient's room and a small portion of a window. If the curtains in my room and the other room were open, I could see if it was light outside.

Friday morning came, and I guessed about what time the campers would be leaving and counselors start heading home. Dad and Sara were given a large stack of get-well cards when they picked up our stuff, but I hoped a few of my counselor friends would visit on their way home. As the clock reached twelve, I estimated that it was a possible time when someone could come. I watched as the next few hours slowly progressed, but it remained Dad and me for the entire day. With most of the counselors from Indiana, I didn't expect anyone to come after Friday. As the day ended, it felt like we were alone and a long way from home.

Over the next few days, nothing changed toward desired progress. My belly was back to normal size, but I still wasn't showing signs of my digestive system working again. The only way I normally eliminated solid waste was through a procedure called digital stimulation. It required a caregiver to use a finger to stimulate the bowel for several minutes and remove anything that was in reach or worked down.

My ICU nurse was not familiar with the procedure and didn't know how to do it. Sara explained how it's done and demonstrated how it should work. After watching, nurse John said he didn't think it would be a skill to list on his résumé. As a registered nurse though, Sara and I informed him it was already assumed.

By Tuesday morning, the schedule of Dad on days and Sara at night had been continuing. However, since I was in the hospital, we knew insurance would not pay for her time so Mom worked out a plan to fly Sara home on Wednesday. The doctors also decided to try removing my NG tube to see if I could try eating something. Pulling the tube out felt very strange, but it didn't hurt. Not long after it was out, my stomach started getting puffy again and began looking like when I came in.

The physician team decided to put the tube back in. I had been sedated when the first tube was placed, but that wouldn't be the case this time. The nurse got a new tube and started pushing it up my nose. Just about an inch in, the pain in my nose was excruciating and I made her stop. She agreed to give me a break but would need to try again. When the second attempt came a few hours later, Sara was helping me for her final shift before flying home. As the nurse shoved the tube up my nose, Sara simultaneously held her hand on my cheek and gave me water to drink. Swallowing was supposed to help the tube go to my stomach instead of my lungs. It hurt going through my nose while feeling like I was being choked and attempting to drink. It was one of the worst things I had experienced, but thankfully it went to the right spot. I was thankful I could at least try to concentrate on Sara's hand and not feel what was being done to me. After an hour with the tube in, an entire suction canister was filled and a second one started. My belly went back to normal size again, but the prospect of getting released would now be much further away.

On Wednesday morning Dad checked out of the hotel and took Sara to the Columbus Airport. After a week in the ICU, the hospital's nurses were becoming familiar. They kept a close eye on me, with my sip and puff call light, during the short times nobody was with me.

Dad returned after playing taxi and said it was up to me as to when we headed home. I increasingly looked forward to being released from my windowless room and getting back to Iowa. While I was in the hospital, I had only been getting fluids through an I.V. and no nutrition. I had barely eaten anything the last few days I was at camp, and I was beginning to show the results of my crash diet. I hadn't gained much weight since my hyperthyroid diagnosis in the fall. What little weight I had was now gone and I was getting quite thin. Another pressure sore had opened on my back. While my body slowly decreased in size, all I could do was watch television. It seemed like most of the commercials were food related. Items I normally wouldn't think about eating started looking good.

Every morning a group of 4-5 doctors would huddle around a mobile computer desk. The group would stand outside each patient's room for a few minutes, sometimes looking through the windowed wall separating each room, and then move on. It was like being on display in a type of zoo or lab experiment.

Since I didn't have anything resembling food, I asked nurse Wendy how they expected me to go to the bathroom. She answered that the prisoners in the concentration camps of World War II weren't given food, but they still pooped. Not only did I feel like a lab experiment, but now I was being compared to tortured prisoners.

With Sara gone, Dad's parents decided to come to help. Mom wanted to come as well, but travel wouldn't be easy with her knee and Dad didn't want two patients. Grandpa and Grandma Vander Molen made the 13-hour drive at one time. A gas station attendant in Iowa helped them program their new GPS system but the screen didn't show a map. The two had to carefully listen to the verbal instructions and they didn't dare turn the system off.

My home night nurse, Mary, called the hospital and talked with Wendy when she helped watch me while Dad went to get lunch. Mary tried explaining my regular routine, that I don't have bowel movements very often and need a lot of stimulation. I was thankful for the effort, but it seemed to not register with anyone.

With more help to watch me, Dad got another room at the same hotel he had been using for the week. With some adjustment of timing, Grandpa and Grandma stayed with me at night while Dad stayed during the day. I had become accustomed to having Sara with me and her knowing how to help without my prompting. Grandma used to watch me one night a week, but that had been over 20 years earlier. My regular cares had become unfamiliar to them, especially in the hospital, and I tried to explain what I needed. I was accustomed to the NG tube at this point, but it was still difficult to speak with it. I was thankful my grandparents had made the 600-mile trip and Dad had some assistance.

Friday came and the physician team decided it was time to take an x-ray to see if there were further problems in my gut. Just before I was taken to x-ray, the nurses got what they had been waiting for. I still had images of my belly taken, but everything looked okay.

After ten days in the hospital, the prospects of release were looking better. The Saturday morning intern huddle wanted to leave my NG tube another day, but the head doctor said to remove it since very little was being suctioned out. This time, I was prepared for the feeling of the tube sliding out my throat and nose, but it still didn't feel good.

My stomach finally behaved and didn't expand like a balloon. By evening I was allowed to have a liquid diet. Plain orange Jell-O didn't seem like a big upgrade from ice and water, but it was something. If everything went well, I could have regular food the next morning and then be released if everything continued to look good.

Grandpa and Grandma came for their night shift and were surprised to see me without a tube sticking out my nose. Grandma said I looked like a new man, and I felt much better. That night, I could finally put a pillow over my face to sleep. It was the only way I could sleep comfortably, but my nose extension didn't work well with a pillow. Without the extension to my face, I could also be fully turned on my side and get off all the sores on my posterior.

Dad arrived early Sunday morning to get me ready to leave and for the drive home. He reminded the nurses that after being released, he and I had a long trip to get back to Iowa. A breakfast tray arrived with a thin slice of ham, hash browns, and other breakfast items. I wasn't sure about starting with this much but had to eat some to get released. Skipping the tough skin of the meat, I ate the majority of what came and didn't feel any problems. As Dad worked on packing, washing my hair, and getting me dressed, another tray was delivered. I wasn't sure how much I was expected to eat, but this seemed a little excessive. Dad ate it while working with me, so he didn't have to go find breakfast.

Just before noon, my food settled, and I felt fine. Even if I wasn't feeling well, I may not have told anyone so I could get closer to home. As we expected, my doctor officially released me from my hospital confines. With paperwork in hand, the nurse came to help get me ready to leave and was surprised to see I was already dressed and ready to go.

Getting in my chair felt strange and good at the same time. I hadn't sat fully upright in over ten days and the last time, I wasn't feeling well. I quickly became familiar with the position and was thankful to be leaving. I drove out to the van in the nearby parking garage and enjoyed feeling the warm summer air. It was a welcome change from being inside and only seeing walls.

Going Home

Dad and I headed west toward home with Grandpa and Grandma following us. As we neared Indianapolis, we stopped at our regular rest area just before the city to do my bathroom routine. I had used the hospital's supplies as a patient but they couldn't provide the unique catheters I used. I had just enough to get home, as long as there weren't more delays.

When I was finished in the restroom, I parked in front of a vending machine full of various candy bars and snack items. Everything looked good and made me want to get one of each, but I settled on a Snickers bar. Back on the road, Dad managed to give me a few bites as he drove through city traffic. It wasn't long before my stomach let me know it didn't like my choice of snack.

By early evening, our two-car caravan made it to eastern Illinois and we stopped at a Culver's restaurant. Dad parked the van in the back of the large parking lot away from most people. I needed my bandages changed for my pressure wounds and my clothing had a distinct hospital smell. Dad laid me on the floor of the van with my chair parked outside. He changed the two dressings on my butt and one on my back before putting on fresh clothes. It wasn't easy to work on me while on the floor but he got everything accomplished. After Dad put me back in my chair, the four of us went inside for supper. Everything on the menu looked inviting as my eyes feasted on the selection. I knew I should probably get something easy to digest, like a shake, but I decided on a cheeseburger. Sitting at our table, I struggled to get through about a fourth of the quarter pound burger before my stomach had enough. Grandma wanted me to eat more but I didn't want to push it.

A few hours later we crossed the Mississippi River into Iowa. Amidst the dark sky, occasional fireworks greeted us on our journey. It was July 4 and I was glad to be independent from Ohio State University and nearing home. Fireworks were eventually replaced by lightning and heavy rain about an hour from home. Dad and I lost track of my grandparent's vehicle behind us, but he kept driving to our destination. About 11p.m., the van pulled into the garage and Mom greeted us as Dad started to unpack. We had originally left for our one-week trip over two weeks earlier. I was exhausted, but glad to be in my own bed and familiar surroundings again.

I hoped the rest of the summer would go smoother and not have more unexpected hospital visits. Now that I was home again, progress needed to be made on my next wheelchair and the possibility of a new form of breathing.

26

REACTIVATION

In Ezekiel 37, the prophet is shown a valley of dry bones that appeared dead and useless. However, God put the scattered pieces together to form a large number of people. He then breathed into them, and they came to life, a vast army. As a quadriplegic, I barely used most of my body and it seemed useless to me. With God's blessing, some of it could function again.

After returning from Ohio, I slowly worked up to eating regular food and started feeling normal again. Cherokee Chairs called to clarify what needed to be adjusted before I could use their chair. A list of four items would be started before another technician came.

My online college classes started in late July with Fundamentals of Programming. The course was an easy introduction to my new method of learning. This was now my third college and third time taking basic computer programming.

The five-week course went by quickly and in August, I started Java Programming. I wasn't very proficient in this computer language, but it was also quite familiar after two previous times in the subject. Because the

University hardly took any credit from my earlier schools, I was required to repeat courses.

With school going well, I continued working toward getting the diaphragm pacemaker. Only a few select hospitals did surgery to implant the system. The closest options were either Lincoln, Nebraska or Chicago, Illinois. I chose to work with Northwestern Memorial Hospital in Chicago. Since it was out of Iowa and my insurance network, it took extra work to get the unusual surgery approved.

My doctors, Synapse Biomedical, Northwestern Memorial Hospital, and I spent the year giving the health insurance company everything they requested to research the DPS. It was up to them to decide if the surgery would be approved. I also continued to do research, along with my friend Bill from Florida. He was also hoping to get approved for the device and reduce his reliance on the ventilator. In conjunction with pacemaker work, I enjoyed helping him read through the Bible in a year and study unfamiliar areas.

In October, the call came that I had been praying for; the surgery was approved. As Evelyn, my case manager, talked about the approval process, I thought about scheduling surgery in the spring and what a change it could be. Evelyn caught my full attention when she said the procedure had to be done within the next three months or I would need to do the entire approval process again. I didn't like to travel in winter and wasn't sure about coordinating a trip to Chicago that quickly, but had to try.

With potentially life-changing surgery ahead, I decided to finish class in October and wait until after Christmas to start again. At church, the high school students needed an extra teacher for Sunday school. To add more responsibilities to my plate, I volunteered for the first few weeks to teach a course from Answers in Genesis. I had benefited greatly from taking the online creation courses and wanted to do the same for the teens. It was fun teaching God's Word and helping the young people understand the world from a Biblical perspective.

It still wasn't certain that the pacemaker would work for me. Testing would need to be done prior to surgery to see if my phrenic nerve worked.

Even if it appeared to work, it was possible that my diaphragm still wouldn't react as needed when the wires were placed in surgery.

The hospital was able to get me scheduled for testing on Friday, November 12. If everything went well, I would have the implant done the following Monday. It only left a few weeks to plan, but at least it would be done before the insurance deadline. As the date approached, Miranda, Sara, and my other nurses speculated how much of a change it would be to not have vent tubes and the ventilator. Transferring to my chair and moving in bed would be easier, but I downplayed the speculation. It was still very possible I couldn't get it and Mom was also very unsure about the prospect of changing everything we had known for so long.

On Sunday, I taught my last class with the high school students before leaving for Chicago. My parents and I didn't ask for prayers or say anything about the surgery, as it might not work, and it would be confusing to explain to most people. I gave a brief explanation to my Sunday school class, but that was the only thing church was told.

Later that week, on Thursday afternoon, my parents and I started the five-hour drive to the large metropolis. Night nurse Mary had lived in Chicago for a few years and still had friends and family in the area, so she easily agreed to help me at nights while in the hotel and to learn about the DPS if it did work for me.

I wasn't used to traveling late in the year and seeing how early the sun set. My parents and I stopped briefly in Rochelle, Illinois to watch trains at the busy intersection of the BNSF and Union Pacific railroads. Eventually, we made it to the city and tried to navigate the multi-lane roads and toll booths. Our new GPS system helped, but Dad often didn't agree with the automated instructions. As he drove, Mom said she couldn't hear my vent making its regular operating noise and wondered if I was okay. I assured her I was fine, and it was working, but to get used to not listening for that sound.

Hotels near the hospital in downtown Chicago were expensive, but Mom found one near O'Hare airport with somewhat reasonable rates. Mary met us at the Country Inn & Suites to find my room and set up my temporary home away from home. I never liked hotel beds very much. They didn't feel like my air mattress at home and only laid flat. However, I managed to get some sleep before the day of testing.

Friday's appointment was in early afternoon, but my parents and I left well before lunch to have plenty of time to find the hospital. Driving through downtown streets seemed strange with buildings higher than I could see through the van's windows. At the hospital, parking wasn't free like in Iowa, but was at least a reduced rate for vehicles with a handicapped parking tag. The three of us ate from a small coffee shop in the lobby before heading into the unknown.

Northwestern Memorial was a rehabilitation hospital for people with spinal cord injuries. When we got to the doctor's office, it was odd seeing other adults in wheelchairs getting checked in. I was normally the only one with a chair in my familiar facilities in Iowa. Mom and Dad sat down and told me to get checked-in on my own. Rolling up to the desk, I noticed it was shorter than usual and I could see the secretary's face instead of just hair over a computer screen. I gave her my name and birthday and was told the doctor was already waiting for me.

I joined my parents but was called back to the patient rooms promptly. Nobody was familiar except a few names I had heard when working to get approval. The first doctor explained much of what I already knew of how the system worked by inserting wires into my diaphragm that would then receive electrical stimulation. He added that the FDA approved the system a little over a year earlier, but only as a humanitarian device. I knew the approval was recent but wasn't familiar with the term. He said it meant that it was a type of trial approval. Once enough people had the system, and it worked well, it would receive full authorization. However, since it was only approved for people with ALS or SCI, it would likely never reach that status due to the low number of patients.

Finally, the doctor said it would take time to rebuild my diaphragm and it may take six months before I would be off the vent and pacing, as he called it, for even an hour. It was also possible that I may never get completely off the vent. Mom was relieved to know it wouldn't be an immediate switch to the pacemaker, but a gradual one. If I understood everything, then I needed to sign paperwork to proceed. Normally, I let my parents sign for me when away from home, but they insisted I sign it myself. While digging a pen out of my portable suction, Dad made sure to point out the clause that long-term effects of pacing were unknown. I was okay with that and with the pen in my mouth, I signed the agreement.

With paperwork complete, the next step was testing my nerve function. My parents and I were taken to a small room that had a machine I didn't recognize. An instructor from the hospital's university was running it and explained it would determine if my phrenic nerve was intact. She would put a slight electrical charge on the left side of my neck and then someone, with their hand on my belly, would try to feel if my diaphragm reacted.

It felt like she tried to fit an entire class into the room to observe. People were crowding around my chair trying to watch. Mom and Dad could barely see me as the test was about to start. I looked around halfway expecting clown costumes and a reenactment of the small car trick.

Sitting in this room in downtown Chicago, I recalled a certain Vander Molen Christmas party. Grandpa received an electric cattle prod to help encourage pigs to move. The device was about three feet long with a trigger on one end and two points shaped like a U on the other. An electric arc traveled between the tips and was meant for the back end of a pig. It also provided some entertainment in the hands of Dad's youngest brother with his siblings sitting around him.

As I sat, a probe came toward my neck that looked exactly like a miniature version of Grandpa's Christmas gift. It was firmly planted on the side of my neck near the appropriate nerve, and a shock applied. Immediately, my head jerked hard to the left without any input from me. One student had her hand on my abdomen but wasn't certain if she felt me take a breath. I didn't know either; all I felt was my head trying to twist off. Therefore, the test needed to be done again to make sure. My neck received multiple jolts as different students shuffled around for the opportunity to see what they could feel on my abdomen. It was hard to tell if I already had air in my lungs from the vent, so shocks had to be between breaths and after I exhaled. I tried to keep my head from snapping to the side, but I was helpless to prevent it. After at least a dozen jolts, my neck was sore, and I was ready to stop playing lab rat. One student, who kept trying to impress the instructor, was confident she felt a reaction. Another one agreed and I was approved to continue toward surgery.

Before the day was done, I had to meet with Dr. Wolfe. I had worked with this pulmonologist over the phone to get insurance approval for the pacemaker and she was the only person I knew. Sitting in yet another office, the specialist introduced herself and asked if I had seen what the pacemaker looked like. None of us had, so she left and soon returned with a medium-size black plastic case. Inside were two off-white boxes that looked a little larger than an old personal digital assistant. They were basic with one small display screen and two buttons. It appeared to be the right size to fit in a pocket and easy to move around.

Dr. Wolfe answered any final questions we had about the process before asking her own questions. She asked, "Carter isn't president anymore, why are you still using an old PLV-100 vent?" It was true that I hadn't gotten a new vent for about ten years since I was at AIB. New LTV 900 vents were available that were much more compact and just a little larger than a laptop. I had been surrounded by them at camp for a few years and felt quite familiar with alternative vent options.

However, as Mom and I explained to the doctor, we didn't like the way new vents operated. For one, the normal operating noise of the LTVs was much louder than mine. Also, the battery life was significantly shorter. With my vent connected to a car battery on my chair, it could go 10-12 hours if fully charged. At camp, the maintenance crew had to constantly swap vent batteries every 3-4 hours for the campers. I could barely get from Pella to Des Moines and back with that time limit. Also, the vent tubes I used were off-white with little color. The tube was obvious on my chest, but not as bad as most of the other bright blue tubes I saw at camp. Campers also used Passy-Muir valves, or speaking valves, which were purple. I liked my white valve that allowed me to talk without pausing and blended in with my other tubes.

I explained that, as a web developer, there were occasions when I was in meetings with clients sitting around an office table. My vent made enough noise already, I didn't want to add to it. Sleeping at night with more noise by my head wasn't appealing either. I also tried to dress well for meetings and church and having bright colored tubes wasn't a fashion statement I enjoyed. New technology worked for some people, but these were a few reasons why I hadn't changed. Dr. Wolfe said she hadn't heard of these objections before but was glad to learn. She didn't give much attention to outfit colors but understood the reasoning and would see if tubes and speaking valves could come in white.

The day at the hospital finished at 4 p.m. Leaving the facility during rush hour on a Friday in downtown Chicago didn't sound like fun. As Dad slowly made progress toward our hotel, the four-lane road was like a parking lot. On the sidewalk, more people were walking than I had ever seen in one place. At street intersections, it looked like a crowd that would nearly equal half my entire high school. Our large van crawled down the road and I watched El trains pass us every few minutes. The tracks were level with the road, and I could see the trains were well utilized.

The sun had set by the time we neared our accommodation and the three of us were exhausted. The only restaurant we knew how to access was KFC. It didn't sound very appetizing but worked well enough.

Sightseeing in Chicago

On Saturday, we met with my cousin Lucas. After college, he and his wife left the Pella area and had been living and working in downtown Chicago for a few years.

Whether testing had been successful or not, we had planned to stay in the city over the weekend and be tourists. Our first destination was the Museum of Science and Industry. After long lines to get in, it was fun to see lightning discharge, a full-size submarine, and a large model train layout. I liked all the different miniature scenes and thought some would be fun to replicate at home. One area of the museum displayed farming practices and allowed kids to feel corn kernels. It seemed odd to have what was familiar to me displayed in a museum, but I guess it was unique for city kids.

After roaming around the museum and catching up with my cousin for a few hours, Lucas became our Chicago tour guide. Driving around the city, we saw more museums before he directed us past President Obama's house, along with armed security. I didn't care for the president's policies for the nation, but his house looked nice. Lucas pointed out the tall red building where he worked, then took us to see his own residence. My cousin's home blended in with a row of attached houses along a small road. We drove around back with the van barely fitting underneath the El tracks.

Off the cramped alley, Lucas pointed out a small garage that went along with their apartment. Apparently, this was a luxury for a house near downtown in the big city. I thought of my aunt and uncle's house in Sully, where Lucas grew up, and how it had large open farm fields on two sides and neighboring houses that were at least 30-40 feet away. I couldn't understand why they would leave the openness of Iowa for this crowded area with so many people, but it was what he and his wife apparently enjoyed.

My parents and I didn't have plans on Sunday and a day of rest was welcome before surgery. Before leaving home, I had found a spot near the hotel where four railroad tracks crossed each other and would likely be a good location to watch trains. Dad found his way to them and a place to sit. After a few hours of sitting, no rail traffic came, but multiple planes flew over from the nearby airport.

Determining train watching a bust, we left the rails and navigated to O'Hare airport. Driving along a service road, Dad found an open gate to an area with luggage carts. He strategically put the van behind the luggage carts to hide us from the road in case parking wasn't allowed. From our vantage point, we could see the intersection of two runways. Smaller planes left the ground in front of us and a few large planes, including 747s, lumbered down the cross-runway before gradually climbing into the sky.

After a late lunch at Red Lobster the three of us returned to the hotel. The following day could either be a day of profound change in my life or nothing at all. I was scheduled to be at the hospital at 6 a.m. on Monday to get checked in for the procedure. It meant a short night ahead, but I was thankful the surgery was at least planned.

Life-Changing Surgery

On Monday, November 15, 2010, Mary got me up early to start my morning routine. Washing my hair in a hotel bed required hanging my head off the side while pouring water over my hair into a trash bag below. It wasn't easy or comfortable, but it got the job done. As usual, for surgery days, I couldn't eat anything, but I wasn't hungry anyway.

Traffic into the city in the early morning was heavy. It would move for a distance and stop again. After a few miles, we saw traffic lights that had been the likely cause of the strange traffic pattern. The outside world was busy, but we arrived at a quiet, early morning, surgery center.

After giving the receptionist my information, I was taken to a waiting room. Dad got me on the bed and changed my warm jeans and sweatshirt to a stylish thin hospital gown. As we waited, Mom and I worked on a crossword puzzle, and I completed my usual hospital activity of counting bumps on the ceiling.

During Friday's meetings, I had talked with an RT and a doctor about not changing my trach for surgery and about the specialized length I used. Despite my requests, the anesthesiologist required me to have a cuffed trach for easier control of my airway. The RT came to our room with an alternate trach in hand. He explained it was a special type and that the length could be adjusted to size four, which I used, or anything I needed.

At home, I was accustomed to changing the trach while sitting up, but the respiratory therapist only allowed me to be perfectly flat. Mom and Dad watched as my cuffless, comfortable, trach was removed, and the required version was chokingly shoved into my throat. During the process,

I remembered that this surgery was my choice but maybe I had made a mistake.

Mom and I resumed our activity after the trach change was complete and we continued to wait. Eventually, we were told that a man had been in surgery before me to get a DPS, but his diaphragm didn't react as required and he couldn't get the system. The unknown man would have been the seventh successful DPS placement at the hospital, but after some other surgical work, he would wake up to learn the news.

About four hours after arriving, I was taken back for my surgery, which had been delayed. Hospital staff explained that a call had been made to our home phone in Iowa to alert us to the delay, but the message wasn't received by us. After all the waiting, I once again felt the familiar induced drowsiness while lying on the operating table. Sometime later, I woke up in an ICU room with nobody recognizable around. Outside the window, it looked like late afternoon, but I wasn't sure. In my throat, I could feel the cuffed trach still in place and inflated. It felt like a large piece of food, or something stuck in my airway that didn't allow me to speak or swallow. Realizing my situation, I immediately felt the need to swallow the liquid in my mouth but had to fight the urge.

I could feel a little something in one lung, but it felt like the usual junk that would eventually need to be suctioned out. Other than that, everything felt normal. A nurse noticed I was awake and asked if I felt okay. I nodded yes. I wasn't very good at mouthing words, but I wanted to know what happened.

I carefully and slowly attempted to mouth, "Was the surgery successful?" The nurse responded, "No, you can't have any ice."

In my head, I thought that was rather obvious since I couldn't even swallow my own saliva. Maybe she thought I wasn't fully aware of my situation or wasn't familiar with post-operative routine. I decided to try again with hopefully an easier phrase to interpret.

I mouthed, "Did it work?" She replied, "Yes, everything went well, and they were able to do the implant."

After so much work to get approval and researching the device, I was thankful to have the desired result. Several minutes later, the RT from the morning came to check on me. The doctor hadn't ordered my own trach to be put back in, but he did negotiate to have the cuff deflated. Taking the water out of the balloon in my throat was a relief and I had a victory swallow to be sure.

Time seemed to move slowly, as it always did in the hospital, but I eventually was allowed to have the foreign object removed from my throat and my own trach put back. Breathing once again felt comfortable with my ventilator and airway restored. Before the day closed, Jeff, an RT from Synapse, came for my first experience at pacing. He had also apparently been with me in surgery and said I had taken some good breaths.

With my parents standing beside me, Jeff plugged a wire into the right side of my chest. Since my back was still curved after my scoliosis surgery, I couldn't move my head to see that side of my body. I now wished I had brought a mirror from home so I could know what was going on.

A gray wire came from my side and was connected to one of the white boxes I had seen a few days earlier. That box was also connected to a larger unit with more buttons. Jeff said in order to change settings on the pacemaker, the battery had to be removed so an access port could be connected to a control unit that could adjust settings. My only starting request was to maintain 15 breaths per minute, the same my vent had given me for over two-and-a-half decades.

Jeff pushed both buttons on the pacemaker simultaneously to turn it on. Four seconds later, with my vent turned off, I took a breath through my nose with my diaphragm activating it. Instantly, I felt a huge amount of pain in my lungs. I cried out in pain and the pacemaker was turned off and ventilator resumed. I again thought, "Why did I do this? Why didn't I listen to Mom and leave everything alone?"

After adjusting some settings, it was time to try again. I was much more hesitant, but I wanted it to work. The next breath was a little sore, but very tolerable and I let the new machine work for a few cycles. At home, when I practiced breathing, I had done it a few times with my trach capped off and, using my neck and throat muscles, could pull air in through my nose. That took a lot of effort, but this new technique was easy on my part and felt natural.

About a minute or two into pacing, my lungs started feeling sore again and I was short of breath. The system was turned off and my familiar vent once again took over my breathing. I listened as Jeff showed my parents how to plug the wire into the side of my chest and then the machine. Carefully listening to the instructions, it sounded like there were also a couple dressings that would need changing.

When the demonstration was complete, trials were done for the day, and everyone was ready to go home for the night. But before they left, Jeff explained that I had to be consistent with progress. If I did two or three pacing sessions for a few minutes one day, I needed to at least do the same the next day. If I decided to take a break and skip an entire day, then I would go back to starting from scratch. Since it had been over 25 years since I last used my diaphragm, it was atrophied and would take time to rebuild.

The nurse said if I lived in one of the suburbs, they would have sent me home for the night. However, since I lived in Iowa, I would stay in the ICU for one night. I had also requested to be able to stay a few days so we could get comfortable with my new breathing device and make sure everything was working correctly. Normally in the hospital, ventilators were connected to a call system so that, if it alarmed, the nurse would be alerted. My vent was too old and didn't have the correct connections. Thankfully, my nurse only had one other patient and would be in my room frequently and I didn't need to change to a hospital approved ventilator.

After surgery, I felt junk in my lungs, and it was increasing as time passed. I was asked if I wanted to try a cough assist device to clear my lungs. I had seen the machines at camp and had heard about them, but never used one. It was supposed to give a large amount of air, then quickly release it and simulate a cough. The process sounded similar to what I did on my own, but stronger. I was already branching out with trying the DPS and thought I would try this as well.

The machine was soon on my trach instead of the vent and started the process. Air kept getting pushed into my lungs, but it wasn't released. I could feel the excess stuff in my lungs get shoved deeper down and starting to hurt. When the air finally released, nothing moved up. Another cycle was tried, but it only got worse. I asked them to stop as the trial was only worsening my problem instead of helping.

At night, I normally did a chest treatment where a vibrating wand was rubbed across my chest and back for several minutes. It helped clear my lungs, but the RT staff was afraid the vibration could dislodge the freshly placed wires in my diaphragm. Therefore, I wasn't advised to use it or to lay on my right side on the port for the pacemaker. It was a long night of running a fever and sore lungs, but finally a bunch of blood and mucus were suctioned out. I was glad to breathe clearly again but wondered about the state of my lungs.

Tuesday morning, Mary came to see me in the hospital and to get trained on the DPS. Jeff returned as well and covered the same points he had with my parents and me the night before. It was starting to sound familiar, and I was able go a few minutes off the vent and just use the pacemaker.

When speaking with the Synapse representative, he had talked about other patients who had used the system. I knew the late Christopher Reeve had used it a short time before his death and I also knew a young boy in Ohio had received one. Jeff confirmed what I said but couldn't share details. He said children were more uncertain due to not testing their nerves prior to surgery. With my experience of nerve testing, I understood why that step was skipped.

As Mary and I caught up on the surgery and how to proceed with training and pacing at home, one of my monitors kept alarming. Mary could see it was alerting about my blood pressure being low. Soon, another doctor, who I had met that morning, came and silenced it. She said that she wished the monitor had a setting marked "quadriplegic" that she could hit. I asked why that would be needed. The younger physician was knowledgeable about spinal cord injuries and explained that with my lack of movement, my blood pressure would always be lower than average. I wasn't aware of that information before and always knew my blood pressure ran low, but didn't know why. Mary asked the doctor about her position in the hospital and how it must be an honor to have it. I got the feeling my night nurse asked the probing questions as a hint to me for flirting.

After Mary left and I was briefly alone with the TV and a sip and puff call light, the alarm sounded again. The female doctor responded promptly and, after it was quieted, I bounced my shoulders as much as I could and said, "Maybe more activity would help." My comment and grin received a small laugh and the physician and I talked a little about my quarter-century experience as a quad.

My parents arrived well before lunch and helped me eat when my meal arrived. My cousin's wife, who was an x-ray tech at the hospital, came and joined us on her break. She worked on Saturday and couldn't come with us on the city tour, but it was fun catching up with her.

Shortly after she left, an ambulance crew appeared at my door. It was time to leave the ICU and go to a room at the rehab hospital where I had initially interviewed. It was all part of Northwestern Memorial Hospital, but the units were in different buildings that were two blocks apart. A tunnel had once existed, but it was no longer available and the only option to change buildings was by ambulance. Dad strongly suggested that for time and expense, it would be better to put me in my wheelchair and drive myself over and help transport my belongings. His idea wasn't an option for my head nurse or anyone else who might listen. My safety was the hospital's responsibility, and an ambulance was the only way to go. As the EMTs transferred my vent and me to the gurney, Dad started packing up. The emergency vehicle was waiting for me and I was soon loaded and on my journey. Upon arrival at the next building, I heard the driver report the travel time: two minutes.

Strapped to the portable bed, I was pushed through the same lobby I had rolled through in my chair a few days earlier. This entrance method felt rather odd, but I tried not to look too perplexed, or healthy, as my arrival caught the full attention of everyone around.

My new room was void of ICU monitors and had a great window view of a brick wall a few feet away. Dad and Mom joined me a few minutes later as Dad had to push my 350-pound wheelchair, with my bag of clothes and new DPS equipment, through the hospital, two blocks of downtown Chicago, and finally up to my room.

Before supper, my parents and I went through another session on the pacemaker with Jeff. Looking at the plugin's location, Dad thought it might hit the armrest on my wheelchair. Jeff said the doctor had looked at putting it on my left side, however, unknown to me, several of my organs were moved to that side. In my early teens, as my body grew and twisted from scoliosis, the process had adjusted organ location. Since it wasn't advised to push wires through a kidney, the port ended up on my right side. Jeff flipped the plugin so it pointed up on my body instead of down, which meant my connection would be backwards from most users, but would be clear of obstacles. Unable to see my side, the conversation didn't make much sense to me, but I trusted Dad and Jeff's judgment.

I tried pacing for a few minutes, but this time Dad hooked everything up. As I experienced more time on the system, my cousin and his wife found us in my room. They wanted to take my parents to a nearby pizza restaurant before we returned home the next day. It was fun to show my new breathing apparatus, but it wasn't long before I returned to my vent.

Soon everybody left, and it was just me, a sip and puff call light, TV, and hospital staff roaming around the halls. The alarm system for my vent was the same in this section of the hospital as it was in the ICU. Since there were fewer nurses, I had to use a different ventilator for the night. Late in the evening, a respiratory therapist came with an LTV 900 on a portable stand. I had seen many campers use them, but I had never been attached to one. I considered requesting to use my pacemaker instead, but thought all night would be too much of a stretch.

I was used to having a humidifier at night but, as the RT changed my breathing, he said none were available. As soon as the vent was turned on, it sounded like a jet taking off a few inches from my head. It was set to the same breaths per minute I was used to but worked differently. On my vent, I would get air for two seconds, then nothing for two seconds. This loaner basically gave air constantly, just in waves of more to less to more. It maybe paused for half a second before continuing the undulation of air. It was miserable.

My lungs were sore from the constant up and down air flow without having a break. Without humidity in the tubes and non-stop breathing, my mouth and upper airway felt like I was chewing on cotton. I didn't like to bother the nurses, and would wait as long as I could, but had to puff on my call light to get drinks. The request was also low priority and it took several minutes before anyone would come to help. I asked if any vent settings could be adjusted, but apparently orders couldn't be changed at night.

By morning, I hadn't slept for more than a few minutes and I was glad when my parents came, and I could get unlimited drinks whenever I wanted. Mom hadn't been around this type of vent before like Dad and I had at camp. She initially thought it was an air pump for a bed mattress, but agreed it was very noisy. Dad soon came to my relief and switched me back to my own machine. The act resulted in the noise maker alarming for a few seconds before it could be silenced. However, nobody responded or checked to see if I had a problem.

After one more test of the DPS and a visit from Dr. Wolfe, my parents and I headed toward home by late morning. The hospital had given me a schedule for the day which interestingly listed me as visiting a psychologist. Dad wondered what I had done that made them think I needed such a visit, but I was released before I found out.

As we headed toward home, my parents and I stopped to eat in Rochelle, Illinois, dining on our fast food by the town's railroad park. I was due for a pacing session and Dad managed to get me hooked up in the van while sitting in my wheelchair behind him. It was a cloudy, damp day with lite rain as we sat by the railroad tracks.

Using a ventilator, I only exhaled through my nose and didn't inhale, so it was rare that I smelled anything. Breathing the moist air with smells around me was a new sensation that most people likely wouldn't notice. After a few minutes, my time off the vent was complete and the three of us drove the rest of the way home. Mary came at 10 p.m. and connected me to the new device for the first time at home. When she brought in my toothbrush, I could smell the toothpaste as soon as she came through the door ten feet away. After more than a quarter-century without use, my smelling ability was very acute.

On Thursday evening we had a training service with all my caregivers while Dad and Mary showed everyone how the DPS worked. Over the next week, I kept increasing my time off the vent and using the pacemaker. I had been told to give a one- to two-hour break between sessions, but no limits on how long to go. I kept pacing until I started feeling short on breath and was able to increase the sessions longer and longer.

A week later was Thanksgiving Day with Mom's side of the family. I wanted to show my new method of breathing without the vent, but wasn't able to go all day. I paced the half-hour drive to Sully, and quickly got inside my grandparents' house to get out of the cold air. A few of my aunts, uncles, and cousins asked about the change and I was happy to share. However, I noticed that while on the pacemaker, I couldn't speak continually like on the vent. Pausing every four seconds to exhale, take a breath, and start again was frustrating. However, I hoped it was just due to learning my new breathing style and I also hoped I could learn to work with it. I pushed my time off the vent a little longer than I would at home, but switched before we started eating. Dad and I moved over to an unoccupied room, and my cousin from Chicago, who had seen me after surgery, followed to see how it was going.

As Dad removed the red decannulation valve that blocked off my trach, he replaced it with the normal hardware that could connect to the vent. Lucas wondered if switching my trach hardware automatically turned the pacemaker on and off, but I had to answer that medical technology wasn't quite that sophisticated. The smells of Thanksgiving food were interesting while pacing, but the experience was gone when back on the vent.

December soon arrived and, six months after the initial visit, another technician from Cherokee Chairs came. Mike had a few parts with him, but not everything for the list I provided in July. One item he did have was an updated box for my vent and its battery connection. However, it still looked like it was done in an early high school welding class and my vent didn't fit.

I let Mike know I was using a new device and that I may not need the vent, but I still needed a place for a backup one. Several years earlier, one of my old ventilators had experienced major motor problems and had to be replaced. Since insurance had purchased it, the defective machine was returned to us with multiple warning labels. Dad gave the large paper weight to Mike to use as a guide to help the process. Since he didn't have any other pieces, Mike left, positive he would be back sometime between Christmas and New Year. I wanted to ask in what year, but I decided to be nice and not say anything.

It had been an eventful year with starting classes at a new school, two surgeries outside of Iowa, and wheelchair progress. I wasn't sure what to expect in 2011, but I hoped it would be more subdued. However, more activities than I anticipated would end, and I would have more projects that were unexpected.

27

LEARN TO BREATHE

"Fear not, for I am with you; be not dismayed, for I am your God. I will strengthen you, yes, I will help you, I will uphold you with My righteous right hand" Isaiah 41:10. Just when you think everything is looking up, it can quickly go down again. Looking to God's strength is how to get through.

As 2011 started, I got back into regular routines and resumed online classes. Being off the vent, pacing became more familiar as I continued increasing my time. Through social media, I was introduced to another quadriplegic, Chuck, who received his injury four years before me. While he also needed total breathing support, he had been using a phrenic nerve stimulator almost all his quad years.

Chuck suggested that instead of going for as long as I could, to set certain time limits, staying with that same duration for a week, then increasing by a few minutes for another week. The method worked well and made it easier to plan when to switch from vent to pacemaker or back.

To have any settings changed on the pacemakers, I had to get one shipped from Synapse's headquarters in Ohio. They would send one with the adjusted settings for me to try, then I had to send one back. By

February, it felt like I wasn't getting a deep enough breath. After corresponding about my experience, I had the pacemaker changed to give me a bigger jolt. The exchange took a few days, but the difference was remarkable. After three hours of using the adjusted machine and then going back to the vent at night, it felt like I was hardly getting any air.

Mary continued as my primary night nurse, but she frequently had health problems. She injured her leg early in February and had to be off for at least a week. The nursing agency couldn't fill the shifts quickly, which meant my parents had to cover the time. It wasn't too unusual, but Mom said they didn't know how much longer they could cover the overnight routine. I had known since high school I would likely be in a nursing home someday, but it felt like that time was approaching.

By early March, I was off the vent more during the day than I was on it. I was also starting my second online class for the year. Management Information Systems was more about understanding technology components than learning the practical use.

Since resuming studies in January, I was primarily only asked about paying tuition. The cost was covered through Vocational Rehabilitation, a Pell Grant, and my own funds. Unfortunately, my educational progress didn't seem to be a concern to my academic counselor, and it soon became frustrating. Repeating much of what I had done in previous classes at other schools didn't feel like I was learning very much. Another student in one of my focus groups was almost finished with his degree and noted that most classes would not be challenging.

As with every class, Management Information Systems concluded with a report done as a group project. Before it was handed in, I warned my group's leader that the paper had several format requirements to fix before submitting it. However, they were not corrected and, along with more errors, the final project received 30 points out of 100. The failing grade drastically reduced my final score from high to very low.

I didn't want to spend a large amount of time and money with little academic challenge and being dependent on classmates for my final grades. Therefore, I decided to stop attending the online university. I had hoped to earn at least my bachelor's degree, but that dream seemed unreachable. Due to skin problems, I couldn't attend regular classes in person multiple days a week, and online options were few and not very good academically. It was a major disappointment, but I was thankful for what I had learned.

Spring came and I continued increasing my time pacing. I was almost completely off the vent during the day, except for a short break in the afternoon. Even with the increased time and practice, I was not happy with my speech quality or with having to stop talking to take a breath. For me, it was most noticeable in church when singing with the rest of the congregation. With the vent and speaking valve, I could sing praise and worship songs with everyone else on cue. While pacing, I had to stop every four seconds and often had to skip sections to keep up with everyone.

In early May, I spoke to second graders at Oskaloosa Christian Grade School. I had been going to the school annually for a few years, but this would be the first time since getting the pacemaker. I decided to use the vent while in class so the students could understand me better. After the 30-minute trip to school, Sara parked in the one accessible parking spot and switched me from the pacemaker to the vent. Even though it had only been several weeks since I worked up to pacing most of the day, it felt odd being on the vent during that time.

I gave my regular presentation about types of disabilities, or different abilities as I said, and adaptive devices that help with everyday activities. As I had done for years, I explained, "The tube on my chest is connected to a machine behind me. My injury means I cannot breathe on my own, so this device breathes for me and allows me to talk and serve God."

Tulip Time in Pella

One week later was the annual Tulip Time in Pella. Seeing food stands set up all around town and people everywhere was typical during the festival. What was not typical is that, for the first time since being injured, I was able to smell the different treats that came from grills and make-shift kitchens.

Before the Friday evening parade, Dad and I went to find supper options while Mom stayed with the van. It was cool for early May, but otherwise a nice evening. As a result, downtown Pella was crowded with locals and tourists from surrounding towns and tour groups, to see the lighted parade and eat Dutch cuisine.

We navigated to one of the brick paved roads that had food booths lining the edge of the street. In the middle of the road, picnic tables were lined up to allow places to eat. This made for tight spaces to get between the benches, booths, and people waiting in line for food or who were trying to pass through. I found a clear spot to park and look over menu options on the various stands.

About two feet from me, a boy sat on a picnic bench poking at his food. My arrival caught his interest, and I noticed him looking at me. It wasn't unusual for kids to stare in my direction. I knew the sight of a lazy man who didn't lift a finger for himself and looked odd wasn't a common sight, so I normally smiled at them, maybe waved with my tongue, and most children then waved or smiled back. This youngster had a stranger than usual look on his face. He waved and said hi, and I responded the same. I wasn't skilled at starting conversations with unfamiliar children, so I tried asking if he'd found any good food options. After awkwardly attempting a short dialogue, a lady sitting across from the boy said to me, "You were in his class last week." I thanked her for the update and a renewed source of conversation. It also explained his confused look. I had told him, along with his class, that I needed the tubes on my chest in order to breathe. A week later, I was sitting beside him, with no vent tubing on, talking without a problem. Before I formulated an explanation of my DPS, Dad was ready to move on and get away from the crowds.

On Saturday my parents and I again had a parking spot for the afternoon parade on another beautiful sunny day, with tulips everywhere. After high school, Kyle and I had kept in touch, but we had mainly moved on to separate interests. Since his wife was busy, my childhood friend came from Des Moines to enjoy Tulip Time with his parents. He found my parents and me at the square and we talked for a while, catching up on life. I told him about getting used to the DPS and especially being able to smell easily.

Growing up together, he hadn't noticed or remembered my lack of ability to smell while on the vent. The missing sense hadn't occurred to me either, or wasn't something I mentioned. However, I did remember a "test" Kyle and I did once. He wondered if people sneezed when breathing pepper and therefore coated my mouth stick with the spice. Putting the blackened pointer in my mouth didn't produce the anticipated result and we assumed the sneeze reaction was false. The experiment would not have worked since I didn't inhale the pepper, but I wasn't willing to revisit the hypothesis.

Volunteering at CHAMP Camp

By the end of May, I had completely transitioned to the DPS while I was awake. I switched to the vent around 11 at night and to the pacemaker again in early morning. I didn't want to try going 24 hours a day due to fear of the insurance company claiming I no longer needed nurses. I was also familiar with using the vent to sleep and didn't want to learn new night habits.

In June, it was time for my volunteer week at CHAMP Camp. Having Dad help during the day and Sara at night had worked well in 2010, but I hoped to skip the hospital stay this time. After 17 years of using Recreation Unlimited near Ashley, Ohio, the camp had moved to Bradford Woods near Indianapolis.

The change meant a decrease of over 200 miles and several hours of driving. Campers and counselors from eastern states weren't fond of the increased travel, but it was nice for us. When our party of three arrived, I looked around the camp's new home. Everything was surrounded by trees and most of the paths were covered in shade. The campers and I wouldn't need to be as concerned about getting sunburned and would have an easier time with heat tolerance.

Along with scenery changes, the buildings were also new to us and were air conditioned, but with much smaller bunk houses. Instead of all the boys housed in two wings of one building, a maximum of six campers could be together. It would allow for easier care of the kids, but socializing with other boys would be harder if friends were in a different cabin.

During counselor training, emergency procedures were covered in case of an illness or injury. My situation and ambulance departure in 2010 was used as an example, but I didn't want to repeat it. Rick, one of the other counselors, said he tried to visit me in the hospital the previous year on his way home. However, he didn't come during visiting hours and wasn't allowed entry. Since he had a two-day drive home, he couldn't wait until visiting time. I was glad to know that at least one camp friend tried to come and check on me.

With several respiratory therapists, nurses, and students as counselors, there was interest in my diaphragm pacemaker system. I gladly showed it to everyone and answered questions. As the orientation time concluded, another counselor wanted to know my secret. He said whenever he saw me, I was surrounded by women wanting to lift my shirt and see my chest. I answered, "You just need to be on a vent for 25 years and then switch to a rare form of breathing. I don't think my method is something you want to try."

My cousin Heidi was in nursing school and she and her roommate also came as counselors. It was fun getting to show them the camp I had enjoyed for so many years and learn the new grounds together. The lake was much larger than we had in Ohio and the campers could get further out on a floating dock for fishing. It was fun helping campers again and seeing them catch largemouth bass as well as bigger fish than in Ohio.

Dad, Sara, and I bunked with the administration team. One evening, one of the counselors from another cabin called over the radio that she had heard from James. I hadn't heard much about him since we were both campers in 1998. Most of the former campers who were fellow quadriplegics had died over the years and I wondered what I was about to hear. Counselor Stephanie gleefully announced James invited her, and all longtime counselors, to his 30th birthday party in a few weeks.

I didn't remember that he was that close to my age but saw the surprised and excited looks from other counselors who remembered him. Several expressed interest in attending the celebration. My 30th birthday was only a few months away and the thought came to me about having a party as well. I mentioned the idea to a few counselors and was told they would love to come.

By the end of the week, everything had gone smoothly, and I didn't have any problems. Most of the veteran counselors agreed we loved the new location but wanted the old buildings. The campers were not able to get together with as many other kids during their downtime, but we did enjoy the air conditioning!

Pacemaker Repairs and Wheelchair Woes

As my favorite months of summer continued, I primarily stayed in bed. The pressure sore on my back healed but two continued to cause problems on my butt. Dr. Abrahamson's treatment was helping, but I needed to stay off them more, so I stayed on my air mattress in bed and, instead of sitting most of the day, started spending more time lying flat.

When August came, it had been nearly three months since I had used the vent during the day and was just breathing with the diaphragm pacemaker. Inhaling allergies increased my need for suctioning, but the system generally made life much easier. Getting in and out of my chair without changing vents and tubes was faster, and moving in bed was less complicated with just one wire and a box.

Near the end of the month, I switched from the vent to the pacemaker as part of my normal morning routine. However, it was not connecting very well and if not positioned carefully, the machine would alarm and not give me stimulation to breathe. After a few days of careful placement, I contacted Synapse Biomedical to see what I needed to do. They said someone would need to come and look at my wires and possibly do some repair work. But before that could happen, insurance would need to approve it and find a place where work could be done.

After several years of helping during the day, and some nights, Miranda decided to start teaching CNA classes at a local college and would no longer be available. Caregivers were hard to find, especially for just two days a week, but my parents and I thought of possibilities. Since I was in Pella again, we reached out to Leah. She had visited a few times but hadn't worked with me since I moved to college in late 2000.

She was working part-time for a nursing agency in Oskaloosa but was available to do two days a week. Sara and I spent a day getting caught up on changes in the previous eleven years, especially with the pacemaker. Leah had changed some from how I remembered, but we were very thankful for her help.

As September started, I contacted my pulmonologist, general physician, and insurance case manager, to get everything arranged for the pacemaker repair. The month continued to progress as I received increasing rejections. Doctors weren't willing to have an outside person do maintenance on the DPS. Finally, when one doctor approved, the facility he worked in wouldn't allow work to be done in their building due to liability. The insurance company would allow repairs but had to first approve payment to a company that was out of network.

While working on the pacemaker, Cherokee Chairs came again to work on my chair. No one had come since May to attempt progress on the wheelchair. Very little had improved since I first received the chair, and I refused to sign paperwork saying I had taken possession of it. Now, Mark came to see what he could do. I sat in the seat, but needed more support to sit straight. Mark had a new chin control system to try that looked similar to what I requested. He had me use the standing feature to see how it worked. I was cautious to stand very far in order not to break anything but went nearly upright. The controls that had been positioned well when sitting were now at my neck and out of reach.

Sara also noted that the back support rubbed a lot as I moved. With the sore on my back healed, we didn't want to open it again. I agreed to do the sitting process once more so a video could be made to show the issue. Once again, only problems resulted instead of progress. As Mark packed up, my parents and I voiced our frustration and how slow Cherokee was on making visits. Mark agreed that over a year was too long to wait and suggested we contact a lawyer for a refund.

By September 30, no progress had been made toward getting repairs on my DPS. As I was switched from the vent to the pacemaker, it completely refused to work. My caregivers had managed to carefully keep it going for over a month, but nothing would connect, and I had to stay on the vent. Sending pictures of the wires to Synapse, they could see the ground wire was damaged as well as one other. A temporary patch could be made, but the wires needed to be fixed if I were to keep pacing.

A few days later I received the patch in the mail and was able to get off the vent again but had to be very careful. I had to slowly get myself used to pacing again after being off for more than a day. More messages and paperwork for a repair kept going, but with no progress. Synapse let me know they were doing training and repair in Rochester, Minnesota, and I could meet them there for work. I didn't want to keep waiting on approvals, so I agreed.

On October 26, nearly two months after I started having trouble, Mom and Dad drove me the five hours toward the Mayo Clinic. I was glad it would finally get fixed, but hoped this wouldn't become a common event. In Minnesota, a respiratory therapist from Synapse looked at the wires coming out of my chest and quickly assessed the situation. I practiced my self-breathing while the pacemaker was disconnected, and she applied something to the wires. After a few minutes, I was again receiving stimulation and could breathe easily.

Before leaving, Dad and I visited a bathroom for my afternoon relief. He took the bag of supplies from the van and started to get set up. Dad searched in every pocket and found everything except the special NG tube. My caregiver said she checked supplies the day before, but apparently missed that catheters were absent. I was over 200 miles from home without supplies. My regular hospital in Des Moines couldn't find the tube I used, and we didn't want to take more time trying to see if Mayo clinic could get one.

Dad sternly voiced his thoughts on the situation as he loaded me in the van where Mom waited. As we started the multi-hour trip home, I began to feel the start of Autonomic Dysreflexia. I normally didn't get too concerned about AD as problems could usually get resolved quickly. Now that it would be several hours before I could cath, I wasn't sure what would happen.

As I continued to AD, my body started to sweat. This was something I normally couldn't do, so I knew I was getting a severe reaction. The three of us stopped for a quick supper and my shirt was damp with perspiration. I attempted to drink as little as possible, but it was a challenge with dry food from a convenience store. Driving south of Waterloo, we passed the care facility where Ken lived. I wondered briefly if they would have something to help, but highly doubted it. At least, I told myself, I could breathe without trouble.

Late in the evening we finally returned home. As Dad put me in bed, he stripped me of my clothes that were completely soaked with sweat. I was feeling miserable, but thankfully did not get bad enough to have a stroke. Nearly fifteen hours after I had last used the restroom, I could again have my bladder drained and body relieved.

With two months of work to get my DPS wires fixed and nearly having a stroke in the process, I wondered if the pacemaker was worth the effort, hoping this would be it for problems. A few weeks later, the wires started getting touchy and only worked in certain positions. With one muscle spasm and my arm hitting the plugin, it stopped functioning and required more work around patches.

November came, along with my 30th birthday. I had kept in touch with Jayde from AIB and talked with her a few times a year. Since her birthday was one day before mine, we decided to have a joint party. I reserved a conference room at a hotel in Pella to have our celebration on Saturday, November 26. It was just two days after Thanksgiving, but I hoped to get a good crowd. I especially looked forward to my camp friends coming as they said in June.

Invitations were sent out early in the month and I waited for replies. When the party came, the room was filled with some of my former caregivers, my relatives, and a few of Jayde's family. Nobody from camp came as I had hoped for the previous five months, but I was still thankful to reach a new decade and to be surrounded by close friends and family.

Back to the Hospital

As 2012 started, I continued dealing with two pressure sores on my upper legs. Staying down more didn't seem to do much more than make it difficult to get web updates finished in a timely manner.

After another two months of paperwork, in early January, I again had the wires on my DPS fixed. This time, I was able to get the work done near Des Moines. Synapse worked with an independent pulmonologist who was willing to do repairs for me and another DPS patient in central Iowa. Driving only an hour was much easier than going to Minnesota. I wasn't sure how often I would need repairs or how many fixes could be done before I needed surgery for new wires.

In late February, I started having trouble with bloating and my gut was not working as well as it should. One Monday morning it was getting very painful, so I had Leah do my bowel routine to see if that would help. It had been several years since she last did the procedure and it took a long time to do. Laying on my side while Leah helped me go, I could feel junk gathering in my lungs. It soon became hard to breathe and when I finally returned to my back, I felt miserable. I was unable to do anything the rest of the day and made an appointment to see my doctor the next day. I kept going back and forth from breathing with the DPS and then the vent. With my lungs and stomach hurting, neither option felt right.

After a long night, my general practitioner didn't think my belly was anything serious and sent me home to see what would happen. Everything continued to get worse until I had my parents take me to the ER in Des Moines.

After a few hours of waiting, the doctors decided I was again having stomach issues like before and opted to put another NG tube through my nose.

I remembered the experience all too well from Ohio in 2010 and wasn't looking forward to it, but I didn't have a choice. It was hoped that the tube would solve the issue and surgery wouldn't be needed. Getting the tube shoved up my nose and down my throat again wasn't any nicer than the previous times. However, since the DPS was unfamiliar to Methodist Hospital, I chose to use my ventilator during my stay. Also having a lot of lung congestion, I was put on breathing treatments to hopefully help clear that up. A few nights into my stay, I was slowly improving. I could feel exactly where the mucus was in my lungs and was careful how I was positioned. I hadn't laid on my right side for two days so I could breathe easier, but thought I needed to try in order to prevent further skin problems.

The nurse and my sitter carefully got me turned so my nose and tube wouldn't get bumped and I was somewhat comfortable. About one minute after the nurse departed, I felt everything from my left lung come up and start to drain into the opposite side. With the shift, the vent couldn't push air into my lungs. The change increased resistance in my lungs, making the machine alarm due to high pressure. When that alarm happened, the vent didn't give me air and exhaled the breath through the machine. After missing a few breaths, I knew I was in trouble. It was nearly impossible to talk, but I managed to click my tongue to get my sitter's attention and croak out the word "suction!"

My oxygen level dropped rapidly without getting air and I was unable to do my self-breathing. The pain in my head was more than I had ever experienced, and I kept fighting to get air. The oxygen monitor alarmed as my numbers plummeted. If I had been on the DPS, I would have received stimulation and taken a breath. Now, I knew I couldn't stay conscience much longer as the pain became excruciating. It took all my concentration to fight for air and try to direct my caregivers.

Standard hospital procedure was for the nurse to call the RT department and they would send someone to suction. I knew I wouldn't last that long, and it was likely not going to be more than a minute, or maybe two, before I passed out. The sitter got my nurse, and they both rolled me to my back, as these thoughts went through my head. Changing positions didn't help my lungs and my head kept increasing in pain as air hunger grew. Every four seconds my hope for air went away with an alarm from the vent.

Thankfully, the nurse recognized I needed immediate help and suctioned me on her own. I prayed she was able to do everything without guidance as I could barely stay conscience. She did very well, suctioned as deep as I normally had to request, and cleared out a lot of junk. As the catheter cleared my trach, she directed the sitter to use my ambu bag. The air pushing into my lungs felt great and rapidly helped my head, but we still had more to get out. After a few minutes, I could breathe easily again and was grateful for a well-trained nurse.

The same scenario came close to happening a few times while in the hospital, but I reacted before I experienced suffocation again. After several days of wondering if I needed surgery, the NG tube was removed, and my gut was back in working order. The doctor warned me to stay away from too much bread and to be careful what I ate. The more often I was in the hospital with the stomach tube, the more frequently I would have problems.

It was a relief to be home again with caregivers who knew me and my equipment. Since I had been off the diaphragm pacemaker for several days, I needed to slowly build my time up again. The process of weaning from the vent and back to the pacemaker was starting to be a regular routine. I really questioned if pacing was a better system than the regular vent, but it did make life easier when I could use it.

Springtime in Pella

In March, six months after the previous visit, Cherokee Chairs again came to work on the chair. This time Sam, the company founder, was the visiting technician. We had exchanged multiple emails, but I hadn't seen him since the summer of 2010 when the system was delivered. He had me try another chin control that mounted on my shoulders instead of laying on my chest.

The change in position was still very similar to the first joystick and it didn't work. I reminded Sam of all the other issues, the backrest rubbing, chair length was too long, a secure vent and battery tray, and more. Sam thought it would be best to take the entire chair back with him so it could be adjusted at their workshop.

Dad and I watched as my chair was pushed up a steep ramp, scraping the footrest on the driveway, into the back of a pickup truck beside another wheelchair. The truck didn't have a tarp or any type of covering to protect the cargo. It was a long trip from Iowa to Arizona and I wondered what weather would have to be endured. I told Sam, "I expect to hear back by April 15th with everything subject to my approval. If it isn't fixed by the next visit on June 15th, I want a full refund." Sam agreed and drove off with my chair.

A few weeks later, it was time to visit my regular grade schools. This year, I decided to try it while using the pacemaker. It was nice not having tubes, but I did not like stopping to take a breath. Trying to explain the system to adults was tricky but attempting to get second graders to understand was even harder.

I would also be visiting Rae's class. The Van Hoerkel family were frequent visitors, and the young lady was used to being around me. I stopped Rae at church a few days before our school encounter and told her I would be visiting, but not to answer all the questions. I wasn't sure what her response would be when Mr. Joel came. I didn't need to worry, though, as she acted as a spokes girl for her shy classmates.

As spring started to feel warmer, I was able to get back on the pacemaker faster than previous times. On May 1, I got my hair cut in the morning and was looking forward to the start of Tulip Time in two days. My church had rented out parking spots at our building, just a few blocks away from the festivities. The young people oversaw it, but I volunteered to monitor the lot and the teenagers for a morning shift.

Sara did my regular afternoon cares of cathing, wound care, looking over my skin, and my stretching routine. Just as we finished a stretch on my left leg, I heard a loud pop. Sara felt it as well and I recognized the sound as when my right femur broke nearly a decade earlier. We weren't sure, but I needed to get my leg checked without using the sling to get me in my chair.

Dad was busy at work and didn't want to come home. After I explained our concerns, he reluctantly came with another coworker to help transport me to Pella Community Hospital. The only other option was to go by ambulance. When the two men came, Dad dug out the standing frame I had last used in junior high. With a few adjustments of the support pads, he made it work as a substitute gurney.

The two guys and Sara slid me onto it from my bed and Dad soon figured out a way to get me secured in the van for the six-block trip to the hospital. The emergency room staff were intrigued by our homemade contraption, which did the trick. Mom joined Sara and me while waiting to see the doctor and to get an x-ray.

Nearly an hour after arriving, I was brought to radiology for leg x-rays. The first scan was taken while laying on my back, but I would need to turn for the next internal picture. Sara watched the technicians' faces as the digital picture came up on their computer screen. She knew immediately by their reaction that our concerns were correct and my leg was broken. A technician said they normally don't diagnose, but the femur was obviously broken, and they didn't want to do further damage by moving me.

A few minutes later, I was talking with the doctor on treatment options. Pella didn't have the ability to do surgery on the break and would need to pass me on to a Des Moines hospital. I knew the bone had to be fixed so I wouldn't have problems like I did with the right leg. Therefore, I could not see Dr. Gunke as I had the last time. Since he refused to do surgery and fix my right leg, I sat improperly and ended up with a pressure sore and further leg damage. The Pella ER contacted Iowa Methodist to see what orthopedist was on call. It wasn't Dr. Gunke, so I decided to give them a try.

Pella ambulance was called to transport me to Des Moines for my second stay at Iowa Methodist for the year. As I laid in the back talking with the EMT, I wondered how this leg break would conclude. I prayed it wouldn't be like the last time and I wasn't sure what to expect. I had an hour-long ride before getting more answers.

28

MISSING

The apostle Paul had much tribulation while spreading the good news of Christ. In Philippians 4:11-12, he told the church he knew what it was like to have plenty and to be in want. When we go from good times to bad, it can be a good learning experience.

When my emergency ride arrived in Des Moines, I was wheeled directly through the ER and into a room in the Intensive Care Unit. My broken leg didn't necessitate the ICU, but it was where space was available, and staff could handle my breathing needs. The skilled care unit meant neither insurance, nor the hospital, would allow a sitter to stay with me. Even though I couldn't use a call light or have my ventilator connected to the alarm system, the hospital thought their monitors were enough. Therefore, my parents, grandparents, and other relatives would need to stay with me while I was in the hospital.

I was still wearing the same clothes I put on before going to the Pella ER. The nurse wanted to cut my shirt off, so she didn't need to turn me and further injure my leg. Looking down, I noticed it was one of my few shirts that fit me and one I liked. Dad demonstrated how to grab behind my neck, partially sit me up, then pull the clothing up high enough to get my arm through the sleeve. The ICU nurse was impressed and hadn't seen such a move before.

After I got checked into my room, a doctor came to consult on plans for my broken femur. Mom and I made sure to emphasize the consequences of not fixing my right leg. The resulting bone infection, pressure sores, and poor circulation could not be repeated, and this break needed to be fixed properly.

The doctor said he would normally put a metal rod in the bone to fix it, but my bones were thin after decades without use, and he didn't think he could find a rod small enough to use. His other option was to secure hardware on the outside of the bone. The concern with this method was not knowing if it would stay in place. Since the rods were fine in my back, I was confident the second option would work. Surgery was planned for the next day and then I would stay another night in the hospital before going home. It was difficult for my parents and relatives to always stay with me, but I could at least continue using the DPS during the day.

Surgery was on Wednesday morning and went well. I was surprised when the anesthesiologist allowed me to keep using my pacemaker during the procedure. I was sent home on Thursday afternoon, less than 48 hours after the break. I didn't need a cast or have any visible signs that there had been a problem. The doctor said I could do my normal activities, but also said I should not put extra stress on my leg for a while.

The first change would be not going out during Tulip Time, which had just started. When he heard about what happened, Pastor Dan and his wife brought me a favorite Dutch treat, funnel cake with strawberries and whipped topping. Even if I couldn't go to the food, it could come to me.

With camp just over a month away, I didn't think it would be a good idea to get lifted in and out of bed by picking up my legs and then be in my chair all day. I reluctantly resigned from my volunteer counselor position in order to prevent further complications. The previous summer had been physically difficult with worsening pressure sores, and I was already questioning if I should keep volunteering. It had been ten years since I had missed a summer at camp, but I wasn't sure it would be the last.

Two weeks later, I had a follow-up appointment with the doctor. After getting an x-ray, the nurse removed the staples in my leg that closed the incision. While he worked, he said that I was a new experience for him. The nurse had seen many bone surgeries in 13 years, but my femur was a purple color instead of the usual off-white. The doctor also said I was the first quadriplegic he had seen that requested the break to be fixed. Anyone else he had treated only wanted to set the bone and have a cast. I was used to being an unusual patient but wasn't aware that even my bones were unique.

Healing continued as the days and weeks passed as I mainly stayed at home working on websites. By late June, I hadn't heard much from Cherokee Chairs since they took my chair in March. Both deadlines of April and June 15 had passed without the promised completed system. I had been asked to send multiple pictures and measurements of my current chair and I had provided everything, but that was the only progress. Therefore, I emailed the owner to see what was going on.

Sam said it wasn't complete yet and they couldn't find a solution for my chin control or the shearing on my back support. I reminded him of our conversation in March and that I had already been waiting over two years. It was time for a refund so I could start looking for a different chair. Sam said he didn't remember agreeing to anything and would only continue trying to make the needed adjustments. This was what I expected, but I had hoped he would honor what we had agreed upon.

In July, I attended a wedding for one of my high school friends, Jana. She had most of our school group in her wedding party. It had been 12 years since our graduation in 2000, and I hadn't seen many of these women since then. In high school, I had hoped to be married and raising a family by this time in life. I was happy to see most of them doing just that, but I felt out of place.

Getting married would mean losing my parents' insurance and would likely end up with me in a nursing home. Because of that, I knew very few quadriplegics with families of their own. A new federal law, the Affordable Care Act, had recently made it so that insurance could no longer have a lifetime spending cap. This made life much easier by not having to worry about the future after hitting my limit, but it also meant I was stuck being dependent on insurance through Dad indefinitely.

As 2012 passed, I continued to work on web development, trying to keep clients happy while maintaining my health. In September, my parents went on a train trip to northern California. For ten days, I was the man of the house and responsible for keeping track of everything. In order for the vacation to work, my caregivers took more hours than usual, and my grandparents helped in the evening.

Using the diaphragm pacemaker, it was easier for my parents to get away. Whoever was helping me didn't have to watch vent tubes or drain water that condensed from the humidifier. They still needed to be careful of the wire connecting me to the stimulator, but it was much less work than the vent required. I also started increasing my time off the vent and kept pacing through part of the night.

Church Volunteering

At church, the Wednesday evening boys' group, Cadets, needed more counselors. Dad had always wanted to help with them and I enjoyed working with kids. Therefore, he and I volunteered to be counselors for Junior Cadets, seven boys with age ranges of first through third grade. I wasn't sure about being in my chair more with two pressure sores or going out on cold winter nights, but I wanted to help.

Through our first few months as counselors, we struggled to learn how we were supposed to work with the boys. A third, more experienced, counselor was going to guide us, but he frequently didn't come and left Dad and me to fend for ourselves. Some nights went okay, and we actually got material covered, but other nights we couldn't wait to be done. Instead of an enjoyable volunteer time, most Wednesday evenings were filled with dread as the clock neared our 90-minute session.

We started helping with Cadets in August, but in October I received a letter from my church council. They wanted to put my name in for selection to be a deacon. My church governing body consisted of two primary roles: elders and deacons. Elders mainly dealt with spiritual concerns in the congregation and deacons with financial needs. Both roles, along with the pastor, made up the church council.

I had been maintaining the church website since starting college in 2000. A few years after moving home with my parents, I took charge of the prayer chain, making sure prayer requests got out to the congregation, and every other month, I worked with two other members to gather articles for the church newsletter. Since I was still figuring out how to work with the boys in Cadets, I wasn't sure I should add another role.

Being a deacon would mean going to meetings every month, along with the full council, to discuss matters of the church. I knew from when Dad had served that they started in early evening and he often didn't get home until after midnight. The commitment would be for three years, longer than anything I had ever agreed to. I wasn't sure how it would work to have someone be with me during meetings without being a council member, or if I should be in my chair longer than usual.

My parents thought we could get a schedule arranged for someone to come with me, but not to be in on the discussions. There was also only a 50% chance I would be selected. Twice the number of people needed were put up for nomination, then names were pulled from a hat. Not having the congregation vote made it close to how the Apostles selected positions in the book of Acts. I was unsure, but decided to leave my name in for selection.

Our congregational meeting was held in November, where we voted on the new budget and selected new council members to replace those whose term was ending. When deacon selection came, the first name pulled and read was "Joel Vander Molen." I briefly dropped my head in a mix of defeat and excitement. I guess I was meant to be used in another role at church.

One month later, in early December, I had my first meeting to learn about everything going on in the church and select my specific role as a deacon. Dad came along as my caregiver but sat in the church basement in one of two places. If I needed to be suctioned, or the DPS had a problem, then someone could get him. Otherwise, I would try to fend for myself and explain what help I needed to my fellow councilmen.

The first task for the three new deacons was to pack bags of candy for the kids to get after the upcoming Christmas program. I couldn't physically help but I talked with the other two deacons who had been selected with me. Generally, deacons were younger men in their 20's and 30's with elders having more life experience. It was nice talking with guys close to my age and to be somewhat on my own. I quickly noticed that more bags of candy were being packed than we had children in church -many more. When I asked about it, I learned they weren't just for the kids. On late nights for deacons, the superfluous bags became sugar fuel for keeping awake. Church council was a volunteer position but did have occasional perks.

Before the bags were finished, the three of us were summoned to the meeting that was already in progress. With some terms ending and new ones beginning, we had to vote on who would hold each position. The current deacon president explained the various roles. Someone would volunteer if interested or a vote would take place if multiple people wanted the spot. I knew I didn't want to be president my very first time in office and I wasn't sure about being the treasurer either. Secretary sounded like a position I could help with and volunteered. One other deacon wanted the position as well, but I was voted to take it.

Each month at our meetings, I would need to record the minutes and everything that happened. Any mail directed to deacons would go through me, and I also had to coordinate each week's offering at church, determining where gifts would go. Coordinating with the deacon president, I was responsible for preparing every meeting's agenda. Finally, I also had to communicate with the church secretary to include any announcements or schedules to the congregation. I wondered if I was taking on more than I should, but everything could be done on a computer. I would need to take my laptop, mouth stick, and table to church for meetings, but it was possible.

Deacons and elders each held separate meetings before coming together as a full body. Between the two sessions, a small supper was served since the night started early. Some confidential discussion topics occasionally continued during mealtime and I, therefore, couldn't have help from anyone outside of council.

Everyone gathered in the church kitchen where food had been brought by a volunteer. There were items to make sandwiches, drinks, and a couple of desserts. I had eaten before I left home, but the freshly made brownies looked good. I parked myself in a corner so people could get around me, and asked Byron, who was nearby, if he would help me eat. I knew him fairly well from our school years and from church and he gladly agreed. It took some initial instruction, but we managed without getting my lap covered in crumbs. I directed him to where Dad had hidden a bag of straws, and getting a drink of pop to wash down the snack was easy.

After supper, both deacons and elders moved upstairs to the council room. I recruited the same man who helped me eat to get us up the elevator to the main level. I waved at Dad as we passed him sitting in the library and then explained how to close the elevator doors for it to work. Byron agreed it was a tight squeeze, but we made it in one piece.

Growing up at Pella II CRC, I had been in the council room a few times. It always had a large table in the middle that was surrounded by chairs. To give me room, the table had been removed and the seats placed against the walls. At the start of every meeting and each church service, all men in council went around and shook hands. With the furniture rearranged, I could drive around the room, nod at each person, and say hello. I wasn't sure how my term would go, but I was thankful I was in a church that worked well with me.

A few weeks later, I was officially installed as a deacon at the first church service of 2013. Both sets of my grandparents came to watch and were glad to see me serve. Normally, the deacons passed the offering plates during the service. I tried to think of a way I could balance the trays on my lap, but my fellow members were willing to take my shift instead.

By spring, I started to get used to being on council and working with the boys in Cadets. For Bible lessons, Dad and I found new books to use and started to feel like we could take the kids another year. I loved teaching the boys and seeing them look to me for guidance as an adult, not just the guy who uses a wheelchair at church. Some nights, I could have taken a boy or two home with me and feel like the dad I had hoped to be. Other evenings, though, I couldn't wait to push them out the door to their parents.

Monthly church meetings became normal as I got into the routine of being secretary. Karen no longer helped me during the day but came most Friday evenings. My parents could get away and spend time together and it made for a good opportunity to work on church paperwork. Karen would open envelopes and lay the contents beside me on a table. I could then reach them with my mouth stick, read the correspondence, and record what was needed to pass along. One to two nights a month usually allowed enough time to keep caught up on everything.

Back to CHAMP Camp

Increasing my hours off the vent and on the pacemaker continued to go well, but it was hard to sleep comfortably with it. If my vent circuits were not positioned correctly, it would push or pull on my trach. Therefore, positioning on my side or back included getting the tubes in the right place. Using the DPS, my trach was capped so I would breathe through my nose and would not have anything attached to my neck. After I was turned, I would still get the feeling of tubes pulling at my throat and feeling the need for them to be repositioned, even though they weren't attached. I heard of a condition called phantom limb where amputees feel pain or sensation in a limb that didn't exist. I had spent the majority of my life with vent tubes, and it sounded similar to that experience. Around 5 a.m. I would change back to the vent and return to pacing before 8 a.m.

I had debated about volunteering at camp in 2012 but didn't go due to the leg break. This year, I applied again to see how it would go. June

2013 came quickly with my second trip to Bradford Woods. Sara did well at night and Dad during the day.

As part of the application, counselors put their preference of what age group to work with. Since I spoke with second and third graders at schools and church, I always put my preference with younger boys. This year, however, I was put with the teenagers, the oldest age group possible. I had been around some of these young men in earlier years but didn't know how to relate with them very well.

Just before camp, the water main for Bradford Woods broke which meant no drinking water in the cabins. As campers arrived on Sunday, so did a large thunderstorm. Unloading ventilators and medical equipment under trees in pouring rain wasn't easy, but volunteers helped keep everything, including campers, dry. The wind from the storm also caused the power to go out while everybody worked to get set up in their bunks.

The administration team kept cabins supplied with bottled water and started getting a count of battery supplies for ventilators. Generators were coming, but not enough for every cabin. I was thankful to say my DPS had enough battery for a few weeks and only using my vent for one hour at night wouldn't take much electricity.

After our four teens arrived, we hung out in the cabin until it was time for our first activity. Energy levels and attitudes of these older campers were much different than I was accustomed to. Most of them had been to camp for several years and everything was routine.

During downtime in the cabin, it was common for music to be belted out from an iPod or some type of device. One of the young men had his favorite sounds playing for all to hear. I tried to listen but could not make out any intelligible words over the noise I assumed was music. Another counselor asked him to turn it down, much to my relief, but I remembered being one of these teenagers looking forward to a week with my friends. Even though this wasn't my regular age group, I would do my best to make sure they enjoyed the week.

Over the next few days, I did all I could to get to know our campers. Now that I used the DPS almost exclusively, I was extra cautious that my right arm didn't spasm and hit my wires. While in the cabin between activities, Sara did extra stretching for my right wrist and arm to keep it lose. One of our teenagers, Mac, was fully able to walk and had fairly good use of his arms and hands but wasn't able to speak verbally. Since he only used a ventilator at night, he didn't have much to do between activities while the other boys had medical treatments.

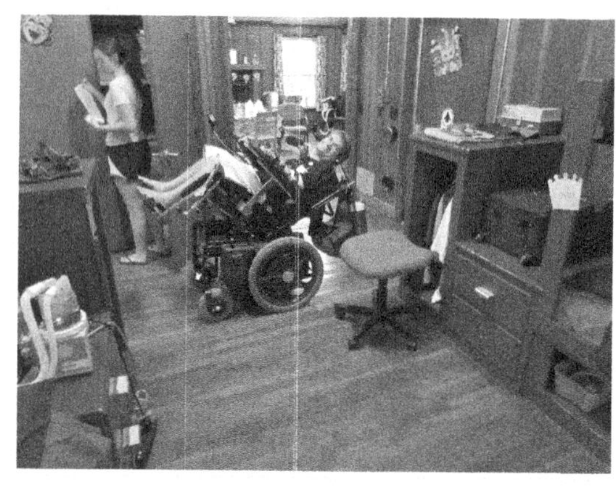

As Sara worked on my right arm, Mac joined us and started copying the same motions with my left hand. I hadn't planned on working with both arms but was happy to see his willingness to help, even when not asked. He quickly learned how to work with my wrist just by watching. I was used to being at camp to encourage the boys and help them, but it was odd and humbling to have the roles reversed.

On a sunny Tuesday afternoon, my trail group's activity was arts and crafts. Dad and I aren't the artistic type, so we never quite knew what to do during this time. In the past, we were glad when it was a morning activity because he and I would be at the lake helping with fishing and could miss the art time, but not this year. Every year, CHAMP Camp held a large fundraiser to help cover expenses. As part of it, various items were auctioned off to the highest bidder. A popular item was the campers' wheelchair art. A large sheet of paper was taped to the ground with paint dropped on it. Kids would then drive their wheelchair over the paint, getting it on their wheels, and leave various patterns on the paper as the camper rolled around. This had been part of the camp's activities for over 15 years, but I had never done it. I knew the paint never completely washed off and Dad wouldn't want me to drive into the house with painted wheels.

Nancy, one of camp's founders, noticed Dad and I weren't doing much and asked if I would do wheelchair art, as it helps raise funds. I had just gotten new tires a few weeks earlier and said I didn't want to get paint on them. She didn't let the excuse slide and continued to ask me to do it. To Dad's dismay, I finally gave in and did wheelchair art. As I spun around in the paint and paper, he captured the event on video. Since it was early in the week, I hoped some of the color would wear off by the time we went home. However, I knew from observing kids in past years that it wouldn't be completely gone.

The water trouble continued for the duration of camp. It was common that cabins were unable to flush toilets and the administration team went from doctors and head nurses to plumbing experts. I was glad I had the opportunity to connect with the older campers. On the last day of activities, it was a full day at the lake. All the campers went to the water for fishing, swimming, boating, canoes, and grilled lunch.

As everybody crowded under the shelter areas to eat, a light rain started. Shortly after, all the campers and counselors were stuffed into the bath houses as strong storms and tornado warnings suddenly came up. A visit from an ice cream truck helped cheer everybody up before we gradually got bused back to the cabins.

With paint still on my wheels, the three of us again packed the van to head home. Before leaving, I talked with my cousin Heidi and her fiancé. They had also volunteered as counselors for the week, but we didn't get much time together. They loved working with the campers as well, even with the extra challenges of the week.

Time Marches On

Returning home after volunteering at CHAMP Camp was always a little depressing. A week of being very active and being surrounded by kids doing amazing things stops, and the real-world returns.

A good thing that happened after camp was that I was able to get off the vent completely and only breathe with the pacemaker. Not switching between the two systems at odd hours of the night was nice. However, I noticed trouble with my nose getting clogged when on my side, making it a challenge to breathe. Since I only used my nose to exhale for more than a quarter century, I figured I had to get used to it.

Every month, my two ventilators received regular service checks. A respiratory therapist would come from Des Moines, check each vent's hours of use, and run a few other tests. Once a year, each machine would also be taken in for an annual check to make sure they were functioning correctly, and no parts needed to be replaced.

I had used the PLV-100 since I was injured in 1985. In college, both vents were replaced with new machines, but the same model. I was used to how they sounded, how to adjust settings, what cues to hear for problems, and how they gave me air. To prepare me, my RT warned me a few times a year that they wouldn't be able to service this model much longer. During the annual evaluation, a test kit of some sort was used. Since these vents were no longer in production and few people used them, the test kits were becoming scarce. When the kits were gone, then the life-sustaining ventilator I had depended on for most of my life could no longer be serviced. I would have no other choice except to get new vents.

Even though I wasn't using them very much, I didn't like the thought of being forced to switch. New models were smaller and lighter, but that's where the advantages ended. It had been at least a decade since I saw anyone else at CHAMP Camp use the same vent as me. All the campers and fellow alumni campers used new vents. As a result, I was quite familiar with them and the problems they experienced.

Camp tech crews were constantly swapping vent batteries for campers as they didn't last for more than a few hours. With one popular model, the LTV-900, I wouldn't even be able to get to Des Moines and back without changing batteries. That scenario didn't only sound inconvenient, but also dangerous if there were problems. The noise of the vents was also a major concern.

Sleeping in the same cabin with the campers, I could hear 4-5 of the machines going simultaneously, all night long. Just being around one sounded like some sort of large creature was huffing and puffing to blow you down. Three years earlier, when I had surgery for the DPS, I had also been on one. The noise and the way it gave me air were very uncomfortable.

Thankfully, although the time hadn't come yet, I was warned it would be soon. Insurance had purchased both vents for the full price over ten years earlier, so I could at least keep the ones I had. If I needed one, I could use it, while ignoring warning labels not to do so. I also wondered if insurance would pay for new vents now that I was using the pacemaker exclusively. Unfortunately, that didn't last long.

By July, it had been several months since I heard from Cherokee Chairs. They had paid for me to get new wheels, but I needed more than cosmetic fixes. My 17-year-old chair was showing signs of trouble with its electronics, and I was getting more concerned that it would soon cease to function. Sam said that they were still working on a solution for my vent's power source. The car sized battery I used was large and it would be better to have something smaller. It was becoming less likely I would need the ventilator in my chair anymore, but it was part of the original order for Cherokee Chairs to include a vent tray. I wanted to stay with what I knew worked and said the current size battery needed to be available. I provided the measurement of the battery I used and tried to get pictures as requested. I was running out of patience with the wheelchair provider, but I tried to be cooperative with what they needed from me.

As time continued marching on, I worked on sites for my web clients fairly regularly, but not as much as I used to. For March, I recorded more than 25 hours of paid work. Including the volunteer hours spent with church and a few other organizations, it kept me very busy. By October, my paid hours of work plummeted to just over five. The extra time allowed me to lay flat and stay off my pressure sores, but it made me wonder if I could continue running VMT much longer.

As for nursing staff, most of my shifts were being covered, but not without problems. Barb, one of my newer night assistants, started not getting along with a day caregiver. They only had to interact a few minutes a day to say how my night went and to pass along any information, but even that was tense. Barb didn't think the day assistant was caring for me correctly. At shift change, she refused to speak to her and just stormed out every morning.

The nursing agency and I tried to arrange schedules so the two didn't see each other, but it didn't always work. Either shift had to sometimes be adjusted unexpectedly, resulting in the two crossing paths. Mom said it felt like dealing with young teenage girls going through puberty.

One evening, as Barb did my regular stretching routine, my arm got stiff as my muscles protested the movement. This was a regular response, but I trained my caregivers to be patient, wait for the spasm to stop, then continue. Instead of waiting, she forced my arm up over my head. I had some sensation of my muscles and could tell if they were stiff, moving, or lose. The little I could feel now obviously hurt because of the movement. I asked Barb to please be careful and not force my limbs against the spasms. For the second round, she did the same thing and the pain increased and lasted for several hours.

With my parents asleep on the other side of the house, I could only pray that the rest of the night would go well, and plan ahead. When she did my bed bath a few hours later, I could tell she was scrubbing much harder than usual, almost to the point I was afraid my skin would tear. It was apparent that Barb's anger issues were not contained to just my daytime staff, and I had to remove her from my case. My agency was having a very difficult time finding backup for when someone called off, so we had tried to resolve the situation, but I couldn't have anyone causing me physical pain and potential harm.

When morning came and I talked with Mom about what had happened, we decided it was time to no longer have Barb come. She had worked with me for about two years several nights a week and did very well but had quickly changed the last few months. I had only requested someone be removed once before, and I hoped it would be the last time.

The situation with Barb made me question again how much longer I could continue to live at home. It was getting harder for my parents to stay up at nights and sometimes made Mom ill afterward. My agency was doing all they could to cover shifts, but nurses were hard to find. Mary was still with me after over 15 years but was having increased illnesses and family trouble and often cancelled her shift. I didn't like seeing the extra burden it put on my parents and wanted to look for an alternative, if needed.

Investigating Alternate Housing

Other than getting married or some other drastic life change, my only other option for relieving my parents was moving into a facility. Unfortunately, very few nursing homes took someone who always required breathing assistance. One option was in Des Moines, near where I used to live. McKinley Manor was close to the airport and within about an hour's drive of Pella. Theoretically, Dad could come and get me and still go to activities at church. It would be more driving, but at least it was an option.

Sara and I made the familiar drive to the city and found the facility not far off the road I used to traverse several times a week. Entering the front door, an alarm sounded as it opened. A nearby delivery driver reached up to a panel near the top of the door jam and silenced the noise. Any time someone went in or out, a code needed to be entered or the alarm would sound.

The facility director showed us around and I asked questions about care needs. She answered my questions, and I didn't notice anything obviously wrong with the place. My acute nose wasn't picking up any foul odors and I didn't see any residents who looked neglected. However, the ones I did see were at least the age of my grandparents and appeared to have severe physical or cognitive challenges. I had always heard bad reports about McKinley Manor but didn't see anything during my brief time. I thanked the director for the tour and hoped I wouldn't need to return, but at least had a possible location if needed.

After a few months of pacing 24/7, my stomach issues returned. I began to look pregnant and overweight. Thankfully, going back to using the vent helped ease the discomfort in my belly. For several days, I was back on my familiar PLV-100 during the night and only on the DPS during the day. Fortunately, I didn't have to go to the hospital, and everything returned to normal on its own. The few days on the vent required me to restart my weaning process at night to get back to the DPS full-time. Was it worth the disturbed sleep, or should I just keep using the pacemaker only during the day? I thought it was better to get back to just using the diaphragm pacemaker and started increasing my time again. I was on the vent for about six hours during the night while I didn't feel well. If I could gain an hour a week, it wouldn't take too long to switch back. At least the process was routine by now.

Trying New Things

With work being slow, I could do other activities during the day. I continued my annual visits to local Christian grade schools and frequently tried to add more to the list. Merely talking about how I did things started to seem like it wasn't enough, and the kids didn't always understand. I had purchased a new camera, a GoPro 3, and was using it to record trains and put videos on YouTube.

Using it to show my daily life and what tools I use was fun, but I needed to think ahead as a director. Starting in early October, it was warm enough to wear shorts while I demonstrated using a mouth stick, ordering inside a restaurant, folding washcloths, and more. It didn't go as quickly as I had hoped, and by November it wasn't finished. The last outdoor item I wanted to include was getting in the van. Students frequently asked how I got into a vehicle, and I wanted to show them.

If I wanted the final product to look like it was done in one day, I had to have on the same clothes. With the camera on my head, my shirt wouldn't be seen, but my legs would. On a 50° day, I braved going on the driveway and got into the van. As I talked about getting on the lift, showing my bare legs and feet, a man rode by on a lawnmower wearing a thick coat and stalking cap. It seemed rather ironic, but I hoped grade school kids wouldn't notice.

Editing and combining the multiple clips into one video was fun, but it forced me to watch and listen to myself. I knew I didn't like hearing my voice, but I didn't realize how noticeable it was when I paused for a breath. Every time the pacemaker stimulated my diaphragm, my shoulders also shrugged, making it look like I was gasping for air. I was happy to finish the video and use it for school visits, but also learned about myself.

I also started visiting college students pursuing various medical disciplines. The bouncing shoulders and breath pauses could be a useful point in teaching, but one I wanted to minimize. A year earlier, I had purchased a language learning program called Rosetta Stone. I had taken a few years of Spanish in high school but didn't remember much of it. I thought it would be beneficial to know Spanish better and to work on my speaking ability. When the lessons became harder, I didn't keep up with it very well and rarely worked on it. I thought the practice had improved my speech quality with the pacemaker, but not as much as I had hoped.

With 2013 nearing completion, I wanted to get final doctor's appointments complete before winter. Visiting with my dermatologist, he confirmed with the nursing agency that my two pressure sores had slightly improved. That was great news, but a third area had opened right on the coccyx bone. In doing my regular skin checks, I had noticed the area was red.

Instead of sitting in bed on my air mattress for 3-4 hours at a time, I decreased my upright time and even tried laying on my side for a while during the day. I couldn't do anything other than watch something online or read, but I hoped it would help. Unfortunately, the red area still broke open. Now, with three pressure sores, I needed to work harder at keeping off my butt.

It hadn't even been a year since I started as a deacon at church, but I wondered if I could complete my three-year term. Cadets were also going well now that Dad and I were in our second year of leading. We were in charge of eight boys ranging from first through third grade.

As fall turned into dreaded winter, life seemed stable and routine. Since August, my parents had been doing several night shifts per week. It wasn't fun but we were getting through by God's provision.

The day before Christmas, we received a letter from the insurance company. It informed us that the insurance plan Dad's employer, Town Crier, was using may not meet the requirements for the Affordable Care Act. Therefore, it would end on March 31, 2014. My nursing care, equipment, doctors, and every medical expense was now in jeopardy of being cut. In another few months, it was possible that I would no longer be able to live at home.

God had filled all my needs before, now would be another time to see where He would lead me.

29

STAY OR GO

"Rejoice always, pray without ceasing, in everything give thanks; for this is the will of God in Christ Jesus for you." (1 Thessalonians 5:16-18) When life is going well, we can sometimes forget to give thanks and pray without ceasing. An uncertain future can quickly bring us back to prayer, as it should.

The start of a new year is often a time of looking forward to a new beginning and what lies ahead. Starting 2014 wasn't that way, I wanted to go back to a more certain past.

Originally, I had liked some of the provisions in the Affordable Care Act, or Obamacare, as it was called frequently. No longer having lifetime caps on insurance spending made my life much easier. I didn't need to constantly watch every cent and wonder what would happen when I reached my limit. I was still careful and kept track of charges, but it did relieve a major burden. I also liked that insurance companies could no longer deny people with pre-existing conditions, like me.

For a brief time, I thought about looking for full-time work again and getting my own insurance. However, I knew it was unlikely I would be able to get the coverage I needed. Now, my nursing care was covered 19 hours or more per day depending on who was working. It had served my family and me very well since our accident 29 years earlier, but it wasn't perfect.

Karen, Sara, and Leah were still hired privately through my parents. Mom paid them for the hours they worked, and insurance reimbursed my parents for what was paid. It used to be that payment would come within a few weeks, but it could now take a month, or even a year, which put financial strain on my family.

Our situation was unusual, and we knew another insurance plan would likely not allow us to hire privately. One reason we could still do it was that it had gone well for many years. Private hired caregivers were also less expensive than having an agency nurse and, therefore, better for insurance.

In early January, I marked one year off my three-year term as deacon at church. I learned a lot in my time and had just started to feel like I knew what I was doing. I also did not have any hospital stays and made it to most of the meetings.

Mom also had a birthday party at our house for her dad. Grandpa Labermen was 86 and still in great physical and cognitive shape. He and Grandma were regular evening caregivers when my parents went on vacation. Mom's parents didn't have monthly lunches for family at their house anymore, but still hosted family several times a year for anyone who could come. It was fun to celebrate Grandpa's birthday, but he was having trouble with a headache. He had fallen on a patch of ice returning books to the Sully Library and was knocked out. The doctor said everything looked okay, but Grandpa wasn't sure.

Insurance Providers and Options

As winter progressed, the Town Crier started looking for insurance options. Dad had been with the commercial printing company for 39 years and was an important part of it. However, only he and one other employee used medical insurance extensively. Everybody else just wanted the cheapest option available.

Mary also continued working as my primary night nurse. She had started working with me in early high school, stayed on through college, and after I moved back with my parents.

I felt selfish for wanting to live at home, and felt that my parents should be free of taking care of me so much. I knew going to a nursing home would mean an end of going to schools or camp, but Mom and Dad would be free of nights with little sleep because of me. They also could go on vacations more easily if we didn't need to find caregivers to help me. Whatever came, I knew God was in control and I would look to Him wherever I went.

It came down to two choices for the Town Crier: a health maintenance organization (HMO) or another plan with the current insurance provider. The HMO was less expensive, but hardly covered anything I needed. Instead of 19 hours a day of nursing care, I could get eight hours per week and would need to change doctors. My family and Dad's one co-worker wanted to keep the current provider. However, the insurance salesman couldn't get specific policy information for the new plan, especially regarding nursing hours.

March soon came and we were still uncertain about what would happen by the end of the month. One evening, Mom asked me if I wanted to try to continue living at home or go to a care facility. She knew I had expressed thoughts about moving to ease their life, but I also enjoyed being active in the community. If possible, I told her I wanted to try to stay home.

The price difference between the two insurance options was the primary deciding point for the Town Crier. Dad agreed he would pay the difference out of his pocket so we could keep the same insurance carrier, with a new plan, but only if it covered my needs for nursing.

For Dad to be willing to pay so much would be a large sacrifice on our household income, but also something not out of character for my family. I was thankful that God had blessed me with a loving family that did so much for me, much more than I deserved.

The Loss of Grandpa Labermen

As the insurance deadline approached, Grandpa Labermen continued to have increasing headaches. Doctors couldn't find the reason but had him try different methods to ease the pain. Finally, he went to the emergency room in Pella to get checked out again. The small-town hospital couldn't do much except send him on to Des Moines for further testing. Mom had been working with the Town Crier to sort out insurance, but she went with Grandma as her dad was moved to a larger hospital. It was discovered that he had blood on the brain and needed surgery to relieve the pressure. At Grandpa's age, the procedure had risk, but it was the only way to stop the extreme pain he was experiencing. Mom's family decided to go ahead with surgery and pray it went well.

On Sunday, March 9, the three of us went to visit Grandpa in the ICU in Des Moines. The procedure was successful in relieving pressure, but he was sedated, unresponsive, and on a vent. Nearly every time I had been in the hospital, I was placed in the Intensive Care Unit. It wasn't because of my health, but due to staff being familiar with my ventilator. For me, it almost seemed like a vacation with new people and new surroundings. However, I was always the patient in the bed who talked with visitors. Reversing the roles was different and I felt out of place.

Just two months earlier, Grandpa had been his normal self in talking with everyone and helping clean dishes for Grandma. Now, he wasn't acknowledging anyone, except to occasionally pucker up for a kiss for Grandma. After more than 60 years of marriage, they still had much love for each other.

A week later, on March 16, Grandpa Labermen passed away at the hospital. It was just a few days after Mom's birthday and two weeks before possible changes for my family. Grandpa was also my first close relative to die.

One of my web clients was a local funeral home. For nearly ten years, I had posted service information for every funeral they managed. Most were older individuals, but some were children, young adults, or babies that had yet to be born. I tried to be prompt getting services online and to be accurate for families mourning the loss of a loved one. Putting my grandfather's service online and listing my family as descendants was a different experience, but I was just as diligent as I had been with every other service.

Sitting at visitation a few days later, many people walked past expressing their sympathy to my aunts, uncles, cousins and me. Several of them were familiar faces, but some were not. Coming up to me, people would thrust a hand in my direction to shake my hand. After a brief, awkward pause, they usually noticed my arms were strapped to my arm rests and didn't move. Some tried to pick up my hand or give a polite tap, both of which frequently caused my arms and legs to shake and spasm. This made the sympathy expresser feel even more strange and they would quickly, but politely, move on. I was familiar with the public not knowing how to interact with me, but I didn't normally interact with strangers this closely. I tried just talking to everyone, thanking them for condolences, and slightly nodding my head as a quad version of greeting.

The next day at the funeral, I wore one of Grandpa's ties and matching blue shirt along with my cousins. Most of my male cousins I grew up with were pallbearers and I was listed as an honorary bearer. After the church service, the family drove out to the cemetery for a brief graveside service. It was a warm, sunny day in mid-March, but the grass was too damp for me to get out of the van.

While Mom and Dad joined the rest of the family, Dad's parents stayed in the van with me. No matter what the situation, I could count on family to help wherever they could. Now that one of my grandparents was gone, that would change.

New Insurance Coverage

Insurance deadlines don't adjust with family tragedies. March 31 was rapidly approaching with no definite answer as to what was coming next. At one point, we were told the new plan wouldn't change anything and we could continue to employ our own nurses and get reimbursed. The next day, that decision would get reversed and private hired help was no longer an option. Eventually, the insurance salesman completely stopped talking to us about what would and would not be covered.

I continued to do my normal activities as much as possible. With three open sores on my butt, I increased my time lying flat in bed, continuing to do web work for The Design Center and my own clients during my sitting times. I also kept attending church meetings and working as the deacon secretary. I didn't know how much longer I would be able to be active and wanted to use the time I had been given.

A few days before the insurance plan would end, it looked like everything would be covered the same as the coverage we already had. It was an answer to the prayers my family, extended family, and church had all been seeking. When April 1 came, I had new insurance cards to distribute and my family's income would be less, but everything else appeared normal. Unfortunately, the relief didn't last very long.

On April 7, 2014, less than a week after starting the new insurance, I received a call from my new case manager. It had been decided that since I no longer used a ventilator, I didn't need to have any nursing services, private hired or through an agency. I explained my diaphragm pacemaker system functioned just like a regular vent and I was completely dependent upon it for air. Just like the vent, someone needed to respond immediately if, and when, something went wrong.

The person on the other end of the line might as well have had the mute button pressed; she didn't care. The last documentation she had of when I used the vent was in December, when I again was able to transition completely back to the DPS. I asked what would happen if I stopped using the pacemaker and went back to just the vent. She replied that nursing would only be covered for the vent if I was recovering from a surgery or similar circumstance and vent use would be temporary. The other allowance would be if I had a diagnosis like ALS and my condition was getting worse and nearing end of life. Using breathing support due to a spinal cord injury did not meet either of those qualifications and nursing would not be covered. The case manager said I could file an appeal when I received the letter confirming the call, but I would be losing coverage for nursing in one month.

It had been a typical Monday. Leah and I were home alone while Mom and Dad were at work. In just a few weeks everything could drastically change again. That night, my parents and I had supper in our usual fashion. I was sitting in bed with Mom and Dad using bedside tables to hold their plates. I waited until we were finished eating before I told them the news. As I expected, they quickly lost what was left of their appetite. We decided when the official letter arrived from insurance, we would file an appeal. The current level of nursing coverage would stay in place during the appeal process, but only until a decision was reached. It wasn't long, but it at least gave us some opportunity to find alternatives.

The next day, Mom talked with my case manager from DHS, and I contacted McKinley Manor in Des Moines. It had been several months since Sara and I visited, but it was a place to start, if needed. Not long after I came home from the hospital in 1985, Mom made a book detailing how to do all my cares. We used it to help with training new caregivers that preferred written instruction and as a reference when needed. I updated it a few years after moving back home from college. The 30-page book detailed every medical item I did. I removed the house rule to put my toys away when I was finished playing and added everything related to the pacemaker. As requested, I emailed the document to the head nurse at McKinley Manor to see if they could take me.

That same day, my nursing agency called to let me know that Mary requested six months off to deal with family problems. For the previous few months, Mary had insisted she couldn't stay one minute beyond her shift so she could get to her daughter's house to help with her grandchildren. My daytime caregivers tried to be sure to come early or Mom watched me a few minutes if needed. However, that apparently wasn't enough. My agency didn't know how they would be able to cover the opening but would do their best.

With possibly only a month remaining to live at home, Dad wondered if Mary could wait until then before leaving. The suggestion didn't change anything, and another difficulty was added to the rapidly growing list.

At least with a one-month warning, I had some time to work on anything I wanted to do while I was living independently. In March, I visited two grade schools and had two more in April. I had originally started speaking at only Pella Christian Grade School but had expanded over the ten years to include a circuit of Christian grade schools and a few colleges. I hoped this wouldn't be the last year I would get to see these students, but knew it was possible.

As April neared its end, I started to get answers on some of the challenges. McKinley Manor looked through my detailed care instructions and concluded they would not be able to take me. My medical needs were too much for them to take on and, therefore, I couldn't be a resident. When my caregivers heard the facility's reasoning, they laughed. I had been told by many nurses I was the easiest patient they ever had. In any case, I would now need to look for alternate living arrangements further from home.

Laura, my DHS case manager, was able to get emergency funding approved for my nursing. Medicaid would cover my night and day nursing when insurance stopped, but only for 60 days. It would allow extra time to find a more permanent solution if, or when, I had no other choice. Days would be covered through something called Consumer Directed Attendant Care, or CDAC. My regular ten-hour shift would be broken into multiple time slots or units. Everything I normally did was given a time estimate; an amount for repositioning, dressing, wound care, and my daily activities. As I understood it, I was limited in how often I could go out and run errands just for fun. Nothing could be documented to say I received help with work, as it could jeopardize my funding. It wasn't ideal, but at least it would buy a few more months.

Laura looked at every available funding option, but there weren't many that applied to me. If I had any type of cognitive disability, then she would have several more possibilities. If we could even show I had a concussion at one point, I could have more flexibility. My parents and I thought back to the day in junior high when Karen tripped, lost control of my manual wheelchair, and I was knocked out when it flipped over. Mom contacted my primary doctor to see if anything had been documented. A note was recorded that a call had been made to the ER about my incident, but that was it. Since I wasn't taken in to be checked out, nothing more was available. If I had gone to the emergency room and documented a concussion, then it would have opened more funding options. Laura suggested trying to find EMS records from when I received my spinal cord injury. Since I was unconscious when they arrived, it may work to show brain damage.

We didn't know where to begin to find records from nearly three decades earlier. She also wondered if Gordon, the man who helped me after the car accident, would be willing to write a statement about how he found me when he came on the scene. However, he no longer lived in Pella and my family wasn't sure where to find him. Mom and Dad knew Gordon had received a lot of ridicule for saving me, and many people said he should have let me die instead of having to live as a quadriplegic. Even though his statement might help, we didn't want to try to locate him and possibly bring back bad memories. It was another avenue that would not work.

I contacted Harmony House in Waterloo where Ken lived. I had visited him a few times and had seen the facility, but I didn't look at it with plans to be a resident. It would be nice to know someone else, but it was a two-hour drive from home. The person who answered the phone seemed nice, but they didn't have any open rooms that would allow them to take me. It wasn't a definite no, but not a yes either.

To add to my stress, the nursing agency was having trouble finding someone to cover Mary's shifts. They were reluctant to hire and train someone if it was only going to be short term. Mary had helped me 4-5 nights a week for nearly 18 years, and we had been through a lot together. Unfortunately, her reliability had become bad, and it didn't look like it would change. I didn't want to, but I told Iowa Health they could remove her from my case. It would make it easier to find a replacement if I had funding and the placement wasn't temporary.

Insurance consulted with my primary doctor to evaluate the level of care that I needed. They did agree I needed regular repositioning to help prevent pressure sores, but that was considered comfort care. My insurance, or any funding source, would not cover that type of care. While evaluations continued, my deadline of May 7 came closer.

When the day arrived, it first got moved back to May 18, then June 7. Working with my doctor meant insurance had to allow more time to reach a conclusion. Living from one day to the next and not knowing what would come was hard, but it gave me more time to live at home and be active.

With long-term prospects not looking good, I decided to resign from my counselor position at camp. I had applied before the insurance policy changed and I was accepted. As usual, there was a waiting list of counselors who had applied but weren't taken due to space. I wanted to give someone else the opportunity to volunteer and not cancel at the last minute.

June started with no answers from funding. Thankfully, as debates continued, time kept passing with full nursing coverage in place. I contacted both of Iowa's senators to see if their influence could help my situation. Senator Charles Grassley's office sent me a reply with a letter from insurance stating what I already knew, they wouldn't cover me since I wasn't on a regular vent. It also reiterated that even if I stopped the DPS and returned to the vent, coverage would not continue.

On June 3, just four days before the next deadline, Senator Tom Harkin contacted me. He had gotten more information and would contact the insurance company that day. By Friday, June 6, I was informed a doctor outside of insurance would review my case and it could be another month until a decision came. I didn't care for politicians or some of Harkin's policies but was thankful for his help. I named my pulmonologist, Dr. Hicklin, as the doctor to work with and prayed he could help return life to normal.

While doctors, politicians, and insurance debated my future, I kept living. With three pressure sores, I continued to decrease how much time I sat in bed and lay flat more. I also frequently laid on my side with nothing on my lower half except a sheet. Laying on my right side, I could read

Trains magazine propped up on my book board. However, it didn't take long before I went cross-eyed.

Taking a Break to Visit CHAMP Camp

Days and weeks kept passing, and it was soon time for CHAMP Camp. I regretted resigning, but felt it was the best decision at the time. Every year one day is designated as visitor time at camp. Camper's families couldn't come, but counselor's families, supporters, or potential campers could come for a half day. Dad and I talked about going, but the idea was brushed aside. On Saturday, I pushed the possibility harder, and he agreed we could visit. A quick call to Sara confirmed she was free, and Monday morning the three of us were in the van headed east. Tilting completely back in my chair, I watched the countryside go by the window and let my mind wander. Going through small towns in Illinois and Indiana, I wondered what life was like in that area.

I had lived in Iowa all my life and only around Pella. Any day, I may have to leave my familiar surroundings and move to a different town where I didn't know the people, surroundings, or churches. After driving a full day, the three of us arrived in Martinsville, Indiana, and found our hotel for the night. This was the camp's fourth year at Bradford Woods, and I had already missed one year. The town near the grounds wasn't very familiar, but we found what we needed.

Tuesday morning, Dad and Sara repacked everything in the van and we headed for camp. Arriving felt like coming home, even if just for a brief time. Several of my long-term counselor friends were surprised to see us, but glad we came. I looked around and spotted the new campers for the year and missed working with them. Another new addition for the year was a zip line. CHAMP Camp, along with Bradford Woods, had set up a zip line through the woods, over a valley, and made it accessible to everyone.

During the two-hour activity block, the three of us quickly visited a couple of trail groups and caught up with friends. After the campers had finished, a call went over the radios to find me and ask if I wanted to try the zip line, but only if I could do it without the vent. Looking down at my tube free chest, that prerequisite was fulfilled. It was an easy yes, and I was soon getting strapped into the special chair made for this purpose. I had brought my video camera along to record trains on our excursion, but it was now on my helmet to record the ride.

After getting in the chair, I was attached to a cable with nothing other than open air before me. After a short countdown, I was flying through the woods with gravity in control. The wind hitting my face and trees going by in a blur was a blast, but the end rapidly approached. Almost as soon as it began, the breaks jolted me to a stop and I was at the platform on the other end, with cheers from my friends. It took over 25 minutes to get in and out of the chair for a trip that took less than 30 seconds. However, it was part of working with counselors dedicated to making every experience possible. It was why I loved volunteering every year and helping kids do things they never thought they could.

I was soon back in my Fortress wheelchair and our small group joined everyone at lunch. As I ate the familiar food-like substance, I looked over the sea of heads. I wanted to capture every second and not let go, but I knew it was about time for it to end. All too quickly, campers and counselors left for their afternoon activities, and we returned to the van. A few friends said they weren't going to let us go, as camp didn't feel right without us. The inevitable had to happen though, and late Tuesday evening, we were back in Pella. It had been 18 hours of driving and one night in a hotel for a four-hour visit. It was gone in a rush, but I was thankful it happened.

The Waiting Continues

Waiting for an answer from insurance didn't take much longer. On July 8, the supervisor from my nursing agency called. My insurance had contacted him to say as of July 14, they would no longer cover any nursing. Instead, they would cover 60 days of an aide from the agency to visit. However, it was not legal for a nursing agency to send a nurse's aide to do the level of care I needed. He said I should be receiving an official letter either that day or the next.

Dr. Hicklin had called me a week earlier after his conversation with the independent doctor from insurance. He only wanted to ask one question: Was the DPS mechanical? My pulmonologist explained that the pacemaker does everything just like a regular ventilator and it's merely a different form. It is an electronic box and wires that can, and did, have problems just like a ventilator. Apparently, it wasn't enough to convince him I still needed nursing care every hour of the day.

With this news, I contacted the staff person at Senator Harkin's office that I had worked with a month earlier. He wanted to know when I had an update and this qualified. I explained that I contacted two nursing homes, and neither one could take me. We had just celebrated the country's independence, but I was about to lose mine due to having a physical disability.

The official letter came in the mail the next day, and I scanned copies of it to email anybody who needed it. The first letter of the four-page document stated that if I had stayed with my previous plan, none of this would have happened. However, that was impossible as it was no longer available.

In a desperate search for options, I contacted more nursing homes. Iowa had six that said they took vent patients, and two had already said no. Contacting one listed in eastern Iowa, I was told the facility was part of a hospital and only took short-term patients and couldn't take me. With another one down, my options kept shrinking. I found another nursing home in Ft. Madison that had a room and would be willing to take me. The small town in the southeast corner of the state was on the Mississippi River and was a busy area for trains. I loved visiting the town as a child and still did as an adult, but it was about a two-hour drive from Pella and took a large portion of the day to visit. If I ended up there, I figured I could at least go train watching when my parents visited.

While Senator Harkin's office worked on further appeals and friends helped with letter editing, my parents, Sara, and I went to visit The

Madison. This was the third nursing home Sara and I had evaluated, but the first for my parents.

A regular point of debate between my parents and me was what I wore on my feet. My caregivers and I had noticed for several years that I had fewer muscle spasms when I was barefoot. I had also seen a lot of research that said shedding shoes had multiple benefits for long-term foot health for people who walked. It didn't pertain to me but did allow me to help educate if someone asked about my naked feet. Going barefoot also helped prevent pressure sores on my feet or damage from shoes being put on incorrectly. Therefore, if it was above freezing, I left footwear at home when Sara and I went out anywhere. Despite repeating all my reasons multiple times, my parents rarely let me go barefoot in public. They were more concerned about appearance and what people thought than if I had more trouble with red areas, stiffness, and spasms.

As Dad unhooked me from the van and I went into the warm summer air, he said, "You want your flip-flops on, don't you?" I quickly and firmly responded, "No thanks." I thought, "If I do end up living here, I need to be seen in control of my own decisions and choosing function over fashion was part of it." Dad uttered a response about first impressions, but I didn't give in.

Mom and Sara got out while Dad retrieved Mom's scooter. Any type of prolonged standing or walking greatly increased pain in her legs, so a three-wheeled scooter helped. Simultaneously, about 50 feet away, someone wearing scrubs pushed an elderly woman in a wheelchair through the facility's front entrance. The woman loudly let out unintelligible sounds as the two entered the building and disappeared from our view.

The four of us made our way to the same door and I heard Dad behind me quietly say to Mom, "Are you ready for this?" I didn't hear her response but guessed she wasn't quite prepared. Our arrival must have been made known, as we were greeted at the door by a man wearing a Hawaiian shirt.

I gave my regular greeting of hello and a head nod toward the greeter and the first words out of his mouth were, "Barefoot! I wish I could go barefoot." I couldn't see my parents behind me, but I had won by making my own decision. The colorfully dressed greeter introduced himself as Donald, the facility director who I had spoken with a few days earlier.

We were ushered into a small meeting room that apparently also served as a church area on weekends. I explained my care needs more thoroughly than I had on the phone and Donald listened along with his head nurse. As I talked about the equipment I have, he asked if the items were owned or rented. I answered that my hospital bed, air mattress, ventilators, and wheelchair had all been purchased by insurance and would come with me.

This was an unfamiliar concept to the director. Medicare and Medicaid always rented equipment. An amount would be paid per item every month as long as it was used. By supplying some of my own needs, he kept commenting about savings and funds that could be used for other necessities. My parents and I thought that my private insurance, through the Town Crier, would still be used even if I were in a nursing home.

Donald corrected us that only state and federal funding would be utilized in my situation. I knew getting equipment like power wheelchairs was hard to do with these programs and often meant getting the absolute minimum a person could use. If I ended up moving, then it would be something else I would need to learn to navigate. It also made it more urgent to replace my wheelchair before losing private insurance.

After completely discussing my needs, we were taken on a tour of the care facility. I would be the youngest resident by several decades and I started to get irritated by frequently being referred to as a kid. Eventually, our group was taken to an empty room that was available in the wing where ventilator patients lived. The featureless white walls made the space feel cold and unfriendly. A bed was in one corner between a window and a bathroom wall. I would be able to see some of the grass outside, but not much else. The bed was also positioned so the occupant couldn't see out the door or into the hallway.

Further questions were asked about my DPS and how it alarmed. Normally, a vent would be connected to a system that notified staff of an alarm. Presumably, the patient would then promptly be checked to see what was wrong. However, my pacemaker didn't have any way to connect to an outside source. Continuing to be a salesman, the director offered possible solutions such as having a child monitor or some other device so I could be heard. He said one nurse, or aide, is responsible for many people and care is not one-on-one.

As soon as the words left his mouth, Mom started quietly sobbing at the idea. Donald tried to offer reassurance, but it was part of the reality of living in a nursing home. Over 29 years earlier, my parents were told that they would be held responsible if anything happened to me and they could even face arrest. Hearing that I wouldn't have anyone who could directly see or hear me made it seem like the years of diligently watching me would end.

The flower shirted man went on to tout how they had worked to wean patients from needing a vent and had healed pressure sores. The facility did not have activities that went out in the community but would consider adding them in the future. However, they did help with hotel costs for visiting family members on weekends. Donald also said that even if I didn't come to live there, he would contact me about doing the facility's website.

With all our questions answered, Sara and my family left The Madison and went to our favorite park by the river. Watching trains, barges, and the swing bridge over the Mississippi provided a sense of calm. This was a place I loved to visit but wasn't sure about being forced to live there. Our group eventually left the rails and made the two-hour journey back home in quiet contemplation.

Senator Harkin's office was able to arrange an appeal to the Iowa Insurance Division to see if they could help. For the third time, I needed to choose a doctor to say why I needed nursing care. This time, I chose Dr. Onders, one of the inventors of the pacemaker system. I had never met him in person but had been corresponding with his office about the trouble I was having. Once again, more time of uncertainty and waiting filled my days.

Down and Out

I made my regular summer visit to the dentist and, as usual, my teeth looked good. I was careful to regularly brush, floss, and take care of my teeth since I used my mouth for everything. The dentist did notice that they were worn down much more than others my age due to stick use, but he assured me crowns could fix it.

My teeth weren't the only thing wearing down. After months of keeping track of appeals, doctors, checking nursing homes, and trying to live, I was wearing down. I trusted completely in God and knew He was in control, but it was hard. My caregivers and nursing agency were also constantly wondering how long they would still have work and if I would be a client much longer.

Thankfully, I had friends to talk with and my church continued to support my family in prayer. Tom and his wife lived near Washington D.C., but we could easily communicate online. One Saturday evening, all three of us played our old, but still fun, game of Starcraft. It had been at least a year since the three of us had taken much time together, but the break from current events helped reenergize me.

As July continued, I did not hear anything on the appeal process with the Iowa Insurance Division. Near the end of the month, my nursing agency didn't want to schedule nurses if they weren't going to be paid. If I was going to be forced into a nursing home and not need nurses, then they could be scheduled with other clients.

Donald from The Madison also called to say they were getting an unusually high number of requests from people using ventilators. If I was going to get a room, I had to reserve it quickly. My guess was other vent users were in the same situation as me and suddenly losing care at home. I wasn't ready to give in and decided to wait a little longer.

Answered Prayer

On July 25, Iowa Home Health needed to get their August schedules finished and had to know whether to include me. My case manager received a call from insurance; they would cover nine hours of nursing at night for a set rate and review again in January. Insurance would no longer cover my privately hired assistants, but they could be paid through the CDAC program that was already set up. It wasn't completely what we had hoped for, but I could continue to live at home.

Most Sundays at church, a short children's message was given prior to the sermon. Kids from preschool and up would gather in the front of church and someone from the congregation would give a quick lesson. It was something I had thought about trying, so I volunteered to be one of the leaders. If I did end up in a nursing home and unable to get out, I thought I had better do everything I wanted while I could.

I was scheduled to lead the children's service on July 27 and planned to teach on being thankful always, whatever the situation. Now that I could stay home for at least another six months, I made the announcement part of my message.

Nearly every week, prayers had been given for my insurance situation and that a good solution would be found. As I started talking to the kids about looking for ways to be thankful in tough times, Rae shot up her hand. The ten-year-old added, "Like now when you could be in a nursing home in two months?" She and her brother remained frequent visitors and had become sort of adoptive grandchildren for my parents. She was aware of the situation and knew that I may not be around much longer.

The congregation quietly laughed at the comment, but I quickly agreed with her and said to keep the comment in mind. After finishing my planned lesson, I concluded with giving thanks for answered prayer and that funding had been secured for nights and that I could remain independent. I stayed sitting with the children in front of me and the congregation behind me. The sound from the unseen crowd was a mix of clapping and cheers for God's provision in my life yet again.

After four months of living with an unknown future, it felt like a lifetime had passed. The increased paperwork and regulations for CDAC during the day would require a lot of careful tracking to make sure everything was correct. It also meant Sara and Leah would get pay cuts, but at least their jobs were secure. I could finally return to the business of living and using the time God had given me.

30

NEW MOVEMENT

Paul wrote in 1 Corinthians 12:15, "If the foot should say, 'Because I am not a hand, I am not of the body,' is it therefore not of the body?" In the body of the church, all members are needed in different roles. In a similar way, I would soon learn the importance of all parts of my body, even if I couldn't control them.

Now that I no longer wondered where I would be living, it was time to get back to regular life. Work on websites with VMT was slow, but I at least had enough clients to allow me to do something useful. I was thankful God had allowed me to go into web development since I could work anywhere I had a computer and internet access. That meant I could be home, in a nursing facility, hospital, or on vacation. However, I wasn't a very good businessperson when it came to charging clients. If it was a small organization that ran primarily, or entirely, on donations, I wouldn't bill them as much as regular businesses.

If two different updates could be combined and round to 15 minutes or less, I would do it. Even if it required adjusting a minute or so of my time, I didn't want to charge more than necessary. The practice meant less time that I could get paid for and less business income, but it also allowed the client to keep more funds for other needs.

Despite doing all that I could to keep my clients, it wasn't enough for some people. One client was aware of my uncertainty with funding. Not long after everything was settled, I learned they had designed and built a new site with a different web developer. The site owner said they loved my work and would recommend me to anyone but didn't want to stay with VMT due to my unstable future.

Being in business, I had always heard you needed to have a lot of resilience and be prepared for anything. This wasn't the first client I lost, but it still hurt every time it happened. I knew everything was in God's hands, but always felt disappointed in myself when a client left.

Along with funding uncertainties, I still had not received my wheelchair back from Cherokee Chairs. I would get infrequent responses from emails and phone calls, but it could be several weeks or over a month between replies. Finally, Cherokee decided they could not make a chair that would work for me. The chin control wouldn't stay in the position that I needed, and it wasn't possible to prevent my back from shearing on the chair's back support when I went from sitting to standing. These were just two items of a long list of problems.

Cherokee had already been paid over $45,000 through my insurance for a chair I never used. I asked them to give the funds to another chair company that had standing systems. However, Sam, the company founder, said any standing chair would have the same problems as his product. Therefore, Cherokee Chairs would provide a wheelchair from a different brand, a TDX.

Further delays continued with trying to get parts for the replacement chair, as well as more time with unanswered messages. Finally, in August 2014, a large crate was delivered containing the TDX. I hoped this long nightmare would finally be over and my aging Action Arrow could be replaced. It had started having electronic issues and would leave me stuck in a tilted position, unable to sit. Every move I made also resulted in creeks and groans coming from somewhere on my wheelchair's frame.

With his battery-operated screwdriver, Dad slowly dismantled the crate around my new TDX chair. Some boards had hardly been secured, but Dad caught them before any fell onto the mobility device. Once the wooden shroud had been removed, we could fully see the TDX as it rested on the shipping pallet. With a brief glance, it was obvious the chair didn't need to move any further. Looking at boxes and parts around the wheelchair, it resembled some type of industrial puzzle. An odd shaped metal box was roughly the size of my ventilator and looked like the same one I had seen before. However, no changes were made to allow for a car battery and I didn't know if my vent would fit. The chin controls were dumped in a box with no instructions on how it could be connected for me to use.

The chair's frame was a dull red, not the blue, or at least black, I had originally selected. Four of the six wheels had an old yellow tinge that made them look ready to disintegrate with any use. No headrest was anywhere to be found, or a user's manual, and the seat was made for an occupant much larger than me. Those were the items we saw with a quick look. Further investigation continued, increasing the list of problems.

Dad found an Invacare serial number on the chair and a different one listed on the packing receipt. The next day, I called Invacare to see if I could find out anything more on my new giant paperweight. I got a helpful person who said the chair had originally been purchased by a company in Florida in June 2009. Now, five years later, it was sent to me in Iowa from a wheelchair provider in Arizona. Invacare wondered how many hours were on the chair but an on switch was one of the missing items and I couldn't check.

After five years of use and apparently changing owners in multiple states, I understood why the wheels looked used. It also meant that this chair was made before I ordered my new wheelchair from Cherokee Chairs. It was not a new chair and I could only speculate how it ended up in its current position. Dad also saw that the length was too long if the backrest was reclined to where I could sit comfortably and not have my head fall forward. Instead of making progress, I would need to return to emails and phone calls. I continued to email and call Cherokee Chairs, but never got a response. My parents and I decided we had been very patient with them, but it was time to seek legal help.

After getting all the documentation together, I contacted the Iowa attorney general with everything that had happened. I didn't want to press legal charges, I just wanted the money returned, or transferred, so I could get a new wheelchair. I wasn't sure how long the process would take, but I needed something done.

With the start of September, I became busy again. I was only sitting upright in bed for a total of six hours a day. Work for VMT was slow, but any site updates seemed to take a long time with my limited hours. Even with few work needs, I started missing emails and not offering a prompt response. Instead of working to improve my service, it felt like I was going backwards.

Volunteer Work

Another year of Junior Cadets started for Dad and me at church. A third counselor also joined us to help with our six active boys. They were all the same kids we had six months earlier, but they seemed older and more mature somehow. Helping our small group of second and third graders let me somewhat experience feeling like a parent.

At some point in the year, every Cadet started off leading the meeting with pledges and concluded with a prayer. Eighth graders went first, and then worked down in age every week until all the boys had opened the meeting. In total, my church only had about a dozen boys in the program, but most felt uncomfortable when it was their turn to lead in front of everyone. I decided to help them prepare for their turn by having one of my boys pray for our small group every week. They needed some prompts on what to say and encouragement to do it, but they started to learn.

Eventually, the turn came for my kids to lead the entire Cadet group. One shy young man went up, did the pledges, then led a prayer that was just as, if not more, clear and heartfelt than his peers. As soon as he said amen, he looked straight at me with a small grin on his face. I smiled back as big as I could and mouthed back to him, "Good job." Coming to Cadets every Wednesday evening felt like a burden some weeks, but moments like that made it all worth it. I got to teach the kids how to know and serve God just as if they were my own. I was thankful God allowed me the opportunity, even if just for 90 minutes a week.

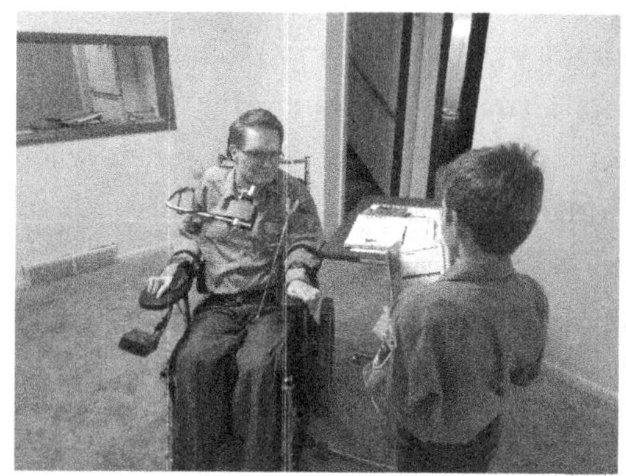

Funding and Medical Concerns

The diaphragm pacemaker made my cares easier, but I was concerned about the wires on the side of my chest getting damaged. When in bed I had everyone put a small pillow on my right side for protection. Then, when my arm had a muscle spasm, it couldn't directly hit the port. It helped, but only if everyone remembered to put the padding in place and be careful when I was being moved around. It was getting close to a year since I had last used the ventilator and I wanted to keep extending my time.

Talking with my doctor, I thought I would try Botox injections to reduce spasms. I was already on the maximum dose of two medicines to calm my muscles, but they didn't completely stop strong bursts of movement in my limbs. It took several tries to find a doctor to give the medicine, but I finally found one.

A rehab doctor in Des Moines who specialized in spinal cord injuries was soon added to my list of specialists. In his office, four full syringes of liquid were carefully injected into different muscles in my right arm. The plan was to completely deaden anything that would pull the arm toward my chest. The toxin would take six weeks to reach full strength and then would need to be updated every three months.

I was hopeful this line of treatment would help. I needed to guarantee my arm couldn't cause damage to the wires and knock out my breathing again. The only other option would be to amputate the arm below my elbow. It would be a permanent solution that would guarantee the limb wouldn't cause trouble, but I wasn't ready for that, at least not yet.

Funding for daytime hours was extended through January, but not guaranteed beyond that. Mom said I would need to look at going onto Medicaid completely at the start of the year as the financial burden for keeping insurance and paying the Town Crier's cost difference was too much to continue indefinitely. That meant I would be back to looking at nursing homes and uncertain of what I could do in the future.

My parents made sure to take a week of vacation while we had coverage. I loved having the house to myself, with caregivers, even though I didn't do much of anything different than when my parents were home. With my day assistants' hours restricted, it was harder to get the evening shift covered. Thankfully, Karen could cover two nights and my extended family could help with the rest.

When Mom and Dad got back, Dad wished he could take a week off by himself and go hiking in the mountains. However, we hadn't planned on it, and I had a church council meeting and we had Cadets to lead. I would need his help with both if I didn't have anyone else planned who could drive the van and stay with me. Moving to a nursing home would be unpleasant for me but would release my parents from the endless burden of my care, allowing them to do what they wished.

Even with all the insurance issues, and with Mary leaving, Iowa Home Health did very well at covering most of my night hours. Even though nurses were hard to find, one from a neighboring town was hired and worked all summer and most of the fall. Unfortunately, staying up at night didn't work for her and another replacement was needed.

The next caregiver was Steph. She seemed to learn quickly during training but, as usual, I knew her first few shifts would need more help to learn my routine. Thankfully, most nights were the same with little change. In mid-December, Steph offered to work when my other experienced night person called in sick. This would be Steph's third shift and she was catching on well.

Shortly after I finished my nightly Bible reading, we noticed my lower abdomen was moving strangely. It would start to expand as I took a breath and then the left side would suddenly bulge out. It looked like pushing on a balloon when one side bulges more than the other. I commented that she had a special treat with something unusual to document. Unfortunately, it wasn't the only oddity she would have to document.

About 1:45 in the morning I suddenly woke up. Junk from either my nose or lungs had collected in the back of my throat, and I couldn't breathe. My pacemaker fired every four seconds to make my diaphragm contract, but nothing could get through my airway. I could just barely start to clear my throat when the next breath would initiate and plug everything up again. My oxygen monitor started alarming that my oxygen was low. Steph noticed the commotion and came to my bed, but I couldn't tell her what to do as I couldn't get air. After further struggle, I was able to croak out for her to turn me on my back. As she did, the mucus moved enough that I could clear my throat and start breathing again.

The entire incident maybe lasted a minute, but it felt much longer, and my heart rate remained high for quite a while. Shortly after, I showed Steph how I point my chin toward my neck to indicate to take the plug off my trach. At least then I could breathe through my throat instead of only my nose and mouth. Insurance wanted to see documentation of why I needed help at all times, and this was exactly one of the reasons.

Not long before the January cut-off, funding for my daytime hours was approved for another six months. My parents and I had started to wonder if it was going to be approved, but it was with only days to spare. It looked like it would be a routine that would be repeated every six months, until private insurance changed, or I no longer lived at home.

Litigation with Cherokee Chairs

January 2015 marked two months since I had contacted the attorney general about Cherokee Chairs. I hadn't gotten a response from anyone and wondered if I needed to find a different lawyer. One evening, the phone rang just before supper. The woman on the other end said she was from Cherokee Chairs. Thinking about our correspondence, her name was vaguely familiar as someone I had talked with before. She said they had been contacted by the Iowa attorney general and were required to offer a solution within a certain time period. The secretary said they were unaware that I still had problems. Sam, the company founder, had reported he was still working with me. I hadn't heard from him, or anyone else, in several months.

As a result of the legal contact and situation update, Sam had been let go from the company. I put my phone on speaker so my parents could also hear the conversation. As we talked, this contact person wanted to know if I still had the same insurance. I answered that I did have the same provider, but with a new plan. The question was odd, and I wondered why she asked. She stated that insurance companies allow a new wheelchair every five years. That time had elapsed since I ordered my first wheelchair and now Cherokee Chairs could provide another one with new insurance money. With that request, my parents and I became extremely agitated. As calmly as I could, I explained my insurance had paid for a chair from her company that we were still waiting to receive. I never signed any paperwork accepting the mobility device, and after five years, a working wheelchair still had not been provided.

The Cherokee representative could not understand why we would not just purchase another chair. After a few more rounds of the same reasoning, we hadn't made any progress. Eventually, the person from Arizona said she would tell the attorney general they offered a solution, but we didn't want it. Cherokee's lawyer would be brought in and informed of the situation. The three of us agreed and tried to calm down enough to eat what Mom had prepared for supper.

A week later, I received a call from someone who said they were with Cherokee Chairs. It was a new name to me, but he said he was an independent occupational therapist who helped the company and wanted to know why the TDX chair didn't work for me.

I went through the list of our findings, missing parts, incomplete work, seat too large, and my investigation into the chair's age. The consultant quickly agreed with my assessment and was equally perplexed as to why the wheelchair had even been sent. Looking at my requirements for the original chair from Cherokee, they were not even close to being fulfilled in what I had received. It was a quick conversation, but it was a nice change to have someone representing the company who wanted to help.

Not much later, Cherokee Chairs called me again, with the same secretary my parents and I had spoken with previously about getting my insurance information. This time, she was much calmer and willing to discuss different options. After consulting with their legal team, they could offer two choices. First, they would get me a new chair without another charge to my insurance and have it finished within six months. Second, the money would be returned to insurance, and I could look for another wheelchair provider. Either way, the TDX sent by Cherokee would need to be returned.

The large wheelchair paper weight had been sitting on its pallet ever since it arrived several months earlier. Returning it and getting it out of the basement would be great. After more than five years of frustration with Cherokee Chairs, I did not want to continue working with them. I easily decided to take the second choice so I would not have to deal with them any longer. My parents agreed with my decision, but now I was back to the beginning of searching for a new wheelchair. Only now, my Action Arrow was 19 years old and in very desperate need of replacement.

As I had done over five years earlier, I returned to Advanced Rehab Technologies near Des Moines. They had last said they couldn't help me anymore, but I hoped that was no longer the case. I still loved the idea of being able to stand and help my bone strength, but I decided it would be best to get a regular chair. It had also been over a year since I last used the ventilator and I just relied on the DPS to breathe. Therefore, I wouldn't include a place on the chair for my vent and battery.

I met with a familiar occupational therapist at Younkers Rehabilitation in Des Moines. Sue and I assessed my needs again and coordinated with Advanced Rehab to find a chair that would work best. They thought a TDX SP from Invacare could fit my needs, similar to what had been sitting on a pallet in my house. However, this time it would be updated to the newest version and ordered to my specifications. The custom molded back support I had been using for nearly two decades would be a challenge, however, Sue soon had a solution of new technology to fix the issue. A seating provider came and mapped my back support with a special pen. Every contour was recorded on a computer, and, in theory, an exact replica would be made.

It was a relief to see rapid progress and working with people close to home. At the last minute, Phil from Advanced Rehab asked if I had a color preference for my chair. I again chose my favorite dark blue, but I wondered if I would get what I wanted.

Time Moves On

February 20, 2015, came as the cold weeks of winter passed. It had now been a full 30 years since my family had been in the car accident that changed our lives. At the time of my injury, my parents would not have guessed that I would be in my third year as a deacon at church. I was also a leader for junior Cadets, did web development, spoke at grade schools, and was quite active. God had allowed us to do a lot and continued to provide all our needs in His timing.

After eight years at Second Christian Reformed Church, Pastor Dan decided to move on to a different role in ministry and help other churches. I had come to know him well in that time, especially in the previous year with funding challenges. As a result of his departure, a pastor search committee was formed to find the church's next minister.

During my ample time lying flat in bed, I started reading a lot of Christian resources on creation, evangelism, outreach, and preaching. I really didn't need to add another activity to my schedule, but a deacon representative was needed on the committee, and I felt my area of study could help. After prayer and talking with my parents, I volunteered to join the group. Looking at previous searches, I didn't think it would be much more than a one-year commitment.

April began a new year for medical insurance. We feared a repeat of the previous year, but nothing happened and monthly rates barely increased. A few months earlier, a different insurance carrier was getting a lot of coverage in the news. The other provider the Town Crier considered was not able to cover their customer's expenses and went bankrupt, leaving everyone without insurance and scrambling to find new carriers. If Dad's employer had gone with them, it would have created problems for his company, staff, and especially me. With this development, my family no longer needed to pay Town Crier's cost difference out of our pocket. It showed how God had taken care of our needs before we knew they existed.

As life moved through various challenges, I continued to communicate with other adult quadriplegics and families with children who had received spinal cord injuries. One of those families had a background that sounded familiar.

The Jordsons lived in Florida and had been on a trip when their SUV was rear-ended by a drunk driver. Oscar, their three-year-old son, received a C2/3 injury and was now a vent dependent quadriplegic. His experience sounded close to my history. About a year after his injury, Oscar also received a diaphragm pacemaker system. While our circumstances were similar, technology and knowledge had greatly changed in three decades. It was encouraging to see how he received physical rehabilitation that wasn't thought of when I was injured, but I also wondered how life would have been different for me.

I continued to keep in contact with Ken in Waterloo, Iowa. Living in the nursing home, he rarely received visitors. I worked with Pastor Dan from church and found a congregation in Ken's area that had a visiting ministry. It took a lot of correspondence to initialize, but the ministry had 6-8 people who regularly visited Ken and helped him learn about Christ.

As Ken's birthday approached in late May, I helped organize a party for him with the church volunteers. When the day came, Sara and I made the two-hour drive north and joined a handful of people in a meeting room at the care facility. A nurse who knew about our plans got Ken in his wheelchair and gave him some excuse to bring him to the room. He was surprised to see birthday decorations, cupcakes, and his friends all waiting for him. Ken had not celebrated a birthday in many years, and I was glad I could help make it happen.

A few weeks later, it was time for another great week at CHAMP Camp, but not for me. I had applied to be a counselor, but not enough room was available in the cabins. Campers' needs came first and staffing counselors who could perform physical cares took priority. Since I was unable to help with medical needs, and took three beds, I didn't make the list. Instead, my parents and I decided to take a regular vacation.

Sara would come to help me in the hotel at night and Mom and Dad would cover the day. Grandpa had died over a year earlier, and Grandma was looking for ways to keep busy. Therefore, she could come along and get away from the house for a while. I had read a lot of material from Answers in Genesis, taken most of their online classes, and really benefited from their ministry, so, our trip would be a visit to the Creation Museum in Kentucky and a visit to camp on our way home, on Grandma's 85th birthday.

The last time all three of us had traveled outside of Iowa on vacation had been ten years earlier, for Tom's wedding. Now with five people in the van, it was stuffed with luggage and every seat was filled. I missed not working with the kids, but I also liked getting to see the ministry that had been helping me study God's word.

It was a full day's drive to our hotel near Petersburgh, Kentucky, but I liked seeing familiar sites as well as new ones as we traveled east. Grandma carefully followed her atlas to track our progress from one state to the next and made sure to get frequent updates. After a night's rest, my parents, grandmother, and I headed to the museum while Sara stayed at the hotel to sleep.

The wet, rainy Saturday morning felt like a good day to be inside. Dad unloaded me from the van in the large parking lot and Grandma and I headed to the building. As soon as I passed a dinosaur replica and approached the main door, it was opened by a smiling gentleman with a gray beard who said, "Hi Joel!"

Grandma was confused how we could be over 500 miles from home and the first person we encountered knew me. A few years earlier, I had taken online apologetics courses with Ron as the instructor. He and I stayed in contact, and he knew I was coming on a weekend that he was giving a presentation at the museum. It was nice to finally meet him in person and we hoped to meet up later.

All who truly repent of their sins and trust in Jesus alone for salvation will be saved.

I knew some of what to expect at the Creation Museum but was still impressed with it. Touring through the main display, we were taken through the Biblical account of a once perfect creation which was now corrupted by sin. At the end, visitors saw how Christ suffered on the cross to take our punishment for sin. All who truly repent of their sins and trust in Jesus alone for salvation will be saved.

After the main walk through the exhibit, the four of us got lunch at Noah's Café and then toured the rest of the museum, watching a 4D movie and Ron's presentation on cursed plants. I was thankful that I could access every part of the museum except a small dinosaur display that was up a flight of stairs.

Sunday morning, our same group of four found a park and watched trains for a few hours. Just after lunch, we picked up Sara from the hotel and returned to the Creation Museum to tour the gardens in the warm Kentucky sun. Since it was Father's Day, I made sure to get pictures of Dad and me together. All five of us watched a few more presentations before finally feeling like we had seen everything. We could have maybe seen it all in one full day if we didn't take much time to read and learn, but I wanted Sara to experience it as well.

Monday morning, we packed the van and started west toward home. A little over two hours after leaving the hotel, our group arrived at Bradford Woods. I had arranged to meet a boy, Aiden, and his mom who lived in the area. He was also a quadriplegic on a vent, and I hoped he would be able to come as a camper.

Visiting camp and acting as tour guide didn't allow much time to visit with my friends. However, I was glad I could show Aiden around. Camp had been something I greatly enjoyed and hoped he could do the same. The morning activity quickly ended, and we were soon all at lunch.

Just like the year before, I looked over the landscape of heads and tables and didn't want to let a second pass by. The camp songs, seeing the new campers, and hearing stories of what had already been achieved in less than a day made me miss it all the more. As soon as it was known it was Grandma's birthday, I was thrust fully into camp mode. The entire room filled with singing happy birthday and then followed by "around the tables you must go!" Grandma wasn't as spry at walking as a few decades earlier, and I was selected to do the celebratory lap around the room.

This wasn't the first time Grandma had seen CHAMP Camp, but it was the first without Grandpa. She didn't say much about it, but I was pretty sure she enjoyed seeing how all the kids could participate in activities, no matter their medical needs.

The moments were quickly gone, and we were soon back on the road to Pella. After dropping Grandma off at her house in Sully, the rest of us were soon home again. Sara had endured four days of little sleep to allow us to go, but I was thankful it worked out to take Grandma and not miss out of everything for summer.

A Bicycle Ride

Working with other quadriplegics allowed me to help them, or their family, learn from my experiences. However, I could also learn and see what they did, especially with the advent of social media. Oscar's parents regularly posted pictures and videos about what he was doing for rehab. I often wondered if this technology had been available when I was injured if I would have regained more function of my body.

Working with other quadriplegics allowed me to help them, or their family, learn from my experiences

One item he used regularly was a Functional Electrical Stimulation (FES) bike which made his legs do a biking motion while stimulating his muscles with electrodes. It had been many decades since my legs did anything coordinated, but I wondered if I could try. When I was evaluated for my wheelchair, I saw that Younker's Rehab in Des Moines had one of these bikes.

Neither my dermatologist nor general doctor thought it was a good idea, but they said I could try the system. A new bone density test showed that after several years of osteoporosis meds, my bones had improved slightly and should be okay for biking. The dermatologist wondered if my skin sores would get worse, but also thought more movement and circulation would help.

Halfway through July, Sara and I went to Des Moines to see if the FES bike would be something I could use. The bike was made by Restorative Therapies, and a representative from the company, and a couple of physical therapists, took us to the machine. The team asked me several questions about my history, what I do for exercise, and how I maintained flexibility. I explained my passive range of motion routine my caregivers did four times a day, but that was all. As one person quizzed me, another started moving my legs. As my knees went higher than I had seen while sitting, I made sure to mention that a few years earlier both femurs had each broken.

My lower half continued to be evaluated by stretching my knees and ankles while everyone watched. One of the therapists asked again to confirm I was thirty years post injury. She was very impressed with the flexibility of my joints, especially my ankles. Most people at this point had frozen or very stiff joints that could hardly move. I contributed it to very good care from my parents, caregivers, and me being particular with exercises, and to God's provision.

Everything seemed to check out, and the therapists continued getting me ready. Sticky pads with a wire on one end were placed very high on my upper legs. I was glad I wore flexible shorts, but started to wonder if everything necessary would stay covered. With four electrodes on each leg, I was then leaned forward, and more electrodes were placed very low on my back, inside my shorts. I thought it looked like I was about to be electrocuted.

The next step was to get connected to the machine, but the representative from the bike company didn't like my lack of footwear. I explained I am always barefoot in order to have fewer muscle spasms and keep a better eye on my feet and prevent problems, which is partly why they were in good condition. She wouldn't hear any of my reasoning and I let Sara put on the backup minimalist shoes I brought for such a scenario.

I couldn't get close enough to the machine with my footrests in place, so I explained how to remove them. I could then park so that my legs could be strapped in, and my feet secured to the bike's pedals. As that was being done, a spaghetti mess of wires were connected to all the electrodes on my legs and posterior. A few more tests and adjustments and everything looked good. One of the therapists programmed some settings on a small tablet computer and then hit a big green "Go" button.

Very slowly, my legs started moving as if they were pedaling a bicycle, but my left knee kept hitting my arm rest. The offending part was promptly removed from my chair with Sara supporting my arm. As minutes passed, the speed of the pedaling quickly increased. It wasn't long before my legs started to spasm and kick against the device they were strapped to. I hoped I didn't have any curled toes or other problems on my hidden feet that may have caused the reaction and would result with more trouble.

Eventually, my body got used to the motion and calmed down. The group standing around me explained that for the first two minutes, the bike's motor did all the work. After that, the electrodes start to stimulate my muscles to do part, and hopefully all, of the work. When the transition started, I didn't have the expected reaction from my limbs. The stimulation lasted for 15 minutes, then the motor would turn off and see if I would do any pedaling with my own muscles.

As I sat and looked at my lower body, everything was moving in a co-ordinated fashion. I wasn't just kicking and spasming as I had seen for the last few decades, they were moving. As I watched, I focused my attention on the small sensation I have of my muscles. I could feel my legs reacting and moving as they should along with the motion. It wasn't a sensation I thought I would ever experience, but it really was happening.

When the motor icon on the computer screen turned off, the pedaling speed rapidly decreased to nearly a full stop before the machine took over again. After 30 years of being lazy, my legs didn't want to give effort on their own. We let the bike work a little longer before turning it off, un-hooking wires, and put my chair back together. I had pedaled 1.26 miles during the workout, more than my legs likely had biked in my entire life.

While electrodes were peeled off my skin, the representative from Restorative Therapies said she was impressed with how well I did. Ideally, I should do 3-5 times a week for it to have much benefit, but the bike came with a price tag of around $14,000 and insurance didn't always cover it. The machine could also work on my arms, but I didn't want to increase strength in my right arm to hit my DPS port. Testing my wrists, they also looked to be frozen in place and unable to do the proper motion.

Once I was sitting as usual, Sara and the therapists checked over my skin. Everything appeared to be fine, but I also made sure to promptly have my footwear removed to check my feet. I scheduled another session in one week and would plan to come every other Thursday as long as I could.

On the drive home, Sara and I talked as we usually did, but I noticed my body didn't twitch. Normally, bumps in the road would make me get stiff and cause my arms and legs to fly around. This trip though, they didn't flinch or show any reaction to anything. Doing my afternoon cares at home, stretching exercises, pressure sore treatment, and cathing, nothing moved. When Dad came home from work, I told him about the bike and my relaxed muscles.

To test my account, he grabbed my feet, raised them about a foot off the bed, and dropped them. Normally, my legs would kick, and my body would react, but they plopped back onto the mattress and didn't even twitch. Just to make sure, he repeated the test a few more times and received the same results. Five hours later, when my 10:00 night nurse came, my body started finally showing signs of life, nine hours after my ride. I thought to myself I could at least reduce my reliance on medication to reduce spasms if this is what the bike did every time. I looked forward to my next trip to see what would happen.

A little over a week later, Sara and I were back in Des Moines at Iowa Methodist Medical Center. Younkers Rehabilitation wasn't an area I normally visited in the hospital, but I knew it would quickly become familiar. This time, I did my normal routine and left my footwear at home. Two of the same people I saw last time greeted me and started showing Sara how to get me connected to the bike. Again, they weren't sure about me biking barefoot, but there wasn't any other choice.

It took about 15 minutes to get everything hooked up, and I was starting to pedal again. This time, I could also see how my feet reacted to the motion. I had read in different studies that when people walk, toes naturally spread out to absorb weight, and regular shoes inhibit that function. Watching very carefully, I could see my feet react to pressure as they should, but very little.

> *Sitting on one edge of a therapy room with other patients around me, I didn't want to miss any of it. Riding a bicycle was a part of childhood I didn't experience. Now, after a thirty-year delay, it was finally happening.*

I wasn't able to get a standing wheelchair and experience life in an upright position; it was also very unlikely that I would ever walk again. This bike was probably the closest I would ever come to doing an activity most people take for granted. However, I could now watch as my lower body went through the motion and responded appropriately. Sitting on one edge of a therapy room with other patients around me, I didn't want to miss any of it. Riding a bicycle was a part of childhood I didn't experience. Now, after a thirty-year delay, it was finally happening.

A New Chair

In late August, after my annual visit to the Iowa State Fair, I returned to Advanced Rehab Technologies. They said my new chair was in and ready for me to get. I presumed some adjustments would be needed and I couldn't take it home immediately, but it was getting close to completion.

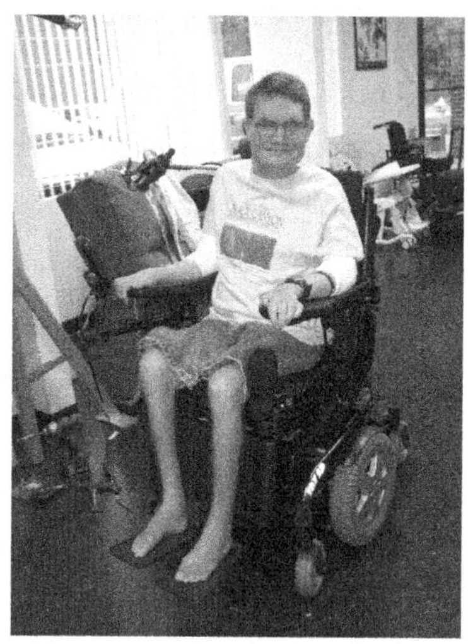

Sara and I waited in a wheelchair display section of the rehab business while my wheels were retrieved from storage in the back. When it was pushed around the corner, it looked like what I ordered. The size appeared correct, chin controls in place, and even the color I requested. However, it looked odd for it to be my chair and not have a shelf for a ventilator.

Using the in-house lift, it wasn't long until I was sitting in my new TDX SP. I had seen several of these models at camp but had never driven one. The chin controls took a little adjusting but were soon in easy reach. My head rest also had buttons that let me move the controls out to the side or in front of me. Phil made further adjustments and I could reach all control surfaces I needed. All that was left was a test drive and for me to learn the driving computer's commands.

As I cautiously moved the stick up to go forward, I warned another customer about a new driver. The chair wasn't as responsive as my Action Arrow, but it still reacted to small inputs correctly. This chair had six wheels, with the main driving wheels in the middle. The different design meant I had a zero-turn radius and could turn on the spot. It was a different sensation, but I liked it.

Phil added arm straps and shortened the metal foot rests to not extend several inches beyond my feet. About an hour after arriving, my new chair was complete and ready to come home with me. I noticed the new back rest didn't quite feel right, but I thought it would just take adjusting. I went back to my old familiar chair to go home, but Sara and the rehab staff got my new mobility aid in the van. The process had only taken four months to go from ordering to having a working chair. After the multi-year nightmare with Cherokee Chairs, it was a relief to have a provider that did good work and genuinely cared about their clients.

Visiting my Friends

With frequent trips to Des Moines for biking, summer soon turned into fall. In September, I made another trip east to Auburn, a small town in northern Indiana. Greg, one of my friends from CHAMP Camp, was having a wedding ceremony and asked me to be his best man. I hadn't communicated with him in a few years and wondered why he wanted me. At first, I was reluctant to ask my parents to take me on another trip, especially to see someone I didn't feel I knew very well. However, Greg was like me and didn't know many people.

Greg had a degenerative muscle condition and had used a ventilator most of his life. When we met as teenagers, he was able to speak on his own, but now could not. Due to using government funded healthcare, Greg and I had very strict regulations on assets and what he could own. Getting married legally meant he would no longer qualify to receive funding for medical needs. Therefore, he and his fiancé were having a wedding ceremony but not signing any legal paperwork. They would be married in their hearts, minds, and the public's eye, but not according to the state.

My parents went on their annual fall trip and returned home a few days before we left for the ceremony. Just Dad and Sara went with me to attend the ceremony in Indiana. I had only been using my new wheelchair for a few weeks and this would be my first extended outing with it. At least my ride would be clean for the ceremony.

Friday evening, we had a short rehearsal at Greg's mother's house and met the small wedding party. Both bridesmaids were friends of Greg that I hadn't met before and who also used wheelchairs. Pastor Dave Powell from CHAMP Camp would conduct the joining of the couple. Greg had originally asked me to preside, but I didn't quite feel comfortable doing so and opted for best man.

Saturday morning, Dad and I left the hotel to allow Sara time to sleep. We found nearby train tracks and happily spent the morning watching trains along a busy CSX main line. By early afternoon, we were back at the hotel, with me dressed in a suit, and off to a rented school for the ceremony. It was a much smaller wedding than I had seen before, but vows were taken before friends and family to be committed to each other for life.

A few hours later, Dad, Sara, and I were back by the tracks before another night in the hotel. On Sunday, as we headed home, I asked Dad to stop in Iowa City at the hospital. Since his birthday in May, Ken had been in and out of the hospital. He was currently in the University of Iowa's ICU recovering from the latest battle with infection.

Finding Ken's room, the three of us talked with him about what had been going on with me and that we were thinking of him. Before leaving, I prayed for recovery soon so that Ken could return to his regular living situation. As we left, Ken started to tear up and thanked us for the visit. I also noticed he had no way of calling a nurse and made sure to address the issue at the nurse's desk. I was assured he would get a call system that he could use.

For our last 100 miles home, I thought about the previous few days and realized I made an inconsiderate error. Ken's immediate family completely ignored him, and he hadn't seen his parents in years. Without asking, I came into the hospital room with Dad helping me, even traveling out of state, so I could help others. As with most families, I didn't agree on every point with my parents, but we were always there for each other.

Dad especially did a lot daily to help with my cares and allow me to stay active. I felt bad I hadn't asked Ken first if he was okay meeting my dad and hearing about him doing so much.

When we got back to Pella and unloaded the van, I made sure to thank my parents for all they did. I took it for granted too easily, but in just a few days I had seen very different lives and how God had blessed me with my family.

A Trach Button

Throughout the year, I kept having pain in my throat. While lying flat in bed, I usually had 2-3 pillows under my head. I couldn't do a lot, but I could at least do some computer work in this position and not waste so many hours. However, my trach would rub the inside of my trachea. I tried to lay differently, but with breathing through the pacemaker, it continued to irritate my throat. I had heard of some long-term quadriplegics with trachs that rubbed a hole through a major artery near their throat. Most ended up losing all their blood very quickly and dying as a result, even if in surgery while trying to fix it.

With this in my head, I consulted with my ENT on what I could do to prevent further complications. It had been nearly two years since I last used my ventilator, and I hoped I wouldn't need it again. However, I still suctioned through the trach a few times a week and I needed to have the connection available if the DPS stopped working, so I didn't want to completely remove my trach and let the hole in my throat close.

I talked with Chuck, another long-term quadriplegic who had been using a different type of diaphragm pacemaker for a few decades. He used something called a trach button instead of a full tracheostomy tube. The button was only a couple inches long and didn't go nearly as far into the throat as my trach. It also had small petals that extended and caught the inside of the stoma. This way, it kept itself in and didn't require trach ties.

My doctor put a small camera down the trach and could see where it was rubbing my throat. He hadn't heard of a trach button before, but I gave him the information I had found from Olympic on different sizes and how to order. Looking it over, Dr. Schulte thought it would stop the rubbing and would work for my needs. While on the pacemaker, I used a plug on my trach that sealed it off. The only time it was uncapped was to clear my lungs or to clean the trach. The button did the same thing, but with a different design.

The new hardware came in late October, and I returned to Dr. Schulte's office for placement. He inspected the device, which he had never seen, and everything appeared fine. As he removed my trach ties, I took a deep breath and blew the trach out of my throat and let it fall to my lap. I no longer left the trach out for short periods as I had with Mary, but it still felt good to have it out. With the open hole in my neck, the doctor took a few measurements, adjusted the button with the provided spacers, and carefully pushed it in. With the outer sleeve in place, the doctor inserted the closure plug to extend the petals.

I expected to feel some discomfort or pain, but it never came. With the plug sealing the hole in my throat, I could talk once again. Everything felt good and I could hardly tell the device was in place. What I did quickly notice was a free neck. After 30 years of trach ties, I was used to having them present. Now, my shirt lightly rubbed where they had been, and it felt like I was being tickled all around my neck.

Back home, it was a typical Friday with Karen staying in the evening so my parents could go out on their weekly date night. I told them I was going to Des Moines for a doctor's appointment but hadn't given any other details. To try and reduce the rubbing on my neck, I wore a shirt with buttons on top and kept it wide open. With my neck fully exposed, I wondered how long it would take them to notice the change.

They returned late in the evening and came to my room to talk about their day. After several minutes of standing a few feet from me, the two departed for other interests without saying anything about my new hardware.

Karen and I glanced at each other and attempted to stifle our laughter. Mom heard us and inquired what was funny, but she still didn't notice.

At Greg's wedding ceremony, I met one of the bridesmaids, Raven. Not long after returning from Indiana, she contacted me on Facebook. Most evenings after her initial contact, she and I spent an hour or two texting through the social media's Messenger program. I sent a picture of my clearly visible neck and kept her apprised of the comments, or lack thereof. My parents went to bed not much later and never noticed the difference.

Saturday morning, Sara was scheduled to work, but called off ill. Before Dad took the sheet off me to do my morning routine, I let them know what the laughter was about the night before. Pulling back the cover and exposing my bare chest, he finally noticed the change. They weren't sure about my decision but knew I had been considering getting the button to relieve the pain.

It had been a busy year with many changes for my entire body. For the first time since I was three, my legs worked in a controlled motion. I had my neck free again and I finally had a new wheelchair. I was ready to enter a period of calm and not have any major problems in life. Such dreams do come true, but they don't typically last long.

31

MOVING ON

Solomon wrote in Ecclesiastes 1:4-5, "*One* generation passes away, and *another* generation comes; but the earth abides forever. The sun also rises, and the sun goes down, and hastens to the place where it arose." God gave him great wisdom, but Solomon realized that each day comes and goes much like the rest with little change. The next few years of my life felt similar, but not completely.

My pressure sores persisted with little change. They didn't get much worse, but not much better either, so I severely limited my amount of time sitting. I would sit upright in bed for 45 minutes, then lay flat for 3-4 hours. It helped my skin but made it nearly impossible to get much accomplished.

For several months, I had been building a new website for a client of The Design Center. The client made several changes that delayed the completion date, but my physical limitations further added to the delay. Before the project started, I was already feeling inadequate to do the work that the web design company asked of me. I would learn a new skill or updated coding technique, but then not have opportunity to use it for a year or more. When the chance finally did come, I had to learn the process again and take longer to finish the project than if I kept up with my knowledge.

After a decade of working with The Design Center, I noticed most of my quotes were being denied and the jobs given to my competitors. When the extended project was finally complete, I wasn't asked to provide any further bids. From a business perspective, I didn't blame them. My work was slow, and I was struggling to keep up with changing technology. No matter the reason, it was still a hard adjustment to make.

Even though I limited time in my chair, I still tried to attend both morning and evening church services each Sunday. After the first service one fall morning, I headed to the corner of the sanctuary near the elevator. A group of elderly people with canes and walkers all waited turns to use the small lift to exit the building. Dad and I usually went last no matter how long it took.

The church sound system recorded every service onto a memory card. When the sound techs finished their duties, I would get the card and use it to put the sermon on the church website the next day. Two ladies with walkers went in the elevator, closed the doors, and went down, but much further than expected. It was obvious they didn't stop on the ground level to exit the building, but we didn't think they wanted to go downstairs. The janitor went to investigate and found the elevator had malfunctioned and went lower than it was supposed to. It wasn't the first time this had happened, but it had been quite a while.

Dad and a few other guys determined it would not be easy to get the elevator working again. They helped the remaining people with mobility challenges down the steps until I was the only one left. Dad said we could leave my chair at church until the elevator was fixed and he would carry me to the van, prop me in a seat, then carry me to bed. Alternatively, the people still at church could carry my chair down the steps, all 400 pounds of it. After some discussion, the second option was determined the best.

A small group followed me to the back of church, to the shortest flight of stairs. Dad laid me on a nearby couch while I listened to events unfold a few feet away. With two men behind my chair and Dad in front, they slowly eased it down the steps. I reminded them it took me eight years to finally get this chair and the price tag was $50,000. Dad was confident they could carefully coax it down the stairway. If not, he would be the first one to get ran over as it crashed down the steps.

As I laid on the couch, I could hear instructions given and a solid thud every time another step was reached. After a few minutes, my wheels were safely at the bottom. When Dad came to retrieve me, he said at only 115 pounds I was much lighter than the chair. When I returned to my regular seat, I thanked the now sweaty volunteers for the help, but didn't plan to return for the evening service.

I was also thankful that God allowed me to be a friend to Ken and to help him come to know Christ. In northern Iowa, he continued to struggle with his health and went in and out of the hospital. Sometimes he was in Iowa City at the University of Iowa Hospital, other times in Des Moines. After rescheduling a few times due to hospital stays, Ken was able to be baptized in November 2015. Just as for his birthday, Sara and I went up to Waterloo and gathered with everyone in the meeting room at Harmony House. The pastor, who had never met Ken before, came with a bowl and a bottle of water. I was thankful I could witness his baptism and coming to God, even with just a small group of a dozen people.

After serving for three years, 2015 was also the year to end my term as deacon. I had held my position as secretary the entire time and was comfortable with leading meetings and helping guide the direction of the deacons. Every year, about a third of our group would change with different men from the church. Some of them I knew well, others I got to know better.

With every new rotation of council members, I continued my practice of asking someone to help me during break time with a snack. The practice allowed my parents to stay out of potentially private conversations concerning church matters and helped me get comfortable in asking more people for assistance.

It was the longest time commitment I had given to anything, including college. However, I was able to stay out of the hospital the entire time and made it to most meetings. The final deacons' meeting was on a Saturday at the end of December. We needed to record the last donations for the year so they could be included in each individual's taxes.

Sara planned to go with me, but it snowed heavily overnight and continued through the morning. Instead of having someone clear a path in the parking lot just for me, I called to say I wouldn't make it. The shoveling had already begun by my fellow deacons, but they understood I didn't do well with cold and snow. I felt bad missing my final time but was glad to be finished with my service.

The cold weather also halted other activities. Over the winter, I did not go to Des Moines to use the FES bike. Sara and I did not want to battle with winter weather just for a half-hour ride. In order to access my legs for the electrodes, I also had to wear shorts or find breakaway pants. I didn't like the thought of wearing shorts in cold temperatures and took a break from exercising. However, when spring came in 2016, I returned to Younkers Rehabilitation to get back into the routine.

Even with visiting every other week, my circulation had started to improve and help my pressure sores. Muscle spasms also decreased on bike days, but nothing like my first session. Now that Sara and I were experienced with setting up a biking session, I also didn't need to schedule a time with a therapist. As long as the bike was available, I could go as often as I wanted and pay a monthly fee. Going to Des Moines, doing a bike ride, and returning home took about four hours and didn't allow time for anything else. However, I still tried to go once a week if possible.

In 2016, after two years away, I was able to return to CHAMP Camp as a counselor. I was thankful I could visit the previous two years, but it wasn't the same as volunteering and working with the campers. There was still no room in the cabin for Dad, Sara, and me, so I was assigned to be with one of the boys' cabins but would bunk with the administration team in a separate building.

Sara and I had a room to ourselves with Dad across the hall with another counselor. During the night, Sara watched me and then slept when Dad and I were gone with the campers. I tried to get going early enough in the morning to help the kids before breakfast, but Dad was content to join them in the cafeteria. I tried to explain to him that I was trying to work with the campers more, but he didn't understand my reasoning. Dad was more concerned about our responsibilities with fishing and getting everything arranged for the campers.

All week, I felt like I was an outsider looking into camp. Dad and I led fishing every morning, joined our official cabin for afternoon activities, and then joined everyone for the evening event. Some nights, Sara and I could follow the kids to the bunk and help with bedtime routines, but it never felt like being part of the group. Sara normally loved helping me and working with the kids but was able to do very little. We easily concluded that if I could return in 2017, I would only do so if I could bunk with the campers.

Volunteering at the State Fair

When August arrived, it was time for my annual visit to the Iowa State Fair. After decades of primarily following Dad as he grazed food booths, I started going with just Sara. It was fun getting to decide where I wanted to go and see, but I ate fewer fair treats as I had to buy them myself.

One display I made sure to visit was the Noah's Ark booth in the Varied Industries Building. Earlier in the year, a request had gone out for volunteers to help staff the booth. A local church had been staffing the booth and paying expenses, but management of the booth had changed to Answers in Genesis. I had already taught on creation apologetics and graduated from the School of Biblical Evangelism. I thought it would be an interesting opportunity where I could use the knowledge God had given me so I volunteered for three days on the three-hour morning shift.

Sara and I arrived on the first day of the fair and found the small hidden handicapped parking area I used for years. We were too early for my shift and looked through farm equipment before my time started. Soon, the two of us navigated through the sea of displays to find our designated area. I prayed with the other volunteers and was ready to go.

Everyone was handing out million-dollar gospel tracts and talking with people as opportunity allowed. Sara was recruited to help with sticker tattoos for kids. While parents waited on their children, I took the opportunity to speak with them. I had Sara put tracts under my hands spread out like a fan. If I could get someone's attention, I would have them pull one out. It took more effort, and my method was slower than the other volunteers, but it worked.

One hour into my shift came my daily time to use the bathroom. However, with my female caregiver, I only knew of one facility I could use on the fairgrounds. Sara and I stopped our duties and headed through the crowds to the correct building. By the time we returned, over 30 minutes had passed. We both concluded that a schedule change was necessary so I wouldn't have to leave my volunteer station for as long.

When 12:00 came, my shift was complete, and I was ready to be done. Whether on the vent or pacemaker, I knew my voice was quiet. To speak louder, I tried bringing in extra air with my breathing techniques. The trick was fine for short durations, but not for several hours.

I came prepared to answer Biblical questions and tell about Christ's work on the cross. The question I heard the most though was, "What?" The atmospheric noises in the Varied Industries Building drowned out my voice. I kept trying to take larger breaths and talk louder but had to remember to exhale every four seconds before my pacemaker gave a pulse, but I didn't always make it and my lungs were sore and my voice was scratchy for several hours.

After helping with two more volunteer sessions, I was more used to the increased air and louder voice. My lungs still ached after my shift, but not as bad as the first time. Not many people would talk with me for long. I wasn't sure why, but was glad God gave me the opportunity to serve.

Saying Goodbye to Ken

All spring and summer, Ken continued to be in and out of different hospitals. One stay in Iowa City was long enough that he lost his room in Waterloo. As a result, Ken had to leave the nursing home he had lived in for 16 years and was placed in another facility in south central Iowa. Ken said the care at the new facility was horrible. One example he gave was using one suction catheter for an entire week. This further increased his need for hospital visits due to getting more infections.

The move meant that Ken was regularly brought to Des Moines for more advanced care. I tried to visit him one to two times a week and coordinate the trips with bike rides. Dad and I also went to visit one weekend and he and Ken shared stories about small-town Iowa. I was thankful I could visit, talk about what I was doing, and try to help any way I could.

By November, Ken had been to the hospital with more major infections and high anxiety at the thought of returning to his new facility. Sara and I visited him but didn't get much response since he was being heavily sedated for healing and a calmer mind. A week later, he was much more alert and laughed at my bad jokes. Unfortunately, that didn't last much longer.

On November 21, six days before my birthday, Leah sat me up in bed after a few hours of lying flat. I had a message from Ken's cousin that he was failing rapidly, and I was the closest one to get to him. Leah wasn't comfortable driving the van, so I called Sara, then Dad, to see if either of them could take me.

Less than two hours later, Dad and I were in Des Moines at Ken's bedside. Four other people were there, Ken's cousins who did occasionally visit and talk with him. Ken's blood pressure was falling, and his body was full of an infection called MRSA. Less than a week earlier, Ken's mother had passed away after battling cancer. Even though they hadn't talked for years, he had hoped to use my van to see her one last time. Ken never regained enough health nor was able to find a caregiver to fulfil his last wish.

Dad was now in his second term as elder at church and had been at the bedside of elderly church members in their final days on earth, but I hadn't. He read some verses from the Bible and prayed for Ken and his family. According to Ken's directives, in such a situation his ventilator was to be removed and he would be allowed to be free of earthly trouble. Our small group surrounded his bed while nurses gave more sedatives to the unconscious man before disconnecting his breathing support.

Minutes after Ken died, one of his cousins opened a document stating who was to get what of his few positions. The six of us at the bedside was the only mention Ken desired, no funeral, memorial service, or any acknowledgement of Ken's life would be made to the public.

The facility Ken had been in only gave to the end of the month to have his belongings removed. I was informed that it was possible that Ken's dad would try to steal anything he could sell for money. My parents took my van and retrieved Ken's sparse belongings a few days later.

I received Ken's nearly new power wheelchair, computer, and a few other items. I knew he had gotten the chair about a year earlier but didn't think he had ever been in it. Dad gave it a thorough cleaning, and the chair did look brand new. Ken and I had discussed what I would do with his belongings if he died before me, and we both agreed on donating whatever I didn't want but could still be used.

A few months later, after making many inquiries, I found an organization in eastern Iowa that took power chairs, fixed them, and sent them to Guatemala. On a sunny spring day in 2017, my parents delivered the chair to the collection center. They were thankful to get a chair in such good condition and said it would be put to good use. My parents said that the man who took the chair prayed for Ken's friends and for my family in giving such a gift of mobility.

Ken was not the first quadriplegic friend that had died, but he was the one I knew the best. We had discussed many points of life and struggles that we both experienced and that were unique for him. I was thankful God gave me the opportunity to see Ken come to Jesus and get regular visits from church. Now, I was sad to lose a friend, but glad that he was free of earthly concerns.

Spring and Summer in Pella

Not long after, it was time for Tulip Time in Pella. Other than eating Dutch treats and watching parades, I hadn't done much during the three-day festival in several years. I saw an announcement that another church was hosting a gospel outreach booth during Tulip Time and needed volunteers. It sounded like something I could easily do and volunteered for two morning shifts. Weather in Iowa in early May can be unpredictable, but I hoped it would be nice enough for me to participate.

When the event came, it was a beautiful week in Iowa and perfect for being outside. Just like at the fair several months earlier, I had Sara put gospel tracts under my hand and I would have people pull one out. Without a lot of noise around, I could be heard and had opportunity to speak with people. One older gentleman rolled nearby in a wheelchair, gladly took a tract, and promptly dropped it.

I offered another in its place, but he carefully, and slowly, leaned over and picked up the million-dollar bill from the ground. We enjoyed talking together for the next several minutes about wheelchair life and coming to God for forgiveness of sins. I was glad I had the chance to meet him and several others.

Friday was my second volunteer morning, but Sara called in saying that she was sick and couldn't come to work. That meant Dad had to take off work to help with my morning routine, and I guessed he wouldn't want to go with me to share gospel tracts. However, Dad surprised me and said he would stay with me at the outreach booth. Throughout the morning, he kept wandering off to nearby antique tractors, but I managed to get him trained to replenish my hand with tracts. It was another busy morning, and I was thankful I could still help, even without Sara.

May quickly turned into June and I was excited for my volunteer week at CHAMP camp. The administrators agreed it didn't work well to have my bunk separate from the campers, so my bed would be in the cabin with the boys while Sara and Dad would sleep in a different building.

I was thrilled to be with the campers again. Some of the kids were in their fourth year of camp, but this was the first time I got to work with them. One boy in my cabin, who went by Batman, was big into pranks, staying up late, and he enjoyed most camp activities. Since he could take care of most of his physical needs and was able to walk short distances, he became the kid I regularly helped.

Batman helped me remember why I enjoyed volunteering with camp by seeing his enjoyment of activities. At school, he didn't always get to participate, but the other counselors and I made sure every camper could be fully involved in everything. Dad and Sara also enjoyed the week more than the previous year since we worked directly with the campers. Sitting in my chair 12 hours a day for seven days deepened my pressure sores, but I knew it was only one week. I figured I had 51 weeks I could lay flat and recover. As Dad and Sara packed the van Thursday afternoon, I confirmed I would volunteer as long as I physically could.

Spreading the Good News

Once home, I resumed my schedule of primarily being flat in bed. While lying down so much, I started reading and watching theologically-based material more than ever. I loved using the time to increase my knowledge of God, His Word, and the world He created. I continued to ingest information, but I hardly let any out. As I heard from one presenter, I was getting spiritually bloated.

While volunteering at the gospel outreach booth in May, I talked with the organizer, Jon, about getting his license to exhort. It allowed him to lead church services and give sermons even though he wasn't an ordained pastor. I thought about getting licensed, too, but wasn't sure of the process or if my parents would approve. It didn't sound difficult but I wasn't sure if I could give the necessary time to prepare and give sermons.

After two years, I was still on the pastor search committee for church. While our search team looked, the pulpit was filled with guest speakers or interim pastors. The current interim, Pastor Tom, was a retired minister, but was a gifted preacher who truly cared for the congregation. I expressed my interest to him in getting licensed and got some tips on how to prepare. After much prayer and thought, when I returned from camp in June, I decided to get tested. Pastor Tom was glad to hear it, but I first needed the approval from my church's council.

It was possible my congregation, Second Christian Reformed Church, was going to merge with two other congregations in Pella and form a new church body. If that happened, the new council would at least partially consist of men who had never met me. I didn't want to go before people who didn't know me or my history to ask for approval. With only a few months to go before voting to merge, this could be my last opportunity before changes occurred. The next meeting was August 7, and I would be one of the first items on the meeting agenda.

As an elder, Dad was also part of the decision makers. He and I went to church together as we had all my life, but this trip felt different. Dad went to the council room to start the evening while I sat several feet away in the empty sanctuary. I prayed for clarity of speech and thought, and that God would use me to help spread and teach His Word.

After a few minutes, Dad called me to join the elders. It had been less than two years since I sat in the same room as a member of council helping decide church matters. Now the situation had reversed, and I was the one asking for a decision from the church.

Most of the men were familiar faces I had seen almost weekly at church for as long as I could remember. They asked various questions that were easy to answer. I wanted to share the knowledge God had given me both through the Bible and life experiences.

Ken, one of the elders, said he remembered me as a two-year-old. Every week at church I would find him and pick a piece of candy out of his pocket.

After my family's accident, he wondered what I would be able to do as a kid who couldn't move or breathe on my own. After a short discussion, Ken and the elders agreed to recommend me to be tested to get my license. I would need to go before the governing board of the area, called classis. I had the choice of either the next meeting in September, or waiting until February.

With the uncertainty of my church's future, I chose to be tested at the next classis meeting. The only problem was, this gave me six weeks to prepare for an exam that most people prepared for in 6-12 months.

Reading the Bible almost daily for 20 years, I felt fairly confident on questions related to scripture. However, the Christian Reformed denomination followed three confessions, or guiding documents, the Belgic Confession, Canons of Dort, and the Heidelberg Catechism. Most teenagers studied the Catechism in Sunday school, but I missed much of it due to trouble with pressure sores. Other than the names and vague familiarity, I never formally studied the other two.

Since finishing my term as deacon, I hadn't had much opportunity to work with our interim pastor. Pastor Tom and I tried to get a schedule together to help with my study, but it was a challenge. I still needed to get to Des Moines weekly to go biking and I volunteered a few mornings at the Ark Encounter booth at the state fair. However, between the busyness, we found a few time slots to get together.

As the pastor and I neared the end of one review and practice time, my nursing supervisor came early for her regular 60-day recertification. No matter what activity I was doing, I always had to juggle it with logistics of living with quadriplegia.

September came quickly along with the time for my test. A few months prior to knowing my test date, my parents had planned their annual fall trip and arranged schedules for me to have caregivers so they could be gone. The time they would be out of Iowa coincided with the day I would be examined.

I needed to be at an unfamiliar church in another town early on a Saturday morning. I had my night nurse, Carolyn, start my morning routine before Sara came at 7:00. When she arrived, I only needed to finish getting dressed and in my wheelchair. Carolyn helped as she could, but she rarely got me ready for the day and I had to instruct her on some of my cares.

Sara and I arrived in time for the meeting, and I started with a short sermon. I was thankful Sara was with me for my test. After years of coming with me to speak at grade schools and colleges, she understood my subtle cues for when I needed a drink or any help. When the message was complete, I was interviewed by two different people. One interviewer and I had gone over his questions beforehand, but I had never met the second person. I was thankful to see that the people testing me sat in a chair for the interview. Instead of looking up their nose as I normally did, I could see them eye-to-eye.

My initial questions were presented by a man whose wife used a wheelchair and was in charge of disability concerns for churches in Pella. I presumed he was responsible for the seating arrangement, but I wasn't sure.

Over 30 minutes later, the audience was allowed to ask me questions directly. Two representatives from churches all over central Iowa and northern Missouri were in attendance and had listened to my message and answers. Turning to my audience, I saw the two familiar faces from my home church and a small sea of other heads looking at me.

One man asked if I was comfortable with speaking to crowds. I responded, "I don't have trouble with talking in front of groups and I get excited the larger the number. After a lifetime of people staring at me when I am in public, and 13 years of presenting at schools, crowds no longer faze me." A few more questions were raised, but none relating to physical challenges.

When everyone was satisfied, Sara and I were ushered out of the room along with Mom's oldest sister and her husband, Dad's parents, and my friend Jon from Pella. After a relatively short wait, I was told I could return to hear the verdict. As I entered the unfamiliar sanctuary, I started to park by the last bench in the back as I always did at my church. After a second, I remembered what I was doing and drove to the front.

If I failed, I could get tested at the next classis meeting in February, but I felt failing would be an embarrassment to my family, church, and myself. If my pacemaker didn't make me take a breath every four seconds, I would have been breathing at a much different rate. As I listened to hear what my future would entail, I was thankful that it was a unanimous vote to approve my license to exhort.

Though I was allowed to preach, I wouldn't be able to offer the sacraments of baptism or the Lord's supper, as well as a few other restrictions. Only fully ordained pastors could offer sacraments, but I didn't know how I could anyway. As I again rolled to the rear of the building, I specifically looked at a few faces I vaguely knew and said thank you.

The next day, my church had their annual outdoor picnic and afternoon service. Brad, the elder who watched my test, told the congregation about Saturday's examination. His evaluation was that I did better than the seminary student who was examined the night before. I was asked to start the service with prayer before lunch was served. I sat in front of the congregation as everyone else stood waiting. I could only actually see a few people but wasn't sure where God would take me next on this new adventure.

Two months later, in mid-November, I was contacted by a church to lead their evening worship service. Planning a sermon didn't feel difficult, but it was different from anything I had done. I knew I couldn't go through pages of notes and could only have what fit on a music stand. I primarily memorized what I would say and typed a few prompts using one sheet of paper. For the scripture reading, I made a PowerPoint presentation to use on the church screen. While displaying the references to the congregation, I could then read it.

When Sunday morning came, I woke up with a sore throat and needed to be suctioned frequently. I attributed it to nervousness as the problem mainly cleared up by the time the church service started. I felt out of place in an unfamiliar congregation, but I was ready to share God's Word.

Part of leading the service meant selecting songs and working with the service coordinator. Sitting at the end of a pew while the congregation sang what I chose felt both odd and cool. After the opening songs and prayers given by the regular pastor, I rolled to the front and started saying what I had planned. I introduced myself, shared a little about my history of speaking and why I was a barefoot preacher. Then, I gave my message of how to respond as Christians during times of suffering.

It was different than speaking at schools. I missed interacting with the people in front of me and resting my voice. The time went by much quicker than I imagined, and I was soon finished. Afterward, several people said they appreciated my message, and I hoped I would have the opportunity to preach again.

Back to the Hospital

My throat kept feeling sore and my lungs congested the following few days. I eventually went to my doctor, and he put me on a strong dose of antibiotics. I hoped the medication would help, but it had the opposite effect. After nearly a week, I was starting to breathe easier, but my stomach didn't get along with the drug.

On Monday night, a week after preaching, my abdomen looked like I was pregnant. My stomach hurt horribly, and it felt like the problems I experienced previously. Tuesday morning, Sara and Mom took me to the ER in Des Moines so I could get help. With the pressure on my lungs, it wasn't easy to speak, but I managed to explain my history and problem without much help from anyone else.

It had been five years since I had been admitted to the hospital. At that time, I was still using the regular ventilator and trach. Now, I only used the pacemaker to breathe and just had a trach button. I knew the NG tube normally made my nose irritated and very stuffy and I wasn't sure how well I could breathe in that situation. Therefore, we would try diet management for a few days and see if that cleared up the issue.

With sitters arranged, Mom and Dad didn't need to come help me, but they still came frequently. I didn't eat anything for over a day and wasn't given the majority of my regular drugs. With no medication to calm my muscles, I was concerned about my arm hitting the DPS port on my chest. However, with my body already stressed from my stomach problem, my arms and legs hardly twitched.

Just lying in the hospital bed, I could barely speak or keep my oxygen level up. Therefore, I was given extra oxygen with a small tube sitting just under my nose. It was something I had seen other people use but had never used it myself. Before, if I needed extra help, the oxygen would have been pumped through my vent.

On Thanksgiving Day, I was feeling some improvement and could increase my diet to liquids. Instead of the turkey and sides I should have been having with my extended family, I slowly ate hot beef broth. It wasn't anywhere close to the same taste, but at least it was something. I still looked much fatter than usual, though, and could hardly croak out words.

At 6:00 Friday morning, the doctor came for his regular rounds to see how I was doing. There wasn't any change or sign of movement in my gut. I would take another day of laxatives, liquid diet, and wait to see progress. As evening came, my belly started getting larger again, and as it did the pain also increased.

Soon, all I could feel was horrendous pain in my belly and I could hardly breathe. My parents were visiting for a few hours, and I had Mom rub my abdomen to try to relieve the pressure. It helped some, but only while she kept rubbing. If I wanted anything, I had to croak my request to Mom who passed the message to my sitter, who couldn't hear me. Near 10:00 p.m., another person took over to help watch me and my parents reluctantly went home. They would be back early the next morning.

My new caregiver resumed rubbing where Mom left off, but not the same. I tried to let her stop and rest her arm but couldn't tolerate her stopping for long. Along with my stomach, I also had severe pain in my neck and head. With every heartbeat, it felt like my veins were ready to burst and I was being hit with hammers. I asked the sitter to have someone take my blood pressure. A few minutes later, a nurse found my pressure was 184/147 with a heart rate well over 100.

With what little voice I had, I tried to explain autonomic dysreflexia to the nurse. I said my normal blood pressure is around 90/50, and this was more than twice that. If the pressure was left untreated, I could easily have a stroke. She relayed the information to a doctor somewhere, but he thought the high blood pressure was good. He said it was my body trying to push liquid into my gut to get it working. I attempted again to explain AD to the nurse, but they had no experience with spinal cord injuries, and my attempt to educate fell on deaf ears.

It was getting close to midnight, and I knew my doctor wouldn't come again until 6:00 a.m. With my pacemaker giving a pulse every four seconds, I took a breath 15 times in a minute. Doing the simple math in my head, that equaled 900 breaths in an hour. I started at 900, then 899 four seconds later, and counted down every breath until starting again the next hour. Each number was a few seconds closer to morning as I waited for the stroke that I knew would be coming. I had just preached on how to respond to times like this, and prayed I would be allowed to live through the night.

While counting, I also prayed for healing for everyone in the hospital with me, and that my fellow patients would come to Jesus for forgiveness of sins while they had opportunity. As my head continued to pound and felt ready to explode with every heartbeat, I also prayed that my parents would be comforted if I died.

Through a very long night of staying awake, counting, and prayer, my doctor came 45 breaths (three minutes) before 6:00 a.m. She was surprised at how much worse I was than the day before and asked if I was ready to try an NG tube. I nodded yes, even though I wasn't sure how well I would be able to breathe through my nose. I had the sitter hold my rarely used cell phone to my ear so I could try to give my parents an early morning update.

A few minutes later, a nurse returned with the now familiar equipment. She found the smallest size tube available on the hospital floor and hoped it would help. Nobody was available to hold their hand on my cheek as the tube was shoved up my nose while I attempted to drink water to get everything in the correct position. I felt every millimeter of it go through my system, but the nurse said I did well. My parents arrived about an hour after my new hardware had been put in my face.

Thankfully, I was able to breathe okay with half my nose completely plugged. It took a few minutes to decide how to hold my breath and not immediately exhale, but I could get air. By Sunday afternoon, four liters of stuff had been sucked out of my body and I was feeling much better. My grandparents also traveled to Des Moines to visit and see how I was doing. Dad's parents came first and started looking through some early birthday cards and messages I had received.

With my stomach size decreased, I could talk more easily, but my voice remained scratchy. My lower abdomen was back to normal size, but I still hadn't cleared out my intestines. By the time Mom's brother and sister-in-law brought Grandma Labermen, I looked like myself. If Grandpa had been alive, they would have come days earlier. However, Mom was glad she waited until later since my skin color had apparently been pale and it may have scared my relatives.

Through every shift change, I explained my diaphragm pacemaker and how to be careful with it. At some point, the IV in my right arm came loose, spilling liquid all over my arm, bed, and near the pacemaker. As long as I drank enough, it was decided, I didn't need the extra fluids and it would be safer to not have anything near my pacemaker port.

Monday morning, my 36th birthday, started another day in the hospital. I received gifts of balloons and email messages, but a special present was having the tube removed from my nose and eating a semi-liquid diet. My birthday supper consisted of strained chicken noodle soup and chocolate pudding with whipped topping. It was the most disgusting soup I had ever eaten, but I had to show I could tolerate food again. Alternating a bite of soup with pudding helped, but I wondered if eating was worth it.

My evening sitter took my blood pressure around shift change, as was required by the hospital. The results came back as 78/45, much lower than a few nights earlier, and too low to be acceptable to the nurses. I promptly had five nurses standing around my bed discussing how to resolve my pressure. Other than being somewhat tired, I explained I felt fine and low blood pressure was normal for quadriplegics. Despite my attempt at education, they decided I needed fluids again. This time, instead of a regular line in my arm, a special technician came and inserted a PICC line directly into the artery. It looked like she was prepping me for surgery, but the procedure was done quickly.

Finally, a week after going to the hospital, I would be released if I could eat solid food. I eagerly ordered eggs and bacon to enjoy an actual breakfast. I also requested to start back on my regular medication in preparation for returning to my normal routine. Just before Dad came to pick me up, the doctor came in. She was concerned about my low blood pressure the night before and wanted to keep me another day for observation. With my gut no longer squeezing my lungs, I had my full voice back. I fully and firmly explained the basics of spinal cord injuries to the doctor.

When I needed a rapid response to high blood pressure, I was ignored. However, I did get complete and unnecessary attention to low pressure. I explained autonomic dysreflexia and why my pressure was lower than most people. Without moving my limbs and being active, my heart doesn't have to work hard. This time she finally understood and allowed me to be released.

During my stay, a few respiratory therapy students I had instructed at a local college recognized me. I was glad they remembered their experience and had been taught about AD, but it was obvious much more education was needed for more medical professionals.

Shortly after my official release, Dad helped the nurses get me dressed and he picked me up and plopped me in my wheelchair. With the sudden change in position, I became extremely lightheaded and felt like I was ready to pass out. The feeling lasted for a minute, but I was not going to say anything and hoped nobody noticed I went silent.

It felt great being home again with my regular nurses who were familiar with my cares and equipment. After a week of receiving laxatives and none of my bladder or muscle control medicines, it took another week to get my body straightened out. I learned again to be careful while on antibiotics and carefully watch how my stomach reacted.

Preaching Opportunities

Thankfully, I didn't have any more medical challenges and was able to volunteer at CHAMP Camp in June 2018. Just like the previous year, my bed was with the boys while Dad and Sara bunked in a different building. Since I was licensed to preach, I volunteered to lead the optional counselor worship service Sunday morning before the campers arrived. Preaching to people I had known well for many years, and would be living with all week, made me more nervous than speaking to a large congregation of people I didn't know.

By biking regularly and staying flat constantly, my three pressure sores had improved. After returning home from my week in Indiana, they got worse, with one doubling in size. I was thankful to help the campers again, but not sure it was worth the physical cost. Mom reminded me that if it's the primary thing I do all year, I can spend the other 51 weeks recovering.

Not long after I was licensed to exhort, Pastor Dave Powell, who I met as a camper at CHAMP Camp, invited me to preach at his church. I wanted to accept, but Dave's congregation was near Louisville, KY. Sara was willing to go and help at night, but I knew it would take a lot of planning and work for my parents. After a few months of deciding how it would work and when, I was scheduled to preach at both morning services the first Sunday of October.

Toward the end of September, as I finished sermon preparation and coordination, my stomach acted up again and I returned to the hospital. It had only been ten months since my previous stay and the experience was fresh in my mind. This time, I didn't wait and allowed an NG tube to be placed in the ER. Three days later, I was home again without any of the blood pressure complications I had before. I needed to reschedule a grade school I had planned to speak at but was determined to preach if God allowed me.

Nine days after getting home from the hospital, my parents, Sara, and I were in the van heading east. Mom wasn't sure about traveling so quickly after having problems, but I convinced her I would be fine. In reality, I wasn't certain myself if I should go, especially with mainly eating fast food while traveling. However, I tried to be careful to only order soft food that was easy to digest and drink plenty of water.

We drove all day Saturday, and I preached the next morning. Pastor Dave was a minister at a Methodist church, and I wasn't familiar with the different routine of their worship service. However, when I finished giving the message, the congregation rose and gave me a standing ovation.

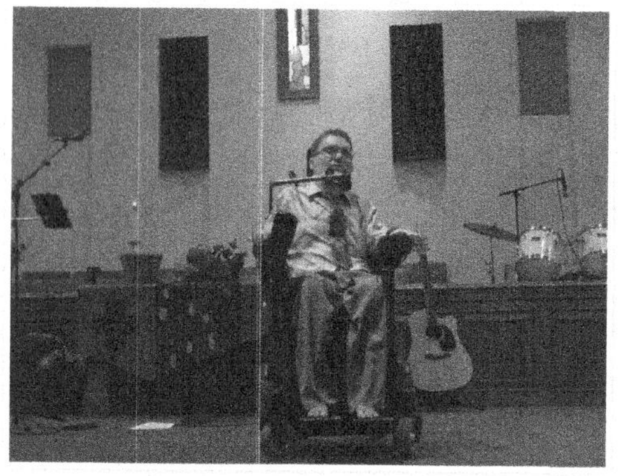

I had now preached six times since getting licensed a year earlier, and never expected such a response. My concern was that I presented God's Word accurately and not just according to my ideas. An hour after the first service, I preached the same message again at the second service. Listening to myself, I could hear and feel how scratchy my voice felt. After having a tube in my throat for a few days and not used to talking much, preaching at both services was a little too much. I was still thankful for the opportunity and prayed my words helped teach.

Late Monday morning, after Sara got some sleep, our group drove another hour east and visited the Ark Encounter. Pastor Dave came with us as well as Karrie, another counselor friend from camp. The last time I did anything with camp friends, outside of camp, was 19 years earlier on my birthday. It was fun going out with them to see the Ark. I had volunteered for three summers at the Iowa State Fair telling about the biblical themed attraction and was finally able to experience it myself.

The ark was built according to the dimensions given in Genesis and I was impressed with how big the structure was and how much room it had inside. The artists' work on crafting animals representing the created kinds was well done. At supper that evening, we tearfully said our goodbyes as everyone headed home. I wasn't sure if I would get to camp and see these friends again. Tuesday was a long day of driving home, along with a rest stop in Missouri to watch trains for an hour.

More Willing Than Able

When 2019 came, I couldn't resist the desire to volunteer for camp one more time. I was accepted, but I was very unsure if it was the right decision. The damage caused to my skin from the previous summer had healed and I didn't want it to get worse again.

For the first time since getting my wheelchair in 2015, I had a pressure map done to identify any problems with my seat cushion. It revealed a large area of pressure directly under one of my sores. After another test, and some rubber bands, the problem was fixed.

As Sara, Dad, and I arrived at Bradford Woods in June, we were greeted with cold, wet weather. On Saturday night, the first day of training, I felt exhausted and didn't feel well. I could tolerate cooler temps better than some quadriplegics I knew, but not for extended periods. Nearly every day rained and stayed well below regular summer temperatures. The buildings at the campgrounds were all air-conditioned as well and were set below 70° during the day and even colder at night.

Every evening, after I got in my bunk, Sara would cover me in all the blankets we had packed. Most nights, my temperature was near 95° and I didn't think I could possibly get through another day. None of the three boys in my cabin were ambulatory and needed total care, just like me. That meant I could only help by talking with them and not by helping them manage their own needs. It felt like I was only there to fill space instead of working with the campers.

At closing ceremonies Thursday morning, I was recognized for my 15th year of volunteering. With just trying to function all week, I didn't feel I deserved the recognition. Heading home a few hours later, with the van's heat running, I finally started to feel better and more awake.

I knew I could no longer physically tolerate the demands of camp and that I had served my final year. I comforted myself with this thought on the long drive home, and was thankful for all the summers I had been able to give. Returning home, I was thankful my pressure sores had not gotten worse during the week. One area did well, even if the rest of me didn't.

Saying Goodbye to Grandpa Vander Molen

Fall 2019 came quickly and I looked forward to celebrating Thanksgiving with my extended family. A week before the holiday, Dad's parents were tearing carpet off of their basement stairs in preparation for new carpet. As they worked after supper, they both fell down the stairway and landed on the cement wall at the bottom. Grandpa hit his head hard on the wall and was rushed to Pella hospital.

After nearly a day of testing and looking at treatment, it was determined little could be done for the 86-year-old and he was put into the care of hospice. Over the next few days, all the Vander Molen family was in and out of the Pella hospice house. Dad came home long enough to help Mom and me when needed but tried to be with his family as much as possible. On November 26, the day before my birthday, Grandpa Vander Molen passed away. I had now lost both of my grandfather's due to head injuries suffered while being fully active.

I was asked to speak at the funeral and give part of the message. I made sure to include how often he and Grandma helped watch me in the evening so my parents could get away.

At one of the evening stays, Grandpa had noticed that I had started to write a book about the life God had given me. At Pella Feed Service a few days later, Grandpa said he hoped he could read it before he died. Unfortunately, that didn't happen, but I became more determined to make sure this book was finished.

32

LOOKING AHEAD

> "When I consider Your heavens, the work of Your fingers, the moon and the stars, which You have ordained, what is man that You are mindful of him, and the son of man that You visit him?" Psalm 8:3-4

On February 20, 2023, I reached 38 years of being a C2/3 vent dependent quadriplegic. Personally, I only know two other people with the same injury level and breathing needs who have reached this anniversary. One man has been injured one more year than me and the other has four more years. A few other friends from CHAMP Camp are a few years behind me and have surpassed three decades.

Statistics have been updated since receiving my spinal cord injury, but they are always a shorter lifespan than what I have already lived. Some of us continue to extend the statistics further with each year we live. Unfortunately, not every quadriplegic I have known has been given as long.

Through CHAMP Camp, the Christopher Reeve Foundation, and friends of friends, I have met many other adults and children with high injury levels. Some have passed away before reaching adult life and others did not get to experience teen years. Several have died around 30 years post injury, but not all.

Some friends I got to know better than others, and their passing was a surprise. I met Aaron in northwest Iowa only once in person, but I still felt close to him as a fellow Iowan. He passed away in early 2019 after nearly 28 years of living with SCI. Living in Florida, I never met Bill in person. However, we researched the diaphragm pacemaker together and compared ideas on book writing. He died in early 2022 a week after a brain cancer diagnosis and a few months before reaching his 25th accident anniversary.

I have also outlived some of my medical team that I had gotten to know and trust very well. My night nurse, Mary, passed away in 2018 after a battle with mental illness. Pulmonologist Dr. Hicklin also unexpectedly died in early 2020 only a few weeks after we had a virtual appointment together.

Somewhere around the time I moved back to Pella after college, Dad and I went train watching in Ottumwa. I don't remember the exact day, year, or even how many trains we saw while sitting beside the tracks. It was an activity we had done many times before, and since, but the conversation this time was different.

About halfway home, Dad spoke up so he could be heard over the noise of the van. He said, "Mom asked me once if I ever apologized for getting you in the accident." His thoughts were briefly interrupted as we drove on a bridge over tracks. He looked left and I looked to the right to catch a glimpse of any rail traffic. A second later, Dad continued, "I'm sorry that I got you and Mom into the car accident. We all wish it hadn't happened, but we don't know how God will use you. I don't know what will happen in the future, but it will be according to His plan." The remaining 15 miles home, we didn't say much. After the excursion, it wasn't mentioned again, and life continued as it always had. However, I won't forget the discussion.

Examining God's Word

God has truly blessed the life He has given me, much more than I, or anyone, deserve. Most people react to this statement with confusion, wondering how someone who has spent most of his life with a severe disability can say such a thing. When I examine myself according to God's Word, it makes more sense. Ask yourself these questions as well, the answer has eternal consequences.

In Exodus 20, God gave Israel the Ten Commandments, also known as the moral law. They are the standard by which God judges all of mankind, including you and me.

The tenth commandment says do not covet, and then gives a list of items that are, or were, frequently coveted. It is easy to see something that someone else has and want it. Advertising is especially geared toward making us covet. For me, I have coveted a different life, one where I could breathe independently, walk, and lead a "normal" existence. Any longing or strong desire for something God has not given breaks this command.

Moving up, the ninth commandment is to not bear false witness against your neighbor, or do not lie. Without much effort, everyone can think of a fib, half-truth, or little white lie we have told. No matter the name, size, or color, it is deceiving someone else and goes against God's standard.

Continuing to exam God's law, the eighth command is do not steal. I haven't robbed a bank but the amount taken isn't the issue. Taking anything, even if it's small, qualifies as theft. Taking music, movies, or anything similar off the internet without purchasing it, or asking for discounts you're not completely qualified to get, breaks the command.

Most people know the seventh command, do not commit adultery. It seems easy, any sexual relations outside of a married man and woman breaks this law. However, Jesus said whoever looks with lust, or sexual desire, commits adultery in their heart. Pretty much anyone who has gone through puberty has had trouble with this, and it doesn't stop as age increases.

Another seemingly simple rule is number six, do not murder. Again, Jesus said whoever harbors hatred toward someone has committed murder in their heart. Dealing with insurance companies, doctors, or clients leaving can trigger thoughts that break the sixth commandment.

The final one I will look at is the third commandment, do not use the Lord's name in vain. In the Old Testament, this was so serious that breaking it received the death sentence. Today, you likely won't be stoned, but it still carries serious consequences. It is common to hear God's name used without complete reverence in movies or in almost anything we watch. Texting phrases with OM- infer God's name and many people use the name of God or Jesus as a common phrase to express disgust, surprise, or in place of a filth word. Any of these cases breaks the command.

God not only sees physical actions, but also our thought life, and will judge every word, action, and thought we have had. I only covered six of the Ten Commandments but, examining myself, I have broken these rules as well as the remaining four.

Revelation 21:8 says, *"But the cowardly, unbelieving, abominable, murderers, sexually immoral, sorcerers, idolaters, and all liars shall have their part in the lake which burns with fire and brimstone, which is the second death."* Jesus also said that no one is good, except God alone (Matthew 19:17).

Therefore, when we see ourselves as sinners, we understand that if God gives us justice, none of us deserve anything other than eternal punishment in hell. No matter how bad something is in this life, cancer, pain, or quadriplegia, can compare to the eternal pain and anguish of hell. However, God so loves the world, that He gave His One and only Son for us (John 3:16).

Whoever truly repents of their sins, turns away from them, and trusts in Christ alone for forgiveness can be made spotless in God's sight. There is no amount of works or actions we can do to earn salvation; it is a free gift to all who come to Him with a humble heart. As David said in Psalm 8, we are nothing but a speck compared to the rest of God's creation, the entire universe. Even so, He cares for us enough to die an incredibly cruel death, to be raised to life on the third day, so that we can live with Him in glory forever.

If you have not given your life to Jesus, I encourage you to do so now. In the quietness of your heart, confess your sins, those secret sins that nobody else knows. God will be found by you if you seek Him, but don't put it off until later. As my family learned on February 20, 1985, life can change in an instant. The change might be an injury, or that your time on earth will be complete. Over 150,000 people die every 24 hours around the world; at some point, it will be your time.

Originally, the world, and universe, were created perfect without cancer, disease, spinal cord injuries, or death. Unfortunately, the parents of all mankind, Adam and Eve, sinned against God and brought a curse on all of creation. As a result, we now live in a fallen world that has a multitude of problems. When a time of trouble comes, I have seen people react by either blaming God and turning away from Him or acknowledging His sovereignty and using the situation to glorify God. Whatever your circumstances, I pray you take the second response, however difficult it might be.

> *When a time of trouble comes, I have seen people react by either blaming God and turning away from Him or acknowledging His sovereignty and using the situation to glorify God.*

This is how I have tried to live the life I have been given. Reading through this book, you have seen times I let life's circumstances get to me and I reaped the consequences. However, as I continue to grow in knowledge of the Bible and God's will, each new challenge makes me rely on Him further. Living as a quadriplegic for most of my life has not been easy, but I try to let it almost become part of the background and see what I'm able to do.

Updates at the Time of this Writing

Every month since high school, I have been responsible for ordering my own supplies for my cares. Daily, I check over my skin for scratches and red areas that I need to watch and make sure they heal. Frequently, problems come up with my wheelchair, nurses call off sick or can't come because of bad weather. It's all part of the routine. If I had written about every instance, if I could even remember them, this would be a much longer book and help put you, the reader, to sleep.

For over two years, Sara and I drove to Des Moines several times a month so I could use the FES bike at Younkers Rehab. In 2017, I received an early Christmas present of my own bike. Instead of using it a few times a month, I now get on it a few times a week. Through increased use, circulation in my legs improved, muscle spasms decreased, and I was able to reduce some of my anti-spasm medication. Finally, after 13 years of dealing with it, one of my pressure sores was declared healed. By fall of 2022, all but one had healed completely.

I have had several occasions when a caregiver quit, and I wondered if a replacement would be found. As the years have passed, it has become increasingly difficult to find help. While I wonder how much longer my parents can cover open shifts, God has always provided another person to help. Having funding and personnel to cover around 19 hours a day is rare, and I know is an extreme blessing.

In November 2021, Sara took off for two weeks for back problems. One day after she returned, she had a seizure and doctors found a tumor in her brain. Thankfully, surgery was able to remove it and cancer treatments were not required. However, she was not allowed to return to work until April 2022. This meant I had several months with three day shifts not covered. It was difficult for my parents to cover an extra 30 hours per week, both physically and mentally.

Thankfully, after trying several ideas to find assistance, a nursing student from Central College in Pella answered our plea for help. She could only do one and a half days a week until the end of the school year, but we were relieved to have her.

After living near Washington D.C. for a few years, Tom, his wife, and two boys moved to Minnesota. He comes to visit in person every few years, but we still meet virtually. It's rare that we get to relive high school years of playing online games together, but we remain close friends.

Not long after my 35th anniversary of SCI in 2020, an event occurred that brought the world to a stop. With an outbreak of a new virus, called COVID-19, schools and businesses were closed and travel was either completely stopped or severely restricted. It was a pandemic that caught the world by surprise and changed lives everywhere.

For the first time since college, I didn't apply to volunteer as a counselor at CHAMP Camp. I knew I could no longer handle the physical demands and it was time to retire. Due to virus concerns, I also couldn't visit grade schools. It was the first time in 15 years I hadn't talked with kids about serving God with a disability, and I missed it, but through virtual meetings I had the opportunity to help teach college students. With mostly everything shut down, it gave me time to make progress on this book. Prolonged health concerns in 2021 also meant CHAMP Camp met virtually and allowed me to volunteer as a counselor without leaving home.

Since we met in late 2015, Raven and I talked almost every night through 2021 and tried dating. However, it was better for us to be friends than a couple. The Van Hoerkels continued regular visits for many years. Rae is now in college pursuing her degree in nursing and James is looking forward to completing high school.

What the future holds for this life, only God knows. My parents are past retirement age and should be looking at slowing down. However, I still receive insurance through the Town Crier. Dad has endured many times of extreme stress and frustration in nearly 50 years with the company. Instead of slowing down, he continues to work more than full-time with no end in sight as long as I need medical insurance. As economies and businesses continue to adjust after the COVID pandemic, the printing industry has much less demand and many print shops have closed. We continue to pray that Dad's employer will be able to stay in business and busy for as long as possible.

I still do some web development work, but it is very little with just a few hours per month. A time will likely come when I can no longer call myself a web developer, but I'm thankful for the decades of work it allowed me to enjoy as well as the multiple friends and connections I made while working with clients.

After getting my license to exhort in 2017, I have preached for multiple congregations. In 2022, I set a personal record of preaching 12 times in one year. Due to weather challenges, I rarely schedule anything between Thanksgiving and St. Patrick's Day. It makes for a busy summer, but I enjoy serving God by teaching His Word.

Mom also continues to work at Pella Feed Service a few days a week. With my daytime hours covered by CDAC, she also does nearly 20 hours of work every week tracking nursing hours and paperwork. She also wants to retire and take social security, but doing so would initiate some hidden regulations and cause me to lose some of my state funding and possibly daytime hours.

Whatever the future holds, be it active and living with my parents or moving to a care facility, I know God is in control. I sometimes have a hard time seeing how I can be active in a different setting but will learn to adapt as needed.

God has given me parents who have done more for me than I can ever repay or say thank you enough. They wanted to start a family earlier, but God waited until they were a little older and could better deal with the challenges to come. I have also been given more caregivers than I can begin to remember. Some of them were mentioned in this book, but many more have been an important part of this life I have been given.

Grandma Labermen said the worst memory of her life was the phone call from the Iowa State Patrol telling her we had been in an accident. She, and all my grandparents, were a big part of helping my family with all the challenges.

Through all these connections, God has allowed me to serve Him in ways my parents or I never imagined. He has enabled me to show that anyone can be active if they choose to be. I have also been given opportunity to speak with many children and adults and help them learn different perspectives. I also was able to write an entire book, just by using a mouth stick.

Occasionally, I wonder what life would have been like for me if I didn't have a spinal cord injury. I think I may have joined the Air Force after high school and then maybe gone into truck driving or become a railroad engineer. Home may have been a small acreage with a pond for fishing, barn to raise sheep, and a large garden. Before it all, would be my wife and kids, teaching them about Christ and the world He has given us.

Sitting in bed, I look at my legs laying out in front of me and wonder what it feels like to walk. I am always barefoot but can only imagine what different textures would feel like under my feet. I look forward to the day I can once again experience a restored body. Until then, I will live through whatever circumstance God has in store for me and look forward to seeing Him face-to-face.

Joel Vander Molen

ABOUT THE AUTHOR

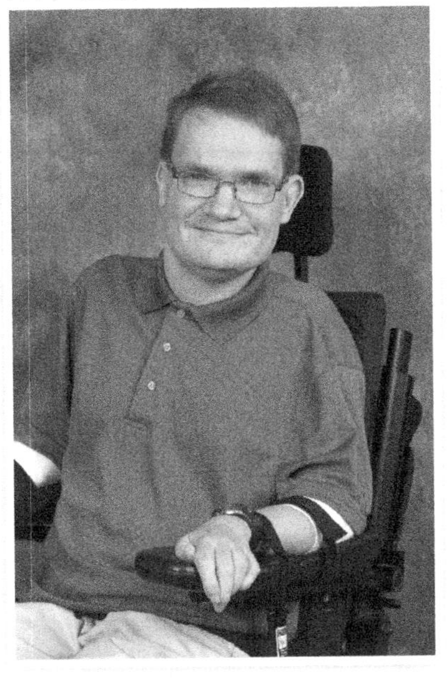

Joel Vander Molen is a disability awareness speaker, web developer, and substitute preacher living in Iowa. At just three-years-old, Joel was involved in a motor vehicle accident and received a high-level spinal cord injury. Unable to breathe independently, feel or control anything below his shoulders, Joel had a challenging life ahead.

Through a loving family, multiple caregivers, and a strong faith in God's plan, these challenges never stopped him. Going through grade school, junior high, and high school, Joel went on to college, even living independently in his own dorm room.

In 38 years as a quadriplegic, life wasn't always easy and circumstances sometimes resulted in poor judgments. However, he learned to look to God first with whatever came and continues to do so while living the quad life.

Made in the USA
Middletown, DE
14 October 2023

40571089R00263